Humanities and Healthcare: Practical and Pedagogical Guides

Humanities and Healthcare: Practical and Pedagogical Guides is a series that encourages the integration of work in the humanities—literature, the arts, music, philosophy, history, popular media, and culture—into the training and practice of healthcare throughout the world. Books in the series will be dedicated to particular topics designed to further biomedical education in healthcare while putting the human experience at the center and contributing to the targets of Sustainable Development Goal 3 Good Health and Well-Being. These textbooks provide practical guidance for postgraduate professional students in healthcare and related areas, undergraduate students in the humanities and pre-health training, practicing healthcare workers, and informal carers. With the goal of bringing local and global concerns together, the series promotes and publishes studies that widen understanding of healthcare, well-being, and systematic care-taking. The aims of the series are to take a broad definition of healthcare and therapeutic practices in regards to physical and mental health in order to highlight practices within and beyond the clinic with a focus on race, ethnicity, class, gender, sexuality, and disability; on healthcare systems and inequitable access to healthcare; on doctor-patient communication; on the landscapes of care work (including domestic care workers and nursing aids and the important diverse group of informal caretakers); on geographies of health and care; and on institutionalized care, aging, gender, neurodiversity, and addiction.

April Patrick

Women's Health in Britain and America

Texts and Contexts

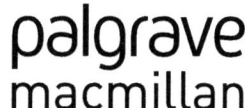

April Patrick
Fairleigh Dickinson University
Madison, NJ, USA

Humanities and Healthcare: Practical and Pedagogical Guides
ISBN 978-3-031-41256-1   ISBN 978-3-031-41257-8 (eBook)
https://doi.org/10.1007/978-3-031-41257-8

© The Editor(s) (if applicable) and The Author(s), under exclusive licence to Springer Nature Switzerland AG 2023
This work is subject to copyright. All rights are solely and exclusively licensed by the Publisher, whether the whole or part of the material is concerned, specifically the rights of translation, reprinting, reuse of illustrations, recitation, broadcasting, reproduction on microfilms or in any other physical way, and transmission or information storage and retrieval, electronic adaptation, computer software, or by similar or dissimilar methodology now known or hereafter developed.
The use of general descriptive names, registered names, trademarks, service marks, etc. in this publication does not imply, even in the absence of a specific statement, that such names are exempt from the relevant protective laws and regulations and therefore free for general use.
The publisher, the authors, and the editors are safe to assume that the advice and information in this book are believed to be true and accurate at the date of publication. Neither the publisher nor the authors or the editors give a warranty, expressed or implied, with respect to the material contained herein or for any errors or omissions that may have been made. The publisher remains neutral with regard to jurisdictional claims in published maps and institutional affiliations.

Cover illustration: FAY 2018 / Alamy Stock Photo

This Palgrave Macmillan imprint is published by the registered company Springer Nature Switzerland AG.
The registered company address is: Gewerbestrasse 11, 6330 Cham, Switzerland

Paper in this product is recyclable.

For Frieda,
who has changed my life and will change the world

Preface

When reading and writing about women's health from the past, whether decades or even centuries ago, it is easy to dismiss the difficulties or the concerns as ones not applicable in our modern lives. We benefit from both medical advances and women's rights; however, women across the US and UK still face significant challenges in accessing the healthcare they need. As I worked on this book, the current realities of medical care for women in the United States became all too clear. In just the matter of a few months, I witnessed and experienced issues related to each of the conditions in this book, all in the lives of relatively young women with significant privilege.

Shortly after the US Supreme Court overturned Roe v. Wade and abortion laws across in many states changed, a friend in Texas recognized the signs of a miscarriage and immediately worried about her ability to access the care she needed because treatment for pregnancy loss can be similar to procedures for surgical abortion. She was eventually able to access care close to home, but many other women have had life threatening complications from miscarriages that doctors can or will not treat. A few months later, another friend gave birth to her first child in a New York City hospital following a mostly healthy pregnancy. Her birth was complicated, but she delivered vaginally and was able to go home on schedule with a healthy baby. She was readmitted less than a week later, however, after her headaches became unbearable. There she learned the doctors had sent her home without mentioning her dangerously high blood pressure—which needed medication for more than a month—along with complications related to her epidural—which can be common but are rarely discussed. Another friend had a similar experience after five days in the hospital following the birth of her first child. Because the doctors failed to discharge her with the necessary medication, she returned to the emergency room a few days later, having to leave her newborn baby at home.

A few months later, a friend and I simultaneously found lumps in our breasts and sought to schedule diagnostic mammograms and ultrasounds separate from our annual checks. I was only able to schedule a mammogram and ultrasound within a week by crossing state lines, while it took my friend over four months to be seen in any facilities in New York City. This delay meant that her doctor's orders for the mammogram had expired and her insurance would not cover the costs, forcing her to pay out of pocket for the care she needed. When my mammogram and ultrasound found the original lump to be a cyst but a suspicious lump in the other breast, it took hours of phone calls and countless tears to get an ultrasound-guided biopsy scheduled for the following week. As I waited for my appointment, I considered that, just half a century earlier, a biopsy would have been a surgical procedure, and without informed consent practices, I would have gone under anesthesia not knowing whether the doctor would perform only the biopsy or continue with a radical mastectomy. During my biopsy, the radiologist was kind and reassuring, describing how each step of the process would feel with helpful detail. After the procedure, she explained that the specificity in her verbal description was only possible after her own biopsy a few years earlier, a powerful reminder of both the value of lived experience and the goals for narrative medicine. If medical professionals cannot directly experience the conditions women patients face, narratives become essential for building empathy and improving both patient experience and outcomes.

Goals of This Book

In preparing *Women's Health in Britain and America, Texts and Contexts*, my primary purpose is to offer a collection of materials that will allow readers of the twenty-first century to understand the historical precedents for contemporary issues. Women's health is a common and politicized topic, but most discussions in popular media or politics consider recent history or developments without the historical contexts. This often-forgotten background is clearly relevant for understanding the fact that the maternal mortality rate is significantly higher for Black women in both Britain and America or when nineteenth-century approaches to abortion are cited in decisions by the U.S. Supreme Court or are used in restricting access to medicine for abortion.

As an educator and researcher, I value the way primary sources help us to explore the complexities of a topic better than any descriptive overview.

Unfortunately, those sources are scattered across a variety of print, digital, and archival locations with few opportunities to cross-reference ideas and issues. Even the sources currently in the public domain are often buried in larger texts with little indication for how to find the specific scene or topic and with the aspects related to women's health as secondary to other topics. By compiling the selections in this volume, I offer access to materials as an opportunity for readers to develop more nuanced knowledge about women's health.

Together, these texts and contexts offer a more complete picture of medical practice in the period, bringing the voices of women, their family and friends, their doctors, and their advocates into conversation. As discussions around women's bodies develop in the twenty-first century, understanding this history and hearing a multiplicity of voices are more important than ever.

Disciplinary approach of this book

My own training in literary studies and teaching in medical humanities and narrative medicine has shaped the structure of this volume and its coverage of these topics. The book's subtitle—Texts and Contexts—suggests the prioritization of narrative texts that comprise a majority of the material. This focus responds, in part, to Monica H. Green's (2008) observations of "blind spots…due to a long tradition in the history of medicine looking from the top down: medical history was the history of medicine of practitioners…and only secondarily of patients" (p. 492). By centering the writing of women or writing intended for them, this collection makes visible those texts that were once a blind spot. To accompany them, the introductory contexts to the chapters and each of the individual texts provide general background information. These serve as a gateway to each of the topics and are meant to complement more specialized resources about the history of medicine, scientific or medical terms, gender studies, and literary analysis.

How to Use This Book

Readers can explore *Women's Health in Britain and America, Texts and Contexts* in several ways. Certainly reading from cover to cover with introductions to each chapter followed by the excerpts would provide a comprehensive understanding of the three main topics addressed—pregnancy and childbirth, contraception and abortion, and breast and gynecological cancers. After a general introduction in Chap. 1, the three main topics are grouped by chapter, each accompanied by a general introduction to the condition or situation, various treatments or approaches to it, social contexts, and risks or complications. Thus the introductions can help to frame readings of the selected texts that follow. Alternatively, readers can read individual chapters or selections in any order, choosing specific medical topics, selection titles, or author names from the table of contents. For this purpose, each chapter and each selection is accompanied by an introduction, offering readers a foundation regardless of where they begin. While this volume is a result of my own teaching and research, it is designed to welcome any reader with an interest in women's health, regardless of their prior knowledge or if they are reading on their own, as part of a reading group, or with the support of a professor.

New York, NY, USA
April Patrick

References

Green, Monica H. 2008. "Gendering the History of Women's Healthcare. *Gender & History* 20.3: 487–518

Acknowledgments

This book is the result of more than sixteen years of work that began with an interest in the poetry of Christina Rossetti, continued with a dissertation and various publications on the narratives of breast cancer in nineteenth-century Britain, and developed into teaching literature and humanities courses that focused on women's health. Long before that, though, my interest in the stories of patients began as a child in the 1980s, spending my summers in Houston, Texas, joining my beloved grandmother as she volunteered with AIDS patients in hospice wards and their homes. Over the time I've worked on this topic both directly and indirectly, a number of wonderful people have supported me.

Since my first email about an idea for an anthology on women's health and our summer 2021 meeting on my university's campus as we emerged from COVID restrictions, Allie Troyanos at Palgrave Macmillan has supported and guided this project and me in so many ways. Thanks, too, to the anonymous readers of the proposal and full draft of this work. Your insightful questions and suggestions have helped to shape this volume.

The inclusion of several texts here is due to the generosity of archivists and descendants of those whose voices are featured here. The memoir by George Wray in Chap. 2 comes from the Carl H. Pforzheimer Collection of Shelley and His Circle, New York Public Library, Astor, Lenox, and Tilden Foundations. From that collection, Elizabeth C. Denlinger and Charles Cuykendall Carter were immensely helpful, and for my in-person visit to the Collection, Charlie enthusiastically pulled related materials, including poems by Wray and a lock of his hair. My inclusion of a short story by Tess Slesinger in Chap. 3 is with the kind permission of her son Peter Davis, who was wonderfully supportive in response to my request. Thanks also to Brad Bigelow who graciously connected me with Peter via email. The journal in Chap. 4 from Lady Helen Selina Blackwood, Baroness Dufferin and Claneboye (later Countess of Gifford) is included with permission from the Dufferin Foundation and with the kind support of Sir Ian Huddleston. This journal has captivated me since I first read a typescript of it in her son's papers at the British Library in 2010. It is an honor to get to share it through this book. Thanks also to Princeton University Press for permission to publish Benjamin Rush's side of the correspondence related to Abigail Adams Smith's breast cancer.

In my time at Fairleigh Dickinson University since 2014, my colleagues and students have brought so much joy to my work. I am greatly appreciative of funding in 2022–2023 through Becton College's Grant-in-Aid program to support the cost of permissions for this volume. Much of my work on this project was developed in a supportive community of scholars in our Becton Faculty Writing Group both during our weekly writing sessions and in our writing retreats. Additionally, ideas for readings and approaches to medical humanities and narrative medicine were explored through my teaching. Thanks to the students in those classes, particularly my Health and Healing classes in both fall 2021 and fall 2023 whose questions about these topics and texts helped me to write the supporting material.

As a graduate student, I was incredibly fortunate to have advisors on my master's thesis and doctoral dissertation that have approached mentorship as a long-term commitment. Linda Hughes has supported my research on women's breast cancer narratives from the start and has encouraged me to find a way to get this work out to the world. Natalie Houston introduced me to Christina Rossetti and helped me fall in love with Victorian studies in 2006, and then fifteen years later, she asked just the right questions that led me to the idea for this book.

In my personal life, I am fortunate to be encouraged through the love and support of my family. Thanks to my mother Mary, my grandfather Fred and late grandmother Helen, and my chosen sisters Amanda and Corrie, who have listened to countless hours of me talking about this topic for more than a decade and asked questions that helped me to refine my thoughts. Eric has been a true partner in life, reading drafts and chatting about my ideas, making me laugh, and ensuring our kid had fun and was out of the house while I finished this project. And my daughter Frieda is the most powerful motivation to explore this topic. I hope the battles we fight today will make the world better for her generation.

Contents

1	**Women's Health and Writing About It**	1
	Introduction	1
	A History of Women's Health and Healthcare	2
	History	2
	Women	2
	Health	3
	Contexts for Women and Medicine	4
	Current Issues in Women's Health	5
	Maternal Mortality Rates	5
	Rates of Women's Cancers	6
	Regressions Around Reproductive and Sexual Health Services	6
	Access to Quality Care for Transgender and Gender Expansive People	7
	Changing Understandings of Mental Illness and Treatments	7
	Reading Representations of Illness by Genre	8
	Life Writing: Narratives from Patient, Family, and Friends	8
	Other Nonfiction: Advice for Women, News Reports, Advocacy	9
	Literary Representations: Novels, Short Fiction, Poetry	10
	Reading These Forms of Narrative Together	11
	Outline of the Remaining Chapters	11
	References	12
2	**Pregnancy & Childbirth**	15
	Introduction	15
	History of Care in Pregnancy and Childbirth	15
	Changes in Birthing Practitioners and Facilities	17

History of Gynecological Research	18
Complications Around Pregnancy and Childbirth	19
Infertility and Miscarriage	19
Pain and Anesthesia	20
Cesarean Section Deliveries and Other Medical Interventions	21
Maternal Mortality	22
Maternal Mental Health	23
Themes and Topics in Selections	23
Maternal Mortality	23
Pain Relief and the Periodical Press	24
Maternal Mental Health	24
Types of Practitioners	24
Poems About Women Who Died in Childbirth (1750–1773)	25
Introduction	25
"On a Lady Who Died in Child-Birth" (*The Ladies Magazine: Or, The Universal Entertainer*, December 1750)	25
"Epitaph, on a Lady Who Died in Child-Birth" by Dr. Templeman (*Monthly Repository for Gentlemen & Ladies*, December 1762)	25
From *Monody to the Memory of a Young Lady Who Died in Child-Bed By An Afflicted Husband* by Cuthbert Shaw (1768)	26
"On Lady Shelley, who died in Childbed Said to be Written by the Rev. Dr. Delap" (*The Gentleman's Magazine: And Historical Chronicle*, August 1772)	28
"On Hearing the Organ Upon First Going to Church, After the Death of The Most Lovely, and Most Beloved Wife, Who Died in Child-Bed of Her First-Born, July 24, 1772" (*Hibernian Magazine, or Compendium of Entertaining Knowledge*, July 1773)	28
Account of and Extract from a New Work (1783)	29
Introduction	29
Account of and Extract from a New Work, Titled, "A Report, Made by Order of Government, of a Memoir, Containing a New, Easy, and Successful Method of Treating the Child bed or Puerperal Fever, made Use of by the Late M. Doulcet, Doctor Regent of the Faculty at Paris, and one of the Physicians of the Hotel-Dieu" (*Hibernian Magazine, or, Compendium of Entertaining Knowledge*, May 1783)	30
Charlotte Temple by Susanna Rowson (1791)	31
Introduction	31
Excerpt from Chapter XXXI: Subject Continued	32

Excerpt from Chapter XXXII: Reasons Why and Wherefore	32
Excerpt from Chapter XXXIII: Which People Void of Feeling Need Not Read	33

Memoirs of the Author of a Vindication of the Rights of Woman by William Godwin (1798) — 36
    Introduction — 36
    Excerpt from Chapter X — 36

Memoirs of a Most Beloved and Affectionate Wife by George Wray (1817) — 42
    Introduction — 42
    Excerpt from *Memoirs of a Most Beloved and Affectionate Wife* — 43

Periodical Coverage of Princess Charlotte's Death in Childbirth (1817–1818) — 56
    Introduction — 56
    Excerpt from "A Memoir of the Life, Death, and Funeral, of Her Royal Highness the Princess Charlotte Augusta" (*The Ladies' Monthly Museum*, December 1817) — 56
    Excerpt from "Brief Memoir of her Royal Highness the Princess Charlotte, with an Account of her last Illness, Death, and Funeral" (*The Literary Panorama and National Register*, December 1817) — 58
    "Death of Sir Richard Croft, Bart." (*Examiner*, 15 February 1818) — 63

"On Men-Midwives" (1819) — 65
    Introduction — 65
    "On Men-Midwives and Particularly on Those Who Practise Medicine as Well as Midwifery" (*The Literary Journal*, March 1819) — 65

"Childbed: A Prose Poem" by Leigh Hunt (1837) — 68
    Introduction — 68
    "Childbed: A Prose Poem" (*Monthly Repository*, November 1837) — 68

The Ladies' Medical Friend by William Hamilton Kittoe (1845) — 69
    Introduction — 69
    Excerpt from Pregnancy — 70

"Etherization in Childbirth" (1848) — 78
    Introduction — 78
    "Etherization in Childbirth" (*Saturday Evening Post*, 23 December 1848) — 79

Periodical Coverage of Queen Victoria and Anesthesia
(1848–1859)   82
   Introduction   82
   "Paradise Regained!" (*The Satirist; or Censor of the Times*, 23 January 1848)   82
   Excerpt from "Ether and Chloroform" (*The Nineteenth Century: A Quarterly Miscellany*, January 1848)   83
   "Secrets from the Palace by a Royal Page" (*The Satirist; or Censor of the Times*, 13 February 1848)   86
   "The Latest Absurdity" (*Trumpet and Universalist Magazine*, 4 March 1848)   86
   "Multiple News Items" (*The Standard*, 22 April 1853)   87
   "Court and High Life" (*Blackburn Standard*, 27 April 1853)   87
   "Chloroform at the Royal Accouchement" (*The Englishwoman's Review*, 8 January 1859)   87
A Popular Manual of Female Diseases by Robert Hall Bakewell (1859)   88
   Introduction   88
   Excerpts from Chapter IX: Pregnancy and Its Diseases   89
   Excerpts from Chapter X: Labour   90
   Excerpts from Chapter XI: Diseases of Childbed   95
Incidents in the Life of a Slave Girl by Harriet Jacobs (1861)   97
   Introduction   97
   Excerpt from Chapter X: A Perilous Passage in the Slave Girl's Life   98
   Excerpts from Chapter XI: The New Tie to Life   99
   Excerpts from Chapter XIV: Another Link to Life   100
"The New Order of Medical Students" (1871)   102
   Introduction   102
   "The New Order of Medical Students" (*The Englishwoman's Domestic Magazine*, June 1871)   102
Far from the Madding Crowd by Thomas Hardy (1874)   107
   Introduction   107
   Chapter XL: On Casterbridge Highway   107
   Excerpt from Chapter XLI: Suspicion—Fanny Is Sent For   112
   Excerpts from Chapter XLII: Joseph and His Burden—Buck's Head   113
   Excerpts from XLIII: Fanny's Revenge   114
The Wife's Handbook by Henry Arthur Allbutt (1888)   115
   Introduction   115

Excerpts from Chapter II: How to Keep the Health During Pregnancy	116
Excerpts from Chapter IV: After Delivery	117
Excerpt from Chapter VI: On Some Complaints of Child-Bearing, and Their Treatment	120
"The Yellow Wallpaper" and "Why I Wrote 'The Yellow Wallpaper'" by Charlotte Perkins Gilman (1892, 1913)	121
Introduction	121
"The Yellow Wallpaper" (*The New England Magazine*, January 1892)	122
"Why I Wrote 'The Yellow Wallpaper'" (*The Forerunner*, October 1913)	135
"La Belle Zoraïde" by Kate Chopin (1894)	136
Introduction	136
"La Belle Zoraïde"	137
"The Curse of Eve" by Arthur Conan Doyle (1894)	142
Introduction	142
"The Curse of Eve"	142
"Progress Made in the Treatment of the Diseases of Women" by Charles Jewett (1895)	151
Introduction	151
"Progress Made in the Treatment of the Diseases of Women" (*The Independent*, 12 September 1895)	151
The Awakening by Kate Chopin (1899)	153
Introduction	153
Excerpt from Chapter XXXVI	154
Excerpt from Chapter XXXVII	154
"Small vs. Large Families" by Ida Husted Harper (1901)	156
Introduction	156
Excerpt from "Small vs. Large Families" (*The Independent*, 26 December 1901)	156
Woman in Girlhood, Wifehood, Motherhood by Myer Solis-Cohen (1906)	159
Introduction	159
Excerpts from Chapter XVI: The Symptoms of Pregnancy	159
Excerpts from Chapter XIX: Preparations for the Confinement	160
Excerpts from Chapter XXI: The Management of Labor	163
"Twilight Sleep in America" by Constance Leupp and Burton J. Hendrick (1915)	166
Introduction	166
"Twilight Sleep in America" (*McClure's Magazine*, April 1915)	167

"Safeguarding American Motherhood" by Anna Steese Richardson (1915)	174
Introduction	174
"Safeguarding American Motherhood" (*McClure's Magazine*, July 1915)	174
"Every Woman's Chance to Serve Humanity" by Anne Martin (1920)	180
Introduction	180
"Every Woman's Chance to Serve Humanity: An Everlasting Benefit You Can Win in a Week" (*Good Housekeeping*, February 1920)	180
"Infant Death Rate Reaches High Mark" (1926)	190
Introduction	190
"Infant Death Rate Reaches High Mark: Nation Compares Unfavorably with Many Others, Children's Bureau Survey Shows. Same is True of Mothers" (*New York Times*, 30 August 1926)	190
Twilight Sleep by Edith Wharton (1927)	192
Introduction	192
Excerpt from Chapter 1	192
References	193
3 Contraception & Abortion	**195**
Introduction	195
History of Methods for Preventing and Terminating Pregnancy	195
Natural Potions, Tools, and Techniques	196
Modern Pharmaceuticals	197
Surgical Methods	199
Legality and Beliefs around Contraception and Abortion	200
Legal History	201
Eugenics	202
Women's Rights and Feminism	203
Themes and Topics in Selections	203
Moral, Social, and Legal Perspectives	203
Fertility Control and Marriage	204
The Perception of Danger	204
Maria: Or, The Wrongs of Woman by Mary Wollstonecraft (1798)	205
Introduction	205
Excerpt from Chapter 5	205

"Fruits of Philosophy" by Charles Knowlton (1832)	208
Introduction	208
Excerpt from Chapter III. Of Promoting and Checking Conception.	208
"Periodical Coverage of Madame Restell" (1841–1878)	212
Introduction	212
Untitled Article (*The New World*, 27 March 1841)	212
"Madam Restell Still in Prison: Ransacking the City to Find a Man Who Will Put His Name on Her Bail Bond" (*The Sun*, 13 February 1878)	213
"The Restell Tragedy" (*The American Socialist*, 11 April 1878)	216
The Ladies' Medical Friend by W. Hamilton Kittoe (1845)	220
Introduction	220
Excerpt from "Abortion or Miscarriage"	221
"Horrible. Death From Abortion." (1846)	221
Introduction	221
Horrible. Death from Abortion. (*National Police Gazette*, 5 December 1846)	221
The Unwelcome Child; or, The Crime of an Undesigned and Undesired Maternity by Henry Clarke Wright (1858)	225
Introduction	225
Excerpts from Letter V: The Wife's Appeal—The Husband's Response	225
"The Evil of the Age" (1871)	231
Introduction	231
The Evil of the Age (*New York Times*, 23 August 1871)	231
Ladies' Guide in Health and Disease: Girlhood, Maidenhood, Wifehood, Motherhood by John Harvey Kellogg (1882)	238
Introduction	238
The Wife: Criminal Abortion	239
The Wife's Handbook by Henry Arthur Allbutt (1888)	247
Introduction	247
Chapter VII. How To Prevent Conception When Advised By The Doctor	247
"Voluntary Motherhood" by Harriot Stanton Blatch (1891)	251
Introduction	251
"Voluntary Motherhood"	252
"The Welcome Child" by Lady Henry Somerset (1895)	258
Introduction	258
"The Welcome Child" (*The Arena*, March 1895)	259

"The Case of Dr. Collins" (1898)   266
    Introduction   266
    The Case of Dr. Collins (*The Speaker*, 9 July 1898)   266
Manual of Health for Women: Plain Advice in Sickness and Health by Peter J. Latz (1906)   268
    Introduction   268
    b. Voluntary Sterility, or the Wilful Prevention of Conception   269
"Waste" by Harvey Granville-Barker (1907)   271
    Introduction   271
    Excerpt from The Second Act   271
    Excerpt from The Third Act   276
    Excerpt from The Fourth Act   278
"A Sunday Morning Tragedy" by Thomas Hardy (1909)   280
    Introduction   280
    A Sunday Morning Tragedy (*circa* 186–)   281
Gloria Gray—Love Pirate by Pearl Doles Bell (1914)   284
    Introduction   284
    Chapter XXVI. A Four Leaf Clover.   284
Harper's Weekly Series on The Control of Births by Mary Alden Hopkins (1915)   287
    Introduction   287
    "The Control of Births" (*Harper's Weekly*, 3 April 1915)   287
    "The Control of Births" (*Harper's Weekly*, 10 April 1915)   288
    "Birth Control and Public Morals: An Interview with Anthony Comstock" (*Harper's Weekly*, 22 May 1915)   292
    "Is Contraception Immoral?" (*Harper's Weekly*, 19 June 1915)   298
Summer by Edith Wharton (1917)   302
    Introduction   302
    Excerpt from Chapter VII   302
    Excerpt from Chapter IX   303
    Excerpts from Chapter XV   303
    Excerpt from Chapter XVII   307
    Excerpt from Chapter XVIII   308
The Crisis: A Record of the Darker Races (October 1922)   310
    Introduction   310
    Excerpt from "Opinion" by W. E. B. DuBois, Birth   310
    "Motherhood" by Georgia Douglas Johnson   311
The Beautiful and the Damned by F. Scott Fitzgerald (1922)   312
    Introduction   312
    Book II, Chapter II, Nietzschean Incident   312

"Mr. Durant" by Dorothy Parker (1924)	314
Introduction	314
"Mr. Durant" (*The American Mercury*, September 1924)	314
"Hills Like White Elephants" by Ernest Hemingway (1927)	323
Introduction	323
Hills Like White Elephants (*transition*, August 1927)	323
"Missis Flinders" by Tess Slesinger (1932)	327
Introduction	327
"Missis Flinders" (*Story*, December 1932)	328
References	339

4 Breast & Gynecological Cancers   341

Introduction	341
History of Breast and Gynecological Cancer Diagnosis and Treatment	342
The Rise of Radical Surgical Treatments	343
The Fall of Radical Surgical Treatments	346
Psychological Effects of Breast and Gynecological Cancer and Treatments	347
Cultural Shifts and the Rise of the Cancer Narrative	348
Themes and Topics in Selections	349
Hiding Cancer and Fear of Surgical Treatment	350
Risks of Some Alternative Treatments	350
Class in Treatment Options	350
"Some Account of a Pamphlet Lately Published" (1761)	351
Introduction	351
"Some Account of a Pamphlet Lately Published, Intitled Observations upon a Treatise on the Virtues of Hemlock, in the Cure of Cancers, Written by Dr. Storck, &c." (*The London Magazine, or Gentleman's Monthly Intelligencer*, July 1761)	351
The Woman of Letters, or The History of Miss Fanny Belton by Maria Smyth (1783)	354
Introduction	354
Excerpts from Letter XVI	355
Letters Relating to Abigail Adams Smith's Breast Cancer (1811)	356
Introduction	356
From Abigail Smith Adams to William Stephens Smith	356
From Abigail Adams Smith to Benjamin Rush	357
From Benjamin Rush to John Adams	358
From Abigail Smith Adams to William Stephens Smith	359

From John Adams to Benjamin Rush	359
From Benjamin Rush to John Adams	360

Account from Paris of a Terrible Operation by Frances Burney D'Arblay (1812) — 361
    Introduction — 361
    Account from Paris of a Terrible Operation—1812 — 361

Letter to Kitty Barry Blackwell by Elizabeth Blackwell (1887) — 374
    Introduction — 374
    Letter to Begin Memoir — 374

The Ladies' Medical Friend by W. Hamilton Kittoe (1845) — 376
    Introduction — 376
    Cancer of the Womb — 376
    Excerpts from "On the Breast and its Diseases" — 377
    Cancer — 379
    Symptoms — 379
    Treatment — 381

"Cancer Said To Be Cured By Mesmerism" (1848) — 382
    Introduction — 382
    "Cancer Said to Be Cured By Mesmerism" (*Chambers's Edinburgh Journal*, 9 December 1848) — 382

Memoirs about Emily Gosse's Breast Cancer by Philip Henry Gosse (1857) and Edmund Gosse (1907) — 383
    Introduction — 383
    Excerpts from *A Memorial of the Last Days on Earth of Emily Gosse* by Philip Henry Gosse — 384
    From *Father and Son: A Study of Two Temperaments* by Edmund Gosse — 393

"Rab and His Friends" by John Brown (1858) — 397
    Introduction — 397
    Excerpt from "Rab and His Friends" — 397

"Extracts from My Case-Book. By an Old Physician" (1858) — 405
    Introduction — 405
    Extracts from my Case-Book. By an Old Physician (*The Englishwoman's Review*, 23 October 1858) — 406

Diary of Helen Blackwood, Lady Dufferin and Claneboye, Countess of Gifford (1867) — 406
    Introduction — 406
    January 1st — 407
    January 4th — 408
    Thursday, January 24th — 410

Thursday, January 31st	411
Saturday, February 2nd	412
Monday, 4th	412
Tuesday, 5th	412
Wednesday, February 6th	412
Friday 8th	413
Saturday 9th	413
Sunday 10th	413
Monday, February 11th	413
Tuesday 12th	414
Friday 15th	414
Saturday, February 16th	415
Sunday 17th	415
Monday 18th	415
Saturday 23rd	415
Monday 25th	416
Tuesday 26th	416
Wednesday, February 27th	416
Thursday, February 28th	416
Friday, March 1st	416
Saturday 2nd	417
Monday 4th	417
Tuesday, March 5th	417
Monday 11th	418
Tuesday 12th	418
Wed. 13th	418
Thursday 14th	418
Friday 15th	418
"The Useful Book. Compiled by Mrs. Warren" (1875)	419
Introduction	419
The Useful Book. Compiled by Mrs. Warren (*The Treasury of Literature and The Ladies Treasury*, 2 August 1875)	419
Ladies' Guide in Health and Disease: Girlhood, Maidenhood, Wifehood, Motherhood by J. H. Kellogg (1883)	421
Introduction	421
Cancer of the Womb	422
Tumors of the Breast	422
Cancer of the Breast	423
"Willie" by Katharine Tynan (1898)	425
Introduction	425

"Willie" (*The Speaker*, 18 June 1898)	426
Articles from *The People's Health Journal of Chicago* (1900–1901)	430
Introduction	430
Free Consultations: Case 60 (*The People's Health Journal of Chicago*, 15 January 1900)	431
Cancer and X-Ray by J. E. Gilman (*The People's Health Journal of Chicago*, 15 November 1901)	431
Manual of Health for Women: Plain Advice in Sickness and Health by Peter J. Latz (1906)	433
Introduction	433
Cancer of the Womb (Carcinoma uteri)	433
Sarcoma of the Womb (Sarcoma uteri)	436
Ovarian Tumors	436
"A Protest Against the Surgical Invasion of Cancers and Tumors" (1917)	437
Introduction	437
A Protest Against the Surgical Invasion of Cancers and Tumors (*Current Opinion*, November 1917)	438
The House on the Bogs by Katharine Tynan (1922)	440
Introduction	440
Excerpts from Chapter X: The Lit House	440
Excerpts from Chapter XII: The Poison of Jealousy	441
Excerpts from Chapter XVIII: Fear	442
Excerpts from Chapter XX: Child's Play	443
"The Prevention of Cancer" by James Ewing (1927)	445
Introduction	445
The Prevention of Cancer (*The Forum*, March 1927)	445
References	449
Index	**451**

1

Women's Health and Writing About It

Introduction

In the past few years, debates in the United States about women's bodies have dominated the news as politicians seek to take decisions about women's health from women and place it into the hands of lawmakers. The maternal mortality rate—especially for Black women—in the United States is one of the highest in the world. Concerns around women's health in the United Kingdom led to the 2022 development of a Women's Health Strategy document and the appointment of the first Women's Health Ambassador, seeking to expand access to contraception, support in miscarriage and menopause, and general support for women's health. Overall, the current state of women's health in the medical, social, and political spheres has led to renewed activism. The current activists build upon a history that extends far beyond when second-wave feminists published texts like *Our Bodies, Ourselves* in 1970 and rallied around the 1967 Abortion Act in the United Kingdom and the Roe v. Wade decision of the American Supreme Court in 1973. Indeed, this current movement is part of more than a century of work toward bodily autonomy and improved healthcare outcomes for women in both Britain and America. This volume offers a history of women's health care in the United Kingdom and the United States since 1750, bringing together the voices of women, their family and friends, their doctors, and their advocates.

A History of Women's Health and Healthcare

Before delving into the medical advances that will provide context for the remaining chapters of this book, some words of definition and introduction about three key words—history, women, and health—are necessary. These definitions offer a sense of the scope for this text and and set expectations for what is included and what is not. They also help to ensure that we begin on the same proverbial page with some shared understandings of how complex words and ideas are being used in this volume.

History

The texts reproduced here represent voices and experiences of people in the United Kingdom and the United States between the years 1750 and 1950; however, the introductions to each chapter include some background before and after that timespan as further context. These two centuries are important for a history of women's health because they illustrate a period of significant change in medical treatment and social structures. The eighteenth century brought many new ideas from the sciences, increasing professionalization of the medical field and wider circulation of print culture. And though the earliest selections in this book were written by people who lived 300 years before our time, many of the broader themes and underlying concerns included in these texts feel relevant today. The latest texts in this volume represent the middle of the twentieth century, even though many medical advances have occurred in the past 75 years. Those more recent experiences are well documented and widely available in anthologies and memoirs as well as through digital media and the internet. The textual evidence from the period included in this book, however, is scattered across various published and archival sources or is discussed in analytical academic texts with limited quotations selected for evidence. In order to offer a different kind of history of women's health for this period than is currently available, this volume combines the telling of secondary sources and descriptive history with the showing of primary texts and archival materials and brings together texts that are not otherwise easy to juxtapose.

Women

The words *woman* or *women* will often mean something different in the selected texts written in the eighteenth, nineteenth, or twentieth centuries than in the introductory overviews written in 2023. The historical material included in this volume reflects a period when the term *women* had a relatively static meaning and primarily referred to cisgender women. Certainly, trans and gender expansive people existed throughout those historical periods, but the texts included in this volume generally refer to cisgender women. Thanks to the research of second-wave feminist scholars, historical narratives from and about women are more readily available and thus their voices and experience have become valued. This is a reminder of both how powerful archival work is in shaping our understanding of our past and the importance of recovering historical narratives and experiences from trans and gender expansive people.

In contrast with the texts selected, this book was written and exists in the twenty-first century when we have more robust language to discuss the broad spectrum of gender identity. In any contextual material written for the purposes of this book, *women* is used in a broader and more inclusive sense to apply to anyone who identifies as a woman, encounters the world as a woman, and/or has embodied experiences of a woman. That can include but is not limited to cisgender women, trans women, trans men, intersex individuals, and nonbinary people. The conditions and medical situations addressed in this book are experienced by many people who do not identify as women. While the word *women* is inadequate, I use it in the hope that a more inclusive meaning allows it to bridge the historical and the present represented on these pages.

Health

Rather than attempting broad coverage of the many conditions that can affect women, this book focuses on three areas to allow for more depth in the consideration of each. Specifically, the conditions covered in the three remaining chapters are pregnancy and childbirth (Chap. 2), abortion and contraception (Chap. 3), and breast and gynecological cancers (Chap. 4). Certainly there are many other conditions that could be included here. For example, in the twenty-first century, heart disease is the leading cause of death for women in both the United States and the United Kingdom, and historically, heart disease appeared in both medical accounts and literary texts.[1] However, heart disease was and is not primarily a gendered condition and was not described in as physical and concrete terms as early or as publicly as the conditions included here.

---

[1] For more on Victorian heart disease in medicine and literature, see Kirstie Blair's *Victorian Poetry and the Culture of the Heart* (2006).

The three conditions in this volume have been prevalent in medical practice and women's lives for centuries, even if understandings of their causes and symptoms and the methods for treating them have evolved. These three are also primarily associated with women, even though they can affect or even afflict men. Additionally, each of these conditions or situations brought women into contact with healthcare, whether in the form of licensed physicians, trained midwives, or other practitioners. Finally, these are all widely represented in the fiction, nonfiction, and life writing of the eighteenth, nineteenth, and twentieth centuries.

Contexts for Women and Medicine

Over the past three centuries, medicine has become institutionalized and has changed dramatically, including larger understandings of physiology and conditions, technology for diagnosis and treatment, approaches to care for various groups. The eighteenth century brought smallpox inoculation and vaccination, forceps and other interventions for childbirth, and the first successful appendectomy. Research from the eighteenth century also led to a number of discoveries and inventions in the nineteenth, including the stethoscope, cellular theory, anesthesia, germ theory and antiseptic practices, the syringe, x-rays, and vaccines for cholera, anthrax, rabies, tetanus, diphtheria, typhoid fever, and bubonic plague. Among other results, these discoveries allowed for longer and safer operations and increased the likelihood of patients surviving during and after surgery. This period also saw the medical field professionalized through the founding of the earliest medical schools in Britain and America in the eighteenth century and the establishment of national licensing and governing bodies for physicians in the nineteenth.

Though women undoubtedly benefitted from these advances, their relationship with the field of medicine was complicated. Women were commonly viewed as weaker or more susceptible to illness than men and the medical profession was male-dominated, so the treatment women received was often limited or discriminatory. Indeed, much of the medical attention paid to women focused on their reproductive health, blaming reproductive organs for their medical issues, shaping their care around their ability to conceive and bear children, and defining them primarily around their role as mothers. Professional roles for women also shifted significantly as licensed physicians began to replace midwives, medical schools and organizations were slow to accept women as physicians, and trained nurses became an important part of the field. Healthcare also offered women a venue for advocacy and activism, from the time that Lady Mary Wortley Montagu fought for smallpox inoculation in the eighteenth century through the work of campaigners for such issues as anesthesia in childbirth and access to birth control and abortion services. This complicated history continues into the twenty-first century, as women still face dismissive or sexist experiences with medical providers.

Current Issues in Women's Health

The texts in the chapters that follow reflect the experiences of women with healthcare between the eighteenth and twentieth centuries, but many of the themes and issues relate to concerns facing women in the twenty-first century. Specifically, a few of these topics include high rates of maternal mortality and women's cancers, regressions in the available care and resources for reproductive and sexual health, and changing understandings of women's mental health. In all of these areas, the difficulties disproportionally affect women from marginalized communities both in their health and in their access to quality healthcare.

Maternal Mortality Rates

Despite advances in healthcare, maternal mortality during pregnancy, childbirth, or the postpartum period continues to be a significant concern in both Britain and America. In Britain, while overall maternal mortality rates have declined, there has been a notable increase in maternal mortality among Black women. In fact, Black women in the United Kingdom are 3.7 and in the United States are 2.6 times more likely to die during pregnancy or childbirth compared to white women, with factors such as inequalities in access to quality care and discrimination playing a role (Knight et al. 2022; Hoyert 2023). In America, maternal mortality rates are some of the highest among high-income countries, with a disproportionate impact on women of color. Factors such as inadequate prenatal care, lack of insurance coverage, systemic racism, and social determinants of health, including poverty and discrimination, contribute to the persistent problem of maternal mortality in both countries (Crear-Perry et al. 2021). This international challenge is the first target in the United Nations Sustainable Development Goal around health, as the organization seeks to "reduce the global maternal mortality ratio to less than 70 per 100,000 live births" by 2030.

Rates of Women's Cancers

The twenty-first century has seen a concerning trend of rising rates of women's cancers. Breast cancer, ovarian cancer, and cervical cancer are among the most common types of cancers affecting women in Britain and America. According to Cancer Research UK, breast cancer incidence rates in Britain have increased by over 50% in the last 25 years, and ovarian cancer rates have also risen. The American National Cancer Institute (2021) reports that breast cancer remains the most common cancer among women, and cervical cancer rates have shown an uptick in recent years, particularly among minority and underserved populations. The discussion about these statistics typically suggests causes related to changing lifestyles, which include delayed childbearing, obesity, lack of physical activity, and exposure to hormonal and environmental risk factors. Efforts toward early detection through screening and prevention strategies, as well as increased awareness and access to healthcare services, have sought to address these alarming rates.

Regressions Around Reproductive and Sexual Health Services

Access to comprehensive reproductive and sexual health services has been limited in recent years. In both Britain and America, funding cuts to or outright defunding of sexual health services, closure of clinics, and changes to policies related to contraception provision have led to reduced access and availability of services, particularly for underserved populations (Waters 2022; Vandevusse et al. 2022). Additionally, the 2022 decision by the US Supreme Court in Dobbs v. Jackson Women's Health Organization overturned two previous cases—Roe v. Wade in 1973 and Planned Parenthood v. Casey in 1992—and ruled that the US Constitution does not confer the right to abortion and returned to the states the power to regulate aspects of abortion not protected by federal law. This led to more interest in forms of medication abortion, which can be distributed through the mail. However, in 2023, some states sought to restrict access to mifepristone and/or misoprostol as part of their restrictions, using the nineteenth-century Comstock Laws as support. Overall, these regressions have implications for public health, including increased rates of unintended pregnancies, sexually transmitted infections, and disparities in access to care, particularly affecting low-income individuals, people of color, and marginalized communities. Additionally, in many states, doctors are limited in providing life-saving care for women experiencing a miscarriage or complications in their pregnancies. Some of the international efforts in this area are supported through the United Nations' Sustainable Development Goals, with targets in two areas working toward "sexual and reproductive health-care services, including for family planning, information and education" (Target 3.7) and "universal access to sexual and reproductive health and reproductive rights" (Target 5.6).

Access to Quality Care for Transgender and Gender Expansive People

For trans and nonbinary people, discrimination, stigma, and inadequate healthcare policies and practices often create barriers to receiving gender-affirming care. Many trans people encounter challenges in accessing hormone replacement therapy, gender-affirming surgeries, and other medical care due to financial constraints, lack of insurance coverage, long waiting lists, and limited availability of specialized healthcare providers. Additionally, lack of cultural competency among healthcare providers can also result in discriminatory or negative healthcare experiences, leading to avoidance or delay in seeking healthcare services. Mental health concerns, including depression, anxiety, and suicidality, are prevalent among trans and gender expansive people, further underscoring the need for comprehensive and inclusive healthcare services (Erickson-Schroth 2022; Sharman 2021).

Changing Understandings of Mental Illness and Treatments

In recent decades, increased awareness and recognition of mental health issues specific to women—including perinatal mental health, postpartum depression, anxiety, and trauma-related disorders—have led to improved screening, diagnosis, and treatment options. Efforts to reduce stigma and increase mental health literacy have also gained momentum, empowering women to seek help and access appropriate care. Advances in research and evidence-based practices have led to more targeted and gender-sensitive interventions for women's mental health concerns. However, challenges remain, including barriers to accessing mental health services, disparities in treatment, and the need for ongoing advocacy and support for women's mental health issues.

Reading Representations of Illness by Genre

While descriptive overviews of the conditions and situations in the chapters that follow will provide helpful background, this volume is largely comprised of narratives from primary and archival sources across a variety of forms and genres. The texts selected for each of these chapters offer a variety of perspectives on each condition or situation, including those of the woman or patient, her family or friends, medical professionals, and activists or advocates working on the topic. Additionally, some of the texts are written by anonymous contributors in magazines and newspapers or novelists representing fictional characters. Regardless of the writer, each of the selected texts reflects either women's experiences in the period or what women could have encountered in popular media or literature. Any texts written by doctors are derived from books or periodicals that target a general audience, which often reframed specialized medical knowledge for women readers. This helps those reading this volume to more fully understand the information a woman would have had about her body, her condition, and/or her situation as she sought to make any medical decisions.

Narratives allow readers to see more depth and more nuance in the experiences of people engaged in the medical system. This is the root of narrative medicine, which "provides the means to understand the personal connections between patient and physician, the meaning of medical practice for the individual physician, physicians' collective profession of their ideals, and medicine's discourse with the society it serves" (Charon 2001). Narrative medicine takes its methods from the humanities, incorporating techniques like close reading and analysis of genre and style. Because readers of this volume may not have training in analyzing the genres and forms represented in the selections, the following sections offer contexts for reading life writing, literary representations, medical texts, and other nonfiction and for analyzing those texts in relationship with one another.

Life Writing: Narratives from Patient, Family, and Friends

The overarching term life writing includes not only published memoirs and autobiographies but also unpublished letters and diaries that reflect the writer's lived experience. This form has a deep connection with representations of health, illness, and disability with many scholars suggesting terms and frameworks for their intersection. Thomas Couser (1997) defines autopathography as "autobiographical narrative[s] of illness or disability" which are "heightening one's awareness of one's mortality, threatening one's sense of identity, and disrupting the apparent plot of one's life" (p. 5). In a study of breast cancer narratives, Mary K. DeShazer (2013) combines Couser's autopathography with autothanatography—"life writing about dying" (p. 10)—to define what she terms mammographies as "a distinctive testimonial and memorial tradition" that has led to "new artistic forms of recounting trauma, celebrating survival, and memorializing the world's dead or dying mothers, daughters, partners, sisters, and friends" (p. 2). Ann Jurecic (2012) analyzes illness narratives—"autobiographical accounts of illness spoken or written by patients" (p. 2)—by reaching outside of literary scholarship to provide what she believes traditional literary criticism does not: "interpretive approaches that enable [critics] to assemble meaning in the face of life's fragility" (p. 4). Each of these descriptions of the intersection of life writing and illness suggests the purposes and effects for these texts as a basis for their analysis.

Charon (2006) proposes reading strategies for this kind of life writing, as she connects the work of the medical doctor in terms that easily apply to analysis of an illness narrative: "listen expertly and attentively to extraordinarily complicated narratives—told in words, gestures, silences, tracings, images, laboratory test results, and changes in the body—and to cohere all these stories into something that made provisional sense" (p. 4). Charon strives to reach this goal, in part, by using autobiographical theory. She expands from the commonly analyzed autobiographical gap—the "space between the narrator-who-writes and the protagonist-who-acts" (p. 70)—to consider what she calls "the corporeal gap," which describes the way "the act of telling separates, momentarily, the teller-who-reports from the body-that-feels" (p. 90). Together, these two gaps create a valuable space for analysis in the life writing from women patients in this volume, while also recognizing that the narratives may not be exact representations of their experience. Instead we can analyze "how writers and readers use narratives of illness to make meaning of the experiences of living *at risk*, *in prognosis*, and *in pain*" (Jurecic 2012, p. 4, italics original).

Other Nonfiction: Advice for Women, News Reports, Advocacy

In popular culture, women encountered a wide variety of nonfiction in books and periodicals, all of which could incorporate information about health and women's bodies more generally. These included the guides or advice manuals directed to women, reports about the medical cases of famous or regular women, and investigative or editorial texts about various conditions or treatments. Outside of verbal communication with friends or family, it was through these texts that many women learned about their bodies, made sense of symptoms they experienced, understood available treatments, and considered medical decisions for themselves and their families. Truly, it is only with awareness about the condition and the various treatment options that a woman could have any control in her own medical care.

By reading the way agency results from information, we can see implicit connections between the historic texts and those of the late twentieth-century Women's Health Movement that provided women with a deeper understanding of their own health. The 1970 publication of *Our Bodies Ourselves* by the Boston Women's Health Book Collective inspired a generation of women to learn about their bodies in order to claim agency over them. As the Collective explains, this text "introduced … ideas into the public discourse on women's health" including the idea "that women can become their own health experts, particularly through discussing issues of health and sexuality with each other." *Our Bodies Ourselves* has remained a revolutionary text for women of the past five decades and, together with the works of the women's health movement it inspired, provides a useful complement to the nonfiction women encountered in before the mid-twentieth century.

Literary Representations: Novels, Short Fiction, Poetry

In addition to the various forms of nonfiction described above, these medical situations are also represented in literature, including sections of novels, short stories, and poems. Some of the poems operate like the life writing above as they memorialize specific women or recall medical situations. Others, however, offer fictional representations of characters, like the novels and short stories, facing health challenges. Like the mid-nineteenth-century fiction of social reform that took "as its subject-matter large-scale problems in contemporary British society" (Guy 1996, p. 3), fictional representations of medical situations addressed the illness, treatments for it, and attitudes and anxieties about it that appear in the nonfiction.

Fiction is an important form for representing health and medical care because it can address critical issues behind the veil of literature. In the selections in this volume, the authors raise important issues in the medical treatment of women, their manipulation or mistreatment, the uncertainties and pain that women endured in their interactions with medicine, and the way class dictated the level of treatment a patient received. As fiction, the texts rely on a protagonist/antagonist construction and focus on conflict to drive the plot. In some fictional representations of illness, particularly those by medical professionals like Arthur Conan Doyle, the male doctor is presented as the heroic protagonist rescuing the woman patient from the clutches of death. For texts that center the woman patient as protagonist, however, her conflict is often directly with the condition or disease she faces, but she may also battle a manipulative or incompetent medical practitioner.

Reading These Forms of Narrative Together

In the chapters that follow, the texts are grouped by condition or situation and then mostly ordered chronologically by publication date. That structure juxtaposes these varying forms and can inspire interesting observations about their relationship with one another. For example, a piece of life writing from the same period as an advice article from a popular periodical could illuminate reasons a woman might fear giving birth in a hospital or seek an herbal abortifacient or hesitate to tell her doctor about finding a lump in her breast. It could also demonstrate cases where a woman or her family were not aware of medical advances that could have changed her experience in some way. Reading for these connections or noting apparent inconsistencies offers the opportunity for analysis and a deeper exploration of the medical history depicted.

Outline of the Remaining Chapters

Each of the remaining chapters includes an overview that provides background on the medical condition and context for the readings followed by a collection of texts in excerpt or in full. The texts are organized chronologically by publication date, except for several clusters of shorter pieces that are connected around a specific theme or style. Each text is accompanied by a brief introduction that provides context about the writer, the situation, the larger work if it is an excerpt, or other aspects that will assist readers in their comprehension and analysis.

Chapter 2 focuses on the most common condition that brings women in contact with medical treatment: pregnancy and childbirth. The overview presents a history of care around pregnancy and childbirth, considering the place of midwives and obstetricians, the development of modern gynecology through exploitative research practices, birthing at home and in medical facilities, the use of cesarean section deliveries, common complications and causes for miscarriage, maternal mortality, and mental health issues that accompany this experience. Chapter 3 continues by considering pregnancies that are prevented or terminated. This overview provides a history of contraception and abortion practices through surgical and nonsurgical methods and the changing legal and social views of contraception and abortion. Chapter 4 centers on cancers most associated with women's bodies, specifically breast, uterine, cervical, and ovarian cancers. The overview considers the methods of diagnosing the cancers, the history of care through surgical and nonsurgical treatments, the rise and fall of the radical mastectomy and hysterectomy as preferred treatments, and psychological effects of treatment.

References

Cancer Research UK. Breast cancer incidence statistics. https://www.cancerresearchuk.org/health-professional/cancer-statistics/statistics-by-cancer-type/breast-cancer/incidence#heading-Zero.

Charon, Rita. 2001. Narrative Medicine: A Model for Empathy, Reflection, Profession, and Trust. *JAMA*. 286:1897–1902. https://doi.org/10.1001/jama.286.15.1897

Charon, Rita. 2006. *Narrative Medicine: Honoring the Stories of Illness*. Oxford: Oxford University Press.

Couser, Thomas. 1997. *Recovering Bodies: Illness, Disability, and Life Writing*. Madison: University of Wisconsin Press.

Crear-Perry, Joia et al. 2021. Social and Structural Determinants of Health Inequities in Maternal Health. Journal of Women's Health. 30: 230–235. https://doi.org/10.1089/jwh.2020.8882

DeShazer, Mary K. 2013. *Mammographies: The Cultural Discourses of Breast Cancer Narratives*. Ann Arbor: University of Michigan Press.

Erickson-Schroth, Laura. 2022. *Trans Bodies, Trans Selves*. 2nd ed. New York: Oxford University Press.

Guy, Josephine M. 1996. *The Victorian Social-Problem Novel: The Market, the Individual and Communal Life*. New York: St. Martin's Press.

Hoyert, Donna L. 2023. Maternal Mortality Rates in the United States, 2021. NCHS Health E-Stats. https://doi.org/10.15620/cdc:124678

Jurecic, Ann. 2012. *Illness as Narrative*. Pittsburgh: University of Pittsburgh Press.

Knight, Marian et al., eds. 2022. Saving Lives, Improving Mothers' Care: Lessons learned to inform maternity care from the UK and Ireland Confidential Enquiries into Maternal Deaths and Morbidity 2018–20. Oxford: National Perinatal Epidemiology Unit, University of Oxford.

National Cancer Institute. 2021. Cancer Stat Facts: Female Breast Cancer. https://seer.cancer.gov/statfacts/html/breast.html

Sharman, Zena. 2021. *The Care We Dream Of: Liberatory & Transformative Approaches to LGBTQ+ Health*. Vancouver: Arsenal Pulp Press.

Vandevusse, Alicia et al. 2022. Disruptions and opportunities in sexual and reproductive health care: How COVID-19 impacted service provision in three US states. Guttmacher Institute. https://doi.org/10.1363/psrh.12213

Waters, Adele. 2022. Sexual health services are at "breaking point" after £1bn in cuts since 2015 *BMJ* 379. https://doi.org/10.1136/bmj.o2766

United Nations. The 17 Goals. https://sdgs.un.org/goals

2

Pregnancy & Childbirth

Introduction

Pregnancy and childbirth represent the most common reason women encounter medical treatment, and for many years, giving birth brought significant risks of ill-health or death for women.[1] This chapter explores birthing from historical understandings of it as a process or series of stages that included pregnancy, delivery, and recovery, rather than a single event (Fox 2022, pp. 1–2). Though birth is often represented as a natural function, the medicalization of this process over the past few centuries has changed women's experiences, along with the types of practitioners they encounter and where they give birth. Still, many of the same concerns continue today, including miscarriage and pregnancy loss, management of pain, medical interventions in difficult births, risks around maternal mortality, and mental health during and after the birthing process.

History of Care in Pregnancy and Childbirth

From the ancient times, practices around pregnancy and childbirth demonstrate a tension between views of birthing as a natural process and potential risks to both the mother and the fetus. Though the surviving medical texts were written by men, women practitioners were central to birthing and shared

---

[1] The use of woman/women reflects the historical language of periods and texts presented here. In 2023, birthing person is more inclusive language to represent that trans and gender-expansive people can be pregnant. For more discussion, see Chap. 1, Women's Health and Writing About It.

their knowledge and experience through oral traditions. Indeed, the crucial role of midwives appears in the works of Hippocrates and Aristotle (Simonds et al. 2002). Interconnected with medical approaches to pregnancy and childbirth are superstitions, religious beliefs, folk remedies, rituals, and ceremonies, some of which remained common beliefs into the early twentieth century (Filippini 2021). The Middle Ages through the seventeenth century brought some advances like the use of instruments however, centuries of obstetric practices were mostly based on trial and error because practitioners had limited understandings of pregnancy and childbirth and of women's bodies more generally.

Most histories of birthing recognize the eighteenth century as a significant turning point in medical practices and cultural attitudes, including the development of obstetric instruments and the emergence of male physicians as primary attendants during childbirth. In Britain, prominent physicians like William Smellie and William Hunter made significant contributions to obstetric knowledge and practice during this period and trained the first American obstetricians. Though midwives continued to play a significant role in American birthing, their practices were increasingly scrutinized and regulated by male physicians. Social and cultural norms influenced childbirth practices, with a focus on modesty, morality, and propriety. Religious beliefs also played a role, with Puritan influences shaping attitudes toward pregnancy and childbirth in both Britain and America. Despite these changes, however, maternal and infant mortality rates remained high due to limited medical knowledge and resources.

In the nineteenth century, medicalization of childbirth continued to increase, with the establishment of obstetric hospitals and the growing influence of male physicians in maternity care. The use of obstetric instruments, such as forceps and anesthesia, became more common. However, this period also saw the rise of midwifery as a profession, with the establishment of formal midwifery schools and the recognition of midwives as important providers of maternity care. Social and cultural attitudes towards childbirth also evolved, with a growing emphasis on cleanliness, modesty, and the role of women as nurturers and mothers (Wertz and Wertz 1989). Still, concerns around childbed or puerperal fever and infant mortality continued, in part because of poor sanitation and limited access to healthcare for certain populations, such as enslaved women and marginalized communities (Rooks 1997).

The twentieth century brought further medicalization and significant technological advancements, with hospital births becoming the norm and obstetricians becoming the primary providers of maternity care (Simonds et al. 2002). The experience of childbirth was transformed by the introduction of electronic fetal monitoring, ultrasound, and cesarean section. The feminist movement and women's rights activism also had a profound impact on childbirth practices, advocating for women's autonomy, informed consent, and natural childbirth. In the later decades of the century, a resurgence of interest in midwifery led to the establishment of midwifery schools and the recognition of midwives as skilled practitioners (Loudon 2000). Alternative birthing options, such as home births and birth centers, gained popularity among some communities, emphasizing personalized care and a more natural approach to childbirth. However, debates around medical interventions, rising rates of cesarean section, and disparities in maternal and infant health outcomes persisted, highlighting the continued complexities of childbirth (Simonds et al. 2002).

Many of the historical changes center on the types of practitioners caring for the mother through pregnancy and childbirth, on the location and environment of birthing, and on gynecological research on women's bodies.

Changes in Birthing Practitioners and Facilities

Through much of history, childbirth and care for pregnant and new mothers was the domain of women, whether relatives or friends of the mother or local midwives. The eighteenth century brought a change to British practice in the form of more professionally trained midwives—often called a man-midwives or *accoucheurs* from their origination in Europe several decades earlier—and the development of obstetrics as a field of medicine. Still, in many cases, a man was only brought in when the mother's or the fetus's life was in danger, and so the early obstetricians were associated with deadly outcomes and thus feared. The development and publication of obstetrical texts in Britain and Europe during the second half of the eighteenth century meant that more of the male practitioners began to understand the anatomy of a woman's body, the differences between a normal and abnormal childbirth, and the appropriate interventions in the latter (Loudon 2000; Fox 2022; Rooks 1997).

The rise of the obstetrics over the midwifery in America occurred several decades later, around the turn of the nineteenth century. The male practitioners had trained in Europe and advertised that knowledge in order to compete with the well-established midwives. Social mores around modesty also limited the male doctors, who were often trained with only models and diagrams and conducted examinations only by touch with the woman's body covered. Still, over time, the masculine practice of obstetrics eventually became the dominant form of care for pregnant and birthing women, in part by centering their practice on the abnormal or risky births and then suggesting ways most births could become abnormal. Additionally, the lack of training and licensure for midwifes complicated their acceptance in the medical field and by middle and upper class families, which eventually limited much of their practice to marginalized communities (Ehrenreich and English 2010; Leavitt 2016; Simonds et al. 2002; Rooks 1997; Loudon 2000). As more women began formal training in medical schools in the nineteenth century, they offered the desired medical knowledge for birthing women without the attendance of an unfamiliar man (Leavitt 2016).

Preferences about the medical practitioner generally connected to the environment and location of the care. For centuries, midwives (and later doctors) visited and cared for birthing women in their homes throughout the period of confinement. These births were social affairs and primarily the domain of women with friends and family members present to support the midwife and birthing woman emotionally and physically. Husbands remained outside of the birthing room but present in the home. The first lying-in hospitals in Britain opened in the eighteenth century, but the concept did not spread widely until the following century. At first, lying-in hospitals primarily provided care for poor or working class women and offered a space for obstetrical observation, training, and practice. These were also spaces where, for many years, puerperal infections spread, creating fear for birthing women who relied on these facilities and leading more privileged women to avoid them. In the early twentieth century, however, as the lying-in hospitals were replaced by the general medical facilities, hospital births grew and became more common among all classes, promising safer options and more comfortable birthing experiences while also serving the increasingly urban populations (Rooks 1997; Wertz and Wertz 1989; Loudon 2000).

History of Gynecological Research

Because of the social expectations of modesty and propriety between the sexes, medical understandings of women's bodies, particularly their reproductive organs, was limited. Thus, much of the gynecological research before the mid-twentieth century was produced through experimentation on and exploitation of women from marginalized communities, particularly the poor women in lying-in hospitals and Black and enslaved women in the American south. Women from marginalized backgrounds were often given less privacy or in their treatment both in the doctor's examination and in the potential audience of medical students and other doctors who might observe. Also, doctors assumed that wealthy white women felt pain more severely than their counterparts from different socioeconomic or racial backgrounds and used that belief to guide their approach to pain management in experimentation and treatment.

One of the best-known examples of this is in the practice of James Marion Sims, who was lauded as the father of gynecology and for his procedure for repairing holes in the vaginal wall that resulted from prolonged and difficult birthing and could be debilitating for women. Though his technique for treating vaginal fistulas benefitted countless women, Sims primarily conduced his research on a group of around ten enslaved women, including three whose names are known, Betsey, Anarcha, and Lucy. He operated on each woman numerous times—Anarcha underwent at least thirty surgeries—without using any of the forms of anesthesia then available. Sims became wealthy and famous for this work, while the fate of the women whose bodies led to his discoveries was erased from the history (Doyle 2018; Epstein 2010).

Complications Around Pregnancy and Childbirth

Though pregnancy and childbirth are considered natural functions of the human body, they are accompanied by potential complications and significant risks for the mother's health from conception through postpartum recovery. From observations and stories about the women around them, birthing women were well aware of the risks of injury or death that accompanied pregnancy, delivery, and recovery (Leavitt 2016). For centuries, practitioners prioritized overcoming these risks for the health and life of the birthing mother, but the falling birth rates in the early twentieth century led to a heightened concern for the fetus (Hanson 2004). These complications include the inability to conceive or to carry a pregnancy to term, the pain that accompanied childbirth, the need for instrumental or surgical intervention during delivery, and the high rates of maternal death that have persisted in spite of medical advances.

Infertility and Miscarriage

Any consideration of birthing must also explore the related concerns about infertility and the loss of pregnancy. Throughout much of western history, cultural expectations of women have linked their femininity to motherhood. Before twentieth-century science produced medical tests and treatments for involuntary childlessness, common practice blamed some combination of divine will and the woman and sought to resolve infertility with folk remedies, superstitious or religious practices, or changes to health and diet. After the rising medicalization of women's health in the mid-nineteenth century, though, gynecologists began to approach involuntary childlessness with surgery (Marsh and Ronner 2019). Similarly, many women used herbal folk remedies to prevent miscarriage, and medical practitioners sought to understand the causes of miscarriage in order to prevent it. However, because of the limited medical technology to confirm early pregnancy, early pregnancy loss was historically difficult to trace. Women suspected pregnancy based on physical symptoms but confirmed it at the point of quickening, when the pregnant woman could feel fetal movement around the third or fourth month of pregnancy (Klepp 2009; Leavitt 2016).

Pain and Anesthesia

In western Judeo-Christian culture, many associated the pain of childbirth with the Biblical story of creation and saw the suffering of women as a necessary punishment for Eve's original sin. Even after the discovery of anesthesia in the middle of the nineteenth century, some believed it immoral for its use in easing the pain women experienced during birth. Other doctors expressed concern that anesthesia would interfere with the natural process of childbirth or was not safe in some way. In spite of this, many doctors began offering anesthesia to birthing women and women began demanding it as part of their birth plans. Famously, in 1853, Queen Victoria was given chloroform as anesthesia during her birth to her eighth child, Prince Leopold, just seven years after William Morton demonstrated its use for dental surgery and James Simpson applied it in obstetrics. Though many contemporary doctors hesitated to adopt the new practice, its use by several famous women helped to spread word of its usefulness and safety. In 1847, Fanny Appleton Longfellow, wife of poet Henry Wadsworth Longfellow, was the first American woman to give birth with anesthesia. Then in the 1848, Queen Victoria's accoucheur Charles Locock consulted with John Snow, a doctor skilled with anesthesia, in advance of the Queen's birth that year, though she waited until 1853 to use it. Word spread through the periodical press; the fact that anesthesia was safe enough for use by the queen led many more women to request it. (Caton 1999; Doyle 2018).

In the early years of the twentieth century, a combination of morphine and scopolamine was developed in Europe and applied in obstetrics as a way to provide both pain relief during birth and amnesia about the experience of birth afterward. As the risks of ether and chloroform had become clear, birthing women and their doctors sought a new solution for the pain experienced during childbirth. In 1914, a group of wealthy and well-connected American women learned of Twilight Sleep, as the German term for it translated, and campaigned for its use in the United States. Many doctors resisted, which led to a public battle on the pages of periodicals that demonstrated physician concerns and some high-profile cases where women died. Those, along with the start of World War I, eventually dissolved the movement (Caton 1999). Still, the option for less suffering in childbirth appealed to women who pushed throughout the twentieth century for safe and effective options for pain management during the birthing process.

Cesarean Section Deliveries and Other Medical Interventions

In the eighteenth and nineteenth centuries, a physician or accoucheur was often summoned to work with or in place of a midwife in particularly complicated or painful deliveries. One common complication was a contracted pelvis that was too small to pass the fetus, which led to a protracted labor and could cause internal tearing and physical trauma for the birthing woman. Another was hemorrhage, which was typically caused by the position or the delivery of the placenta. The interventions in these cases relied on instruments like the crochet, forceps, or vacuum or surgery through a Caesarean section.

The earliest interventions in difficult births sought to bring the fetus out, as doctors and midwives understood that protracted labor was likely to result in the death of the birthing woman. This sometimes meant pulling or squeezing the fetal head hard enough to cause damage or death or dissecting the fetus in the uterus to have pieces small enough to be delivered or removed. Instruments for doing this included the crochet and scissors, which were used to dismember the fetus and went out of fashion in the nineteenth century. The preferred instruments of most obstetricians were the forceps, which were used to pull the fetus and took many forms based on the preferences of the doctor and the medical situation. Critics of obstetrics observed that the use of instruments like forceps varied widely in the skill of the physician using them and that they were often used too early in the birthing process and too frequently in the practice of many obstetricians (Leavitt 2016; Fox 2022).

Though doctors attempted to perform Caesarean section surgeries as early as the sixteenth century, they were rarely successful at saving lives until the nineteenth century when reliable anesthesia and antiseptic surgical practices were available. By the early part of the twentieth century, the Caesarean section was preferred over forceps in cases where fetal head was not yet in the pelvis to avoid the danger of injury to both the birthing woman and the fetus. Eventually, the Caesarean section has come to represent a significant portion of births in America and Britain. Though all of these interventions came with significant risks, they were used in attempts to prevent the all-too-common maternal mortality.

Maternal Mortality

Childbirth was a risky process that could result in maternal and fetal death for a variety of reasons. British maternal mortality rates in the second half of the seventeenth century were between 150 and 210 maternal deaths per 10,000 births and mostly dropped over the following century as more births were attended by a trained midwife or physician. Though maternal death is a portion of the many possible causes of death in pre-industrial Britain, it was a particularly notable one, as it resulted from something most women experienced at some point in their lives rather than specific illnesses or accidents. Additionally, because birth rates were higher in the eighteenth and nineteenth centuries, not including the number of miscarriages and stillborn infants, women were pregnant more often and thus facing this risk frequently through their childbearing years (Loudon 2000; Leavitt 2016).

In addition to risks described above that were addressed with medical instruments or surgical intervention, the most common cause of material death was postpartum infection and sepsis, which was called child-bed or puerperal fever. For the centuries prior to the acceptance of antiseptic surgical practice, there were no efforts to prevent infection during the birthing process. A physician or midwife would attend a birth in their regular clothes without cleaning their skin or clothing, arriving directly from other births, dissections, or other patients. During the delivery, bacteria from a practitioner's hands or tools would infect the uterus, and the resulting infection could kill the woman in as little as a day or two or as late as a week after the birth. This led to frequent outbreaks in villages or neighborhoods and in the lying-in hospitals and the entirely preventable deaths of countless birthing women (Loudon 2000; Leavitt 2016).

Maternal Mental Health

With the risks of serious complications and death facing birthing women, it is no surprise that maternal mental illness was a factor for many and was a topic of interest for physicians. Though women had experienced mental illness during pregnancy and after birth for centuries, the term "puerperal insanity" was introduced by physician Robert Gooch in 1820, and the ensuing medical discussion focused primarily on extreme behaviors, whether violence, delirium, or melancholia. In some cases, women recovered shortly after birth, but in others, they never fully recovered or progressively declined after each birth. Some of the temporary delirium could be associated with the infections and high temperatures from puerperal fever; in other cases, the misunderstood hormonal imbalances in pregnancy or the postpartum period triggered significant responses. Much of the postpartum mental illness was dismissed by physicians as a result of the delicacy of women in the period. In the late nineteenth and early twentieth centuries, treatment for women with "puerperal insanity" ranged from home care until they recovered enough to resume their domestic duties to the asylums that isolated and cared for women using the popular approaches of the period. Over the course of the twentieth century, medical and psychological understandings of pregnancy and childbirth developed to offer a much more nuanced perspective on women's mental health, recognizing much less severe symptoms and exploring more effective treatment options (Loudon 2000; Marland 2004; Hanson 2004).

Themes and Topics in Selections

Across the texts presented in this chapter, several key ideas recur and offer the opportunity for comparison.

Maternal Mortality

The most common topic in this chapter is maternal death, primarily as a result of puerperal infection. This is represented in memorials by those grieving, guides warning women of the signs and symptoms of puerperal fever, suggestions about which type of practitioner or birthing location has the best outcomes, medical texts advocating for safer practices in childbirth, social texts raising awareness about the widespread problem, and fiction about the risks. Nearly every text in this chapter considers the risk and the fears of women and their family and friends, even if the woman does not die in childbirth.

Pain Relief and the Periodical Press

Approaches to managing the pain and trauma of childbirth are central to many of the representations of the experience, and each of the approaches was presented and debated on the pages of periodicals. Popular magazines and newspapers were often a way for women to learn about medical advances and to use those to advocate for themselves and their treatment. Starting in the middle part of the nineteenth century, discussion focused on anesthesia through ether and chloroform with particular coverage about Queen Victoria's births, while the early twentieth century brought interest in twilight sleep as a way to both reduce and forget the pain of childbirth. The doctors writing medical advice books were generally in favor of the use of anesthesia to reduce the suffering of their patients and the shock of childbirth.

Maternal Mental Health

As discussed above, mental health concerns related to pregnancy and childbirth were commonly misunderstood by practitioners and by society at large. Beyond the general fears around maternal mortality, specific issues with mental health are addressed in part in Bakewell's *A Popular Manual of Female Diseases* and Allbutt's *The Wife's Handbook* and are fictionally represented in the protagonists of both Gilman's "The Yellow Wallpaper" and Chopin's "The Belle Zoraïde."

Types of Practitioners

The evolution of care from local midwives to licensed obstetricians has included significant debate about which practitioner is best suited to care for women in pregnancy and childbirth. "On Men-Midwives" and "The New Order of Medical Students" both specifically consider moments in this history. Each of the included advice books for women was authored by a licensed medical practitioner, and so they tend to emphasize the necessity of a licensed doctor for the birthing process.

Poems About Women Who Died in Childbirth (1750–1773)

Introduction

Memorial verse was popular in England in the mid-to-late eighteenth century as seen in the incredibly popular "Elegy Written in a Country Churchyard" by Thomas Gray. The poems collected here follow similar patterns in remembering women who died in childbirth, particularly in their recognition that the infant's life seems to replace the mother's or that she sacrificed her own life in bringing forth the child. These memorials emphasize the unique nature of grief following maternal mortality and idealize the women who died.

"On a Lady Who Died in Child-Birth" (*The Ladies Magazine: Or, The Universal Entertainer*, December 1750)

> The Breath which this resigns, while that receives,
> One comes into a World the other leaves.
> His Cares are all to come, her's are all past,
> The Son's first Moment proves the Mother's last.
> His Life, her Death; her Death his Life supplies,
> He kills in Birth, and she in bearing dies.

"Epitaph, on a Lady Who Died in Child-Birth" by Dr. Templeman (*Monthly Repository for Gentlemen & Ladies*, December 1762)

> Beneath this humble stone, now rest inshrin'd,
> Alas! What once inclos'd the purest mind.
> Yet, while she leaves us for her kindred skies,
> See from th' expiring flame a Phœnix rise!
> By the same hand, severely kind was giv'n
> To us a cherub, and a saint to heav'n.
> Adieu, blest shade; alas, to early fled!
> Who knew thee living, but laments thee dead?
> A soul so calm, so free from every stain,
> So try'd by torture, and unmov'd by pain!
> Without a groan with agonies she strove!
> Heav'n wond'ring snatch'd her to the joys above.

From *Monody to the Memory of a Young Lady Who Died in Child-Bed By An Afflicted Husband* by Cuthbert Shaw (1768)

IX.
How shall I e'er forget that dreadful hour,
When feeling Death's resistless pow'r,
My hand the press'd, wet with her falling tears,
And thus, in falt'ring accents, spoke her fears!
"Ah, my lov'd lord, the transient scene is o'er,
"And we must part (alas!) to meet no more!
"But oh! if e'er thy Emma's name was dear,
"If e'er thy vows have charm'd my ravith'd ear;
"If, from thy lov'd embrace my heart to gain,
"Proud friends have frown'd, and Fortune smil'd in vain;
"If it has been my sole endeavour, still
"To act in all, obsequious to thy will;
"To watch thy very smiles, thy with to know,
"Then only truly blest when thou wert so:
"If I have doated with that fond excess,
"Nor Love cou'd add, nor Fortune make it less;
"If this I've done, and more--oh then be kind
"To the dear lovely babe I leave behind.
"When time my once-lov'd memory shall efface,
"Some happier maid may take thy Emma's place,
"With envious eyes thy partial fondness see,
"And hate it for the love thou bore to me:
"My dearest S---- forgive a woman's fears,
"But one word more (I cannot bear thy tears)
"Promise--and I will trust thy faithful vow,
"(Oft have I tried; and ever found thee true)
"That to some distant spot thou wilt remove
"This fatal pledge of hapless. Emma's love;
"Where, safe, thy blandishments it may partake,
"And oh! be tender for its mother's sake.
"Wilt thou?-----
"I know thou wilt—sad silence speaks assent;,
"And in that pleasing hope thy Emma dies content."
XVIII.
And thou, my little cherub, left behind,
To hear a father's plaints, to share his woes,
When Reason's dawn informs thy infant mind,

And thy sweet-lisping tongue shall ask the cause,
How oft with sorrow hall mine eyes run o'er,
When, twining round my knees, I trace
Thy mother's smile upon thy face?
How oft to my full heart halt thou restore
Sad mem'ry of my joys--ah now no more!
By blessings once enjoy'd now more distrest,
More beggar by the riches once possest

XIX

My little darling!—dearer to me grown
By all the tears thou'st caus'd—(O strange to hear)!
Bought with a life yet dearer than thy own,
Thy cradle purchas'd with thy mother's bier:
Who now shall seek, with fond delight,
Thy infant steps to guide aright?
She who, with doating eyes, wou'd gaze
On all thy little artless ways;
By all thy soft endearments blest,
And clasp thee oft with transport to her breast,
Alas! is gone—Yet shalt thou prove
A father's dearest, tend'rest love:
And O! sweet senseless smiler (envied state!)
As yet unconscious of thy hapless fate,
When years thy judgment shall mature,
And Reason hews those ills it cannot cure,
Wilt thou, a father's grief t' asswage,
For virtue prove the Phœnix of the earth?
(Like her, thy mother dy'd to give thee birth)
And be the comfort of my age?
When sick and languishing I lie;
Wilt thou my Emma's wonted care supply?
And oft, as, to thy list'ning ear,
Thy mother's virtues and her fate I tell,
Say, wilt thou drop the tender tear,
Whilst on the mournful theme I dwell?
Then, fondly stealing to thy father's side,
Whene'er thou see'st the soft distress,
Which I wou'd vainly seek to hide,
Say, wilt thou strive to make it less;
To sooth my sorrows all thy cares employ,
And in my cup of grief infuse one drop of joy?

"On Lady Shelley, who died in Childbed Said to be Written by the Rev. Dr. Delap" (*The Gentleman's Magazine: And Historical Chronicle*, August 1772)

> Tears, such as angels weep, should now diffuse
> Around this hallow'd earth, their holiest dews,
> Where rest fair Wilhelmina's last remains.
> She for her infant bore a mother's pains,
> And died to give it life. In beauty's bloom
> Heav'n snatch'd its fav'rite to an early tomb,
> Its gent'lest, best belov'd, who seem'ed design'd
> To shew how far a meet and modest mind,
> With its own simple pow'rs and native grace,
> Could mend the features of the fairest face;
> How fix a friend's, a brother's, a husband's love,
> Beyond, alas! the pow'r of death to move.
> Self tutor'd thus, above all rules of art,
> This Child of Nature play'd her blameless part,
> And sunk with that unsullied soul to rest,
> Which Heav'n first breath'd into her infant breast.

"On Hearing the Organ Upon First Going to Church, After the Death of The Most Lovely, and Most Beloved Wife, Who Died in Child-Bed of Her First-Born, July 24, 1772" (*Hibernian Magazine, or Compendium of Entertaining Knowledge*, July 1773)

> Here while religion's power to try,
> With earnest prayer to Heav'n I cry,
> That it would deign to ease a part
> Of the distress which wrings my heart.
> Hark! how the pealing organ plays,
> To celebrate Jehovah's praise!
> See! where the Seraph Mary floats,
> On the harmonic swelling notes,
> Exulting in her bless'd abode,
> Full in the presence of her God,
> Who lent her just to grace the earth,
> Till ripen'd into second birth,
> A saint he snatch'd her, which while here,
> Her sinless soul approach'd so near;

But, to sweet mercy still inclin'd,
Her life-bought babe she left behind.

Shall then the doating husband mourn,
And wish she could to earth return?
Would he from sordid, selfish ends,
Bring her to earth, tho' now she bends
Her well pleas'd maker to adore,
Where time, and pain, and death's no more?
Where this world's transitory toys,
Are drown'd in unexpiring joys?
Be still my soul—reject the thought—
Let me bear sorrow as man ought,
Nor murmur at the wholesome rod,
Inflicted by the parent god.
Let me train up her helpless young,
Worthy the angel whence it sprung;
Let me, by her example, sir'd,
By her bright excellence inspir'd,
Endeavour by each act in this,
To reign with her in worlds of bliss!
Sunday, Aug. 9th, 1772

Account of and Extract from a New Work (1783)

Introduction

This review essay covers John Whitehead's English translation of a work by Denis Doulcet. The suggested treatment is based more on humoral theory and focuses on removing putrid elements (seen in pus from the misunderstood infection) from the body through the use of a medicine made from ipecacuanha, which would induce vomiting. The treatment was developed through Doulcet's work in Paris at Hôtel-Dieu, the oldest hospital still operating in France and perhaps in the world. The translations, followed by the review article, bring this knowledge to those in Britain directly caring for woman in childbirth.

Account of and Extract from a New Work, Titled, "A Report, Made by Order of Government, of a Memoir, Containing a New, Easy, and Successful Method of Treating the Child bed or Puerperal Fever, made Use of by the Late M. Doulcet, Doctor Regent of the Faculty at Paris, and one of the Physicians of the Hotel-Dieu" (*Hibernian Magazine, or, Compendium of Entertaining Knowledge*, May 1783)

The fatality of the puerperal fever, which certainly occasions the death of most of those women who die in child-bed, is so well known, and its consequence has been so much dreaded by the most skillful of the faculty, from the want of. Any known adequate remedy, that every attempt to facilitate and render certain the cure of this rapid and alarming disease, cannot fail to merit the attention and regard of the publick.

As the success of the proposed remedy is said greatly, it not wholly, to depend on its timely exhibition, we shall give a description of the commencement and progress of this terrible disease, verbatim from the report.

"This disease comes on suddenly, without any previous symptom to announce its approach; and this often happens after a pregnancy the most exempt from accidents, and after the most happy delivery. It commonly appears the third day after the woman is brought to bed; sometimes sooner, seldom later. In its commencement, the belly is affected with considerable distention, and becomes extremely painful, without any diminution of the *lochia*, which still continue to flow. The breasts, which ought to swell with milk, become flaccid, and the natural course of this nutritious fluid is in general suspended. The patient is affected with a fever, which however is not very high; the pulse is small, contracted, and quick; and the strength sinks. These first signs, which essentially characterise the disease, are common to all the women attacked with it; but they are often, though not always, accompanied with many other symptoms, such as rigor and shivering more or less violent, which is perceived on the first attack; with vomiting of a green matter, or slightly tinged with yellow, though more frequently there is nausea without vomiting; a diarrhea in which the stools are milky and extremely fœtid. The eyes sparkle; the countenance is discoloured; the tongue is commonly moist, but covered with a thick white fur, which is sometimes yellow or greenish towards the root.

All these symptoms come on the first day of the disease; they increase with, rapidity, and in a short time the pains of the belly become insupportable. This violent state is succeeded, towards the end of the second day, by a fallacious calm, which is followed by a cold viscid sweat, with stools and evacuations intolerably fetid, with a tremulous weakness, delirium, and lastly with death, which often closes the scene about the end of the third or beginning of the fourth day.

It appears from this Report, that "the method of cure at present established in the Hotel-Dieu, and which has never yet failed of success since it was applied, consists in taking the advantage of the moment of attack, and giving, without losing an instant of time, fifteen grains of ipecacuanha in two doses, at the distance of an hour and an half from each other, and repeating them again the next day in the same manner, whether the violence of the symptoms be abated or not; and if the disease should continue much the same, they are repeated again the third, and even the fourth day, according as the case may require. In the intervals between the doses, the effect of the ipecacuanha is kept up by a potion composed of two ounces of oil of sweet almonds, one ounce of syrup of marsh-mallows, and two grains of kermes mineral. The common drink is linseed tea, or an infusion of scorzonera root, edulcorated with syrup of althea; and towards the seventh or eighth day of the disease the patient takes a mild purgative, which is repeated three or four times according to the exigency of the case."

Dr. Whitehead recommends that the nurses in our hospitals, being always present, should administer the remedy above prescribed; and for the safety of private families, wishes every midwife and nurse to be made acquainted with this simple and successful method of cure; which he is of opinion, would at least be thus far useful, that, by exhibiting the proper dose of ipecacuanha on the first appearance of the disease, time might be allowed to call in more proper assistance.

Charlotte Temple by Susanna Rowson (1791)

Introduction

This novel presents the story of a British girl seduced by a British officer and taken to America, where he abandons the pregnant Charlotte. She finds kindness in a neighbor named Mrs. Beauchamp and writes to her parents in England about her plight. In the scenes excerpted here, Charlotte is alone in New York and has sought help but been rejected by Mrs. Clayton, a friend of her seducer. She has been taken in by one of Mrs. Clayton's servants. *Charlotte Temple* was one of the first popular novels in America and follows the common tropes of the eighteenth-century seduction novel.

Excerpt from Chapter XXXI: Subject Continued

…

John,[2] assisted by his fellow-servant, raised and carried her down stairs. "Poor soul," said he, "you shall not lay in the street this night. I have a bed and a poor little hovel, where my wife and her little ones rest them, but they shall watch to night, and you shall be sheltered from danger." They placed her in a chair; and the benevolent man, assisted by one of his comrades, carried her to the place where his wife and children lived. A surgeon was sent for: he bled her,[3] she gave signs of returning life, and before the dawn gave birth to a female infant. After this event she lay for some hours in a kind of stupor; and if at any time she spoke, it was with a quickness and incoherence that plainly evinced the total deprivation of her reason.

Excerpt from Chapter XXXII: Reasons Why and Wherefore

…

Charlotte had now been three days with her humane preservers, but she was totally insensible of every thing: she raved incessantly for Montraville[4] and her father: she was not conscious of being a mother, nor took the least notice of her child except to ask whose it was, and why it was not carried to its parents.

"Oh," said she one day, starting up on hearing the infant cry, "why, why will you keep that child here; I am sure you would not if you knew how hard it was for a mother to be parted from her infant: it is like tearing the cords of life asunder. Oh could you see the horrid sight which I now behold—there there stands my dear mother, her poor bosom bleeding at every vein, her gentle, affectionate heart torn in a thousand pieces, and all for the loss of a ruined, ungrateful child. Save me save me—from her frown. I dare not— indeed I dare not speak to her."

Such were the dreadful images that haunted her distracted mind, and nature was sinking fast under the dreadful malady which medicine had no

---

[2] Servant to Mrs. Clayton.
[3] Bloodletting, whether by a scalpal or leeches, was common through the nineteenth century as part of treatments based on the humors.
[4] A friend of Charlotte's seducer.

power to remove. The surgeon who attended her was a humane man; he exerted his utmost abilities to save her, but he saw she was in want of many necessaries and comforts, which the poverty of her hospitable host rendered him unable to provide: he therefore determined to make her situation known to some of the officers' ladies, and endeavour to make a collection for her relief.

When he returned home, after making this resolution, he found a message from Mrs. Beauchamp, who had just arrived from Rhode-Island, requesting he would call and see one of her children, who was very unwell. "I do not know," said he, as he was hastening to obey the summons, "I do not know a woman to whom I could apply with more hope of success than Mrs. Beauchamp. I will endeavour to interest her in this poor girl's behalf, she wants the soothing balm of friendly consolation: we may perhaps save her; we will try at least."

"And where is she," cried Mrs. Beauchamp when he had prescribed something for the child, and told his little pathetic tale, "where is she, Sir? we will go to her immediately. Heaven forbid that I should be deaf to the calls of humanity. Come we will go this instant." Then seizing the doctor's arm, they sought the habitation that contained the dying Charlotte.

Excerpt from Chapter XXXIII: Which People Void of Feeling Need Not Read

When Mrs. Beauchamp entered the apartment of the poor sufferer, she started back with horror. On a wretched bed, without hangings and but poorly supplied with covering, lay the emaciated figure of what still retained the semblance of a lovely woman, though sickness had so altered her features that Mrs. Beauchamp had not the least recollection of her person. In one corner of the room stood a woman washing, and, shivering over a small fire, two healthy but half naked children; the infant was asleep beside its mother, and, on a chair by the bed side, stood a porringer and wooden spoon, containing a little gruel, and a tea-cup with about two spoonfulls of wine in it. Mrs. Beauchamp had never before beheld such a scene of poverty; she shuddered involuntarily, and exclaiming—"heaven preserve us!" leaned on the back of a chair ready to sink to the earth. The doctor repented having so precipitately brought her into this affecting scene; but there was no time for apologies: Charlotte caught the sound of her voice, and starting almost out of bed, exclaimed—"Angel of peace and mercy, art thou come to deliver me? Oh, I know you are, for whenever you was near me I felt eased of half my sorrows; but you don't know me, nor can I, with all the recollection I am mistress of, remember your name just now, but I know that benevolent countenance, and the softness of that voice which has so often comforted the wretched Charlotte."

Mrs. Beauchamp had, during the time Charlotte was speaking, seated herself on the bed and taken one of her hands; she looked at her attentively, and at the name of Charlotte she perfectly conceived the whole shocking affair. A faint sickness came over her. "Gracious heaven," said she, "is this possible?" and bursting into tears, she reclined the burning head of Charlotte on her own bosom; and folding her arms about her, wept over her in silence. "Oh," said Charlotte, "you are very good to weep thus for me: it is a long time since I shed a tear for myself: my head and heart are both on fire, but these tears of your's seem to cool and refresh it. Oh now I remember you said you would send a letter to my poor father: do you think he ever received it? or perhaps you have brought me an answer: why don't you speak, Madam? Does he say I may go home? Well he is very good; I shall soon be ready."

She then made an effort to get out of bed; but being prevented, her frenzy again returned, and she raved with the greatest wildness and incoherence. Mrs. Beauchamp, finding it was impossible for her to be removed, contented herself with ordering the apartment to be made more comfortable, and procuring a proper nurse for both mother and child; and having learnt the particulars of Charlotte's fruitless application to Mrs. Crayton from honest John, she amply rewarded him for his benevolence, and returned home with a heart oppressed with many painful sensations, but yet rendered easy by the reflexion that she had performed her duty towards a distressed fellow-creature.

Early the next morning she again visited Charlotte, and found her tolerably composed; she called her by name, thanked her for her goodness, and when her child was brought to her, pressed it in her arms, wept over it, and called it the offspring of disobedience. Mrs. Beauchamp was delighted to see her so much amended, and began to hope she might recover, and, spite of her former errors, become an useful and respectable member of society; but the arrival of the doctor put an end to these delusive hopes: he said nature was making her last effort, and a few hours would most probably consign the unhappy girl to her kindred dust.

Being asked how she found herself, she replied—"Why better, much better, doctor. I hope now I have but little more to suffer. I had last night a few hours sleep, and when I awoke recovered the full power of recollection. I am quite sensible of my weakness; I feel I have but little longer to combat with the shafts of affliction. I have an humble confidence in the mercy of him who died to save the world, and trust that my sufferings in this state of mortality, joined to my unfeigned repentance, through his mercy, have blotted my offences from the sight of my offended maker. I have but one care—my poor infant!

Father of mercy," continued she, raising her eyes, "of thy infinite goodness, grant that the sins of the parent be not visited on the unoffending child. May those who taught me to despise thy laws be forgiven; lay not my offences to their charge, I beseech thee; and oh! shower the choicest of thy blessings on those whose pity has soothed the afflicted heart, and made easy even the bed of pain and sickness."

She was exhausted by this fervent address to the throne of mercy, and though her lips still moved her voice became inarticulate: she lay for some time as it were in a doze, and then recovering, faintly pressed Mrs. Beauchamp's hand, and requested that a clergyman might be sent for.

On his arrival she joined fervently in the pious office, frequently mentioning her ingratitude to her parents as what lay most heavy at her heart. When she had performed the last solemn duty, and was preparing to lie down, a little bustle on the outside door occasioned Mrs. Beauchamp to open it, and enquire the cause. A man in appearance about forty, presented himself, and asked for Mrs. Beauchamp.

"That is my name, Sir," said she.

"Oh then, my dear Madam," cried he, "tell me where I may find my poor, ruined, but repentant child."

Mrs. Beauchamp was surprised and affected; she knew not what to say; she foresaw the agony this interview would occasion Mr. Temple, who had just arrived in search of his Charlotte, and yet was sensible that the pardon and blessing of her father would soften even the agonies of death to the daughter.

She hesitated. "Tell me, Madam," cried he wildly, "tell me, I beseech thee, does she live? shall I see my darling once again? Perhaps she is in this house. Lead, lead me to her, that I may bless her, and then lie down and die."

The ardent manner in which he uttered these words occasioned him to raise his voice. It caught the ear of Charlotte: she knew the beloved sound: and uttering a loud shriek, she sprang forward as Mr. Temple entered the room. "My adored father." "My long lost child." Nature could support no more, and they both sunk lifeless into the arms of the attendants.

Charlotte was again put into bed, and a few moments restored Mr. Temple: but to describe the agony of his sufferings is past the power of any one, who, though they may readily conceive, cannot delineate the dreadful scene. Every eye gave testimony of what each heart felt—but all were silent.

When Charlotte recovered, she found herself supported in her father's arms. She cast on him a most expressive look, but was unable to speak. A reviving cordial was administered. She then asked in a low voice, for her child: it was brought to her: she put it in her father's arms. "Protect her," said she, "and bless your dying—".

Unable to finish the sentence, she sunk back on her pillow: her countenance was serenely composed; she regarded her father as he pressed the infant to his breast with a steadfast look; a sudden beam of joy passed across her languid features, she raised her eyes to heaven—and then closed them for ever.

Memoirs of the Author of a Vindication of the Rights of Woman by William Godwin (1798)

Introduction

In this biography of Mary Wollstonecraft, her husband William Godwin details Wollstonecraft's life, concluding with her death ten days after childbirth with their daughter, author Mary Shelley. The memoir is direct in its representation of Wollstonecraft's life, including her love affairs, a previous illegitimate child, and the vivid details of her decline and death from puerperal infection. Godwin's grief is evident in the text overall and in this excerpt about Mary's final days. His narrative demonstrates the escalation in practitioner, from midwife to physician, in the case of complications in childbirth. It is an interesting parallel to the memoir by Wray that follows.

Excerpt from Chapter X

I am now led, by the course of my narrative, to the last fatal scene of her life. She was taken in labour on Wednesday, the thirtieth of August. She had been somewhat indisposed on the preceding Friday, the consequence, I believe, of a sudden alarm. But from that time she was in perfect health. She was so far from being under any apprehension as to the difficulties of child-birth, as frequently to ridicule the fashion of ladies in England, who keep their chamber for one full month after delivery. For herself, she proposed coming down to dinner on the day immediately following. She had already had some experience on the subject in the case of Fanny; and I cheerfully submitted in every point to her judgment and her wisdom. She hired no nurse. Influenced by ideas of decorum, which certainly ought to have no place, at least in cases of danger, she determined to have a woman to attend her in the capacity of midwife. She was sensible that the proper business of a midwife, in the instance of a natural labour, is to sit by and wait for the operations of nature, which seldom, in these affairs, demand the interposition of art.

At five o'clock in the morning of the day of delivery, she felt what she conceived to be some notices of the approaching labour. Mrs. Blenkinsop, matron and midwife to the Westminster Lying in Hospital, who had seen Mary several times previous to her delivery, was soon after sent for, and arrived about nine. During the whole day Mary was perfectly cheerful. Her pains came on slowly; and, in the morning, she wrote several notes, three addressed to me, who had gone, as usual, to my apartments, for the purpose of study. About two o'clock in the afternoon, she went up to her chamber,—never more to descend.

The child was born at twenty minutes after eleven at night. Mary had requested that I would not come into the chamber till all was over, and signified her intention of then performing the interesting office of presenting the new-born child to its father. I was sitting in a parlour; and it was not till after two o'clock on Thursday morning, that I received the alarming intelligence, that the placenta was not yet removed, and that the midwife dared not proceed any further, and gave her opinion for calling in a male practitioner. I accordingly went for Dr. Poignand,[5] physician and man-midwife to the same hospital, who arrived between three and four hours after the birth of the child. He immediately proceeded to the extraction of the placenta, which he brought away in pieces, till he was satisfied that the whole was removed. In that point however it afterwards appeared that he was mistaken.

The period from the birth of the child till about eight o'clock the next morning, was a period full of peril and alarm. The loss of blood was considerable, and produced an almost uninterrupted series of fainting fits. I went to the chamber soon after four in the morning, and found her in this state. She told me some time on Thursday, "that she should have died the preceding night, but that she was determined not to leave me." She added, with one of those smiles which so eminently illuminated her countenance, "that I should not be like Porson," alluding to the circumstance of that great man having lost his wife, after being only a few months married. Speaking of what she had already passed through, she declared, "that she had never known what bodily pain was before."

On Thursday morning Dr. Poignand repeated his visit. Mary had just before expressed some inclination to see Dr. George Fordyce,[6] a man probably of more science than any other medical professor in England, and between whom and herself there had long subsisted a mutual friendship. I mentioned

---

[5] Dr. Louis Poignand was a French physician and accoucheur who was a member of the Royal College of Physicians andlicensed in midwifery.

[6] Dr. George Fordyce was a Scottish physician and a member of the Royal College of Physicians. He was more well-known than Poignand but not a specialist in maternal health or midwifery.

this to Dr. Poignand, but he rather discountenanced the idea, observing that he saw no necessity for it, and that he supposed Dr. Fordyce was not particularly conversant with obstetrical cases; but that I would do as I pleased. After Dr. Poignand was gone, I determined to send for Dr. Fordyce. He accordingly saw the patient about three o'clock on Thursday afternoon. He however perceived no particular cause of alarm; and, on that or the next day, quoted, as I am told, Mary's case, in a mixed company, as a corroboration of a favourite idea of his, of the propriety of employing females in the capacity of midwives. Mary "had had a woman, and was doing extremely well."

What had passed however in the night between Wednesday and Thursday, had so far alarmed me, that I did not quit the house, and scarcely the chamber, during the following day. But my alarms wore off, as time advanced. Appearances were more favourable, than the exhausted state of the patient would almost have permitted me to expect. Friday morning therefore I devoted to a business of some urgency, which called me to different parts of the town, and which, before dinner, I happily completed. On my return, and during the evening, I received the most pleasurable sensations from the promising state of the patient. I was now perfectly satisfied that every thing was safe, and that, if she did not take cold, or suffer from any external accident, her speedy recovery was certain.

Saturday was a day less auspicious than Friday, but not absolutely alarming.

Sunday, the third of September, I now regard as the day, that finally decided on the fate of the object dearest to my heart that the universe contained. Encouraged by what I considered as the progress of her recovery, I accompanied a friend in the morning in several calls, one of them as far as Kensington, and did not return till dinner-time. On my return I found a degree of anxiety in every face, and was told that she had had a sort of shivering fit, and had expressed some anxiety at the length of my absence. My sister and a friend of hers, had been engaged to dine below stairs, but a message was sent to put them off, and Mary ordered that the cloth should not be laid, as usual, in the room immediately under her on the first floor, but in the ground-floor parlour. I felt a pang at having been so long and so unseasonably absent, and determined that I would not repeat the fault.

In the evening she had a second shivering fit, the symptoms of which were in the highest degree alarming. Every muscle of the body trembled, the teeth chattered, and the bed shook under her. This continued probably for five minutes. She told me, after it was over, that it had been a struggle between life and death, and that she had been more than once, in the course of it, at the point of expiring. I now apprehend these to have been the symptoms of a decided mortification, occasioned by the part of the placenta that remained in the womb. At the time however I was far from considering it in that light. When I went for Dr. Poignand, between two and three o'clock on the morning of Thursday, despair was in my heart. The fact of the adhesion of the placenta was stated to me; and, ignorant as I was of obstetrical science, I felt as if the death of Mary was in a manner decided. But hope had re-visited my bosom; and her chearings[7] were so delightful, that I hugged her obstinately to my heart. I was only mortified at what appeared to me a new delay in the recovery I so earnestly longed for. I immediately sent for Dr. Fordyce, who had been with her in the morning, as well as on the three preceding days. Dr. Poignand had also called this morning but declined paying any further visits, as we had thought proper to call in Dr. Fordyce.

The progress of the disease was now uninterrupted. On Tuesday I found it necessary again to call in Dr. Fordyce in the afternoon, who brought with him Dr. Clarke of New Burlington-street,[8] under the idea that some operation might be necessary. I have already said, that I pertinaciously persisted in viewing the fair side of things; and therefore the interval between Sunday and Tuesday evening, did not pass without some mixture of cheerfulness. On Monday, Dr. Fordyce forbad the child's having the breast, and we therefore procured puppies to draw off the milk. This occasioned some pleasantry of Mary with me and the other attendants. Nothing could exceed the equanimity, the patience and affectionateness of the poor sufferer. I intreated her to recover; I dwelt with trembling fondness on every favourable circumstance; and, as far it was possible in so dreadful a situation, she, by her smiles and kind speeches, rewarded my affection.

Wednesday was to me the day of greatest torture in the melancholy series. It was now decided that the only chance of supporting her through what she had to suffer, was by supplying her rather freely with wine. This task was devolved upon me. I began about four o'clock in the afternoon. But for me, totally ignorant of the nature of diseases and of the human frame, thus to play with a life that now seemed all that was dear to me in the universe, was too dreadful a task. I knew neither what was too much, nor what was too little. Having begun, I felt compelled, under every disadvantage, to go on. This lasted for three hours. Towards the end of that time, I happened foolishly to ask the servant who came out of the room, "What she thought of her mistress?" she replied, "that, in her judgment, she was going as fast as possible." There are moments, when any creature that lives, has power to drive one into madness. I seemed to know the absurdity of this reply; but that was of no consequence. It added to the measure of my distraction. A little after seven I

---

[7] 'Chearing' was the contemporary spelling of 'cheering'.
[8] Dr. John Clarke was a member of the Royal College of Physicians and licensed in midwifery.

intreated a friend to go for Mr. Carlisle,[9] and bring him instantly wherever he was to be found. He had voluntarily called on the patient on the preceding Saturday, and two or three times since. He had seen her that morning, and had been earnest in recommending the wine-diet. That day he dined four miles out of town, on the side of the metropolis, which was furthest from us. Notwithstanding this, my friend returned with him after three-quarters of an hour's absence. No one who knows my friend, will wonder either at his eagerness or success, when I name Mr. Basil Montagu. The sight of Mr. Carlisle thus unexpectedly, gave me a stronger alleviating sensation, than I thought it possible to experience.

Mr. Carlisle left us no more from Wednesday evening, to the hour of her death. It was impossible to exceed his kindness and affectionate attention. It excited in every spectator a sentiment like adoration. His conduct was uniformly tender and anxious, ever upon the watch, observing every symptom, and eager to improve every favourable appearance. If skill or attention could have saved her, Mary would still live. In addition to Mr. Carlisle's constant presence, she had Dr. Fordyce and Dr. Clarke every day. She had for nurses, or rather for friends, watching every occasion to serve her, Mrs. Fenwick, author of an excellent novel, entitled Secrecy, another very kind and judicious lady, and a favourite female servant. I was scarcely ever out of the room. Four friends, Mr. Fenwick, Mr. Basil Montagu, Mr. Marshal, and Mr. Dyson, sat up nearly the whole of the last week of her existence in the house, to be dispatched, on any errand, to any part of the metropolis, at a moment's warning.

Mr. Carlisle being in the chamber, I retired to bed for a few hours on Wednesday night. Towards morning he came into my room with an account that the patient was surprisingly better. I went instantly into the chamber. But I now sought to suppress every idea of hope. The greatest anguish I have any conception of, consists in that crushing of a new-born hope which I had already two or three times experienced. If Mary recovered, it was well, and I should see it time enough. But it was too mighty a thought to bear being trifled with, and turned out and admitted in this abrupt way.

I had reason to rejoice in the firmness of my gloomy thoughts, when, about ten o'clock on Thursday evening, Mr. Carlisle told us to prepare ourselves, for we had reason to expect the fatal event every moment. To my thinking, she did not appear to be in that state of total exhaustion, which I supposed to precede death; but it is probable that death does not always take place by that

---

[9] Dr. Anthony Carlisle was a member of the Royal College of Surgeons and professor of anatomy. He remained a friend of the Godwin family and of the daughter born in this scene, Mary Shelley, for many years. 'Intreated' was the contemporary spelling of 'entreated'.

gradual process I had pictured to myself; a sudden pang may accelerate his arrival. She did not die on Thursday night.

Till now it does not appear that she had any serious thoughts of dying; but on Friday and Saturday, the two last days of her life, she occasionally spoke as if she expected it. This was however only at intervals; the thought did not seem to dwell upon her mind. Mr. Carlisle rejoiced in this. He observed, and there is great force in the suggestion, that there is no more pitiable object, than a sick man, that knows he is dying. The thought must be expected to destroy his courage, to co-operate with the disease, and to counteract every favourable effort of nature.

On these two days her faculties were in too decayed a state, to be able to follow any train of ideas with force or any accuracy of connection. Her religion, as I have already shown, was not calculated to be the torment of a sick bed; and, in fact, during her whole illness, not one word of a religious cast fell from her lips.

She was affectionate and compliant to the last. I observed on Friday and Saturday nights, that, whenever her attendants recommended to her to sleep, she discovered her willingness to yield, by breathing, perhaps for the space of a minute, in the manner of a person that sleeps, though the effort, from the state of her disorder, usually proved ineffectual.

She was not tormented by useless contradiction. One night the servant, from an error in judgment, teazed her with idle expostulations, but she complained of it grievously, and it was corrected. "Pray, pray, do not let her reason with me," was her expression. Death itself is scarcely so dreadful to the enfeebled frame, as the monotonous importunity of nurses ever-lastingly repeated.

Seeing that every hope was extinct, I was very desirous of obtaining from her any directions, that she might wish to have followed after her decease. Accordingly, on Saturday morning, I talked to her for a good while of the two children. In conformity to Mr. Carlisle's maxim of not impressing the idea of death, I was obliged to manage my expressions. I therefore affected to proceed wholly upon the ground of her having been very ill, and that it would be some time before she could expect to be well; wishing her to tell me any thing that she would choose to have done respecting the children, as they would now be principally under my care. After having repeated this idea to her in a great variety of forms, she at length said, with a significant tone of voice, "I know what you are thinking of," but added, that she had nothing to communicate to me upon the subject.

The shivering fits had ceased entirely for the two last days. Mr. Carlisle observed that her continuance was almost miraculous, and he was on the watch for favourable appearances, believing it highly improper to give up all hope, and remarking, that perhaps one in a million, of persons in her state might possibly recover. I conceive that not one in a million, unites so good a constitution of body and of mind.

These were the amusements of persons in the very gulph[10] of despair. At six o'clock on Sunday morning, September the tenth, Mr. Carlisle called me from my bed to which I had retired at one, in conformity to my request, that I might not be left to receive all at once the intelligence that she was no more. She expired at twenty minutes before eight.

Her remains were deposited, on the fifteenth of September, at ten o'clock in the morning, in the church-yard of the parish church of St. Pancras, Middlesex. A few of the persons she most esteemed, attended the ceremony; and a plain monument is now erecting on the spot, by some of her friends, with the following inscription:

> MARY WOLLSTONECRAFT GODWIN,
> AUTHOR OF
> A VINDICATION
> OF THE RIGHTS OF WOMAN.
> BORN, XXVII APRIL MDCCLIX.
> DIED, X SEPTEMBER MDCCXCVII.

The loss of the world in this admirable woman, I leave to other men to collect; my own I well know, nor can it be improper to describe it. I do not here allude to the personal pleasures I enjoyed in her conversation: these increased every day, in proportion as we knew each other better, and as our mutual confidence increased. They can be measured only by the treasures of her mind, and the virtues of her heart. But this is a subject for meditation, not for words. What I purposed alluding to, was the improvement that I have for ever lost.

Memoirs of a Most Beloved and Affectionate Wife by George Wray (1817)

Introduction

This narrative details the final days of Caroline Wray and the grief of her husband Reverend George Wray, who dedicates his text to his child born in the birth detailed here. The selection is excerpted from a handwritten manuscript by George Wray that is held in the Carl H. Pforzheimer Collection of Shelley

---

[10] 'Gulph' was the contemporary spelling of 'gulf'.

and His Circle at the New York Public Library. The story bears many similarities to Godwin's *Memoirs* of Wollstonecraft, though the style is more raw than Godwin's published version. Here, too, the husband's grief about the loss of his wife is evident throughout.

Excerpt from *Memoirs of a Most Beloved and Affectionate Wife*

The anxiety which pressed upon her mind regarding the issue of her approaching confinement was extraordinarily great – It was indeed a subject in itself naturally calculated to make her anxious; – but she had an indistinct apprehension of something that alarmed her. – No one ever took more pains to obviate every difficulty attending to her situation or to avert the evils commonly resulting from it. – In the use of coercive she was constant. – In the care & management of her person she was studious & exact: - in adopting the advice that was given her she was most particular: - yet the liveliness of her apprehensions – tho they seldom depressed her spirits except for the moment – were often mentioned by her. – It was but a short time before her confinement that she said to me with most uncommon tenderness – "Do you think I shall get well over it" – I answered her "I have no fear" – She replied with emphasis – "But I have." Wonderful are all the ways of Divine Providence – but perhaps in nothing more than preparing the mind for those great changes which cannot be foreseen nor turned away. – We know not how the Almighty works. – We cannot tell how his Holy Spirit acts upon our spirits, - tho' we are sure it does act upon them, & are conscious of its influence. – May not the soul be made sensible to impending danger when great trials are preparing for us - & may not this sensibility excited our fears and teach us caution tho' we know not why we feel so – nor can assign any cause for the use of our apprehensions?

--Equally wonderful & inscrutable are the ways by which the Almighty prepares & executes his purposes. – The whole plan is laid long before - - it is carried on in secret - & things seemingly of the most trifling or casual kind – contribute most surprisingly to its final accomplishment. – Thus it was in the case before us. – There were events apparently of no moment at the time - & and in the determination of which we were left to our own discretion – yet we were almost guided by necessity in the course we took - - though they either caused or completed the sad sad catastrophe. Such was the choice of a nurse.

It has been a source of real satisfaction to me – that neither of us ever planned the name of the child – or any particulars relating to it. – Doubtless the same motive governed us both, & our reserve was the effect of a perfect correspondence of sentiment. – We did not think it propoer. – Our conversation was continually upon the subject – yet all that ever passed on this interesting particular – was in these few words. – Expecting a hope in her safe delivery Caroline said to me – "I should like my Father & your mother to be Godfather & Godmother" – To which I announced "That is exactly my own wish, & what I meant to have proposed." – It is clear that the name of the child was not even so much as contemplated till the moment of its birth. – My only wish was that it should resemble herself.[11]

Mrs. Wainman came to us on Monday the 22' Sep. – My beloved wife's health was excellent - & except frequent faintings – she could not have been better. – Thus she continued till Friday Oct' 3rd assiduously expecting the important time - & relieving any little depression of spirits by saying – "If I have but my Doctor & my Nurse I shall do." –.

Friday Oct 3rd. – She seemed much as usual & walked about in the garden – but on going to bed- she said with rather a forced smile – "You only laugh & joke, but I feel very queerly." – How little do we know what is coming upon us – Neither she nor I suspected that this was the last time she would ever go to bed. --- Shortly afterwards when I went to her, she told me she thought the event was coming on - & so it proved. – Her doctor & nurse were sent for - & when I went to announce the arrival of one of the nurses, she said to me in an agony of pain "O! pray for me – I shall never survive it." – Her sufferings were uncommonly severe - & Mr. Chorley was apprehensive for her safety. – When I had occasion to go into the dressing room & she heard me speak – she called to me in the most piteous & affecting tone "My Husband! Is that my Husband"--!!!! Mr. C-- immediately said "Don't see him – you had better not see him—" and she acquiesced at once saying – "very well."—.

At 5 o clock in the morning her delivery was accomplished – She brought forth a fine boy. - - Mr. C—called it a severe & distressing labor – that he scaresly ever knew so short an one at the first child – that it should have been double the time - & that some circumstances which he stated had aggravated its severity –.[12]

When she had got a little composed I went to see her. After rejoicing with her that all was happily accomplished, she said with great tenderness – "Is not it one of the right sort? I am glad it is born perfect – It was the first thing I asked. – I thought it would have been too much for me – but when I heard it cry, I made a great effort – Tell my dear father that when I first heard it cry – I

---

[11] The adjoining paragraph was written under feelings which made it gratifying to show, that there were no presumptuous expectations formed with respect to the issue of the birth.

[12] The nurse told me some years afterwards that it was the most distressing labour she had ever witnessed in all her life. 1822.

thought at that moment I should like it to be called William & him to be a Godfather."

All went on well thro' the remainder of this day.

Sunday Oct 5. – I did my duty as usual. – My afternoon sermon was from these words – "The time is short—" 1Cor. 7C. 29v. – The subject of this discourse which I had borrowed from an unknown but eloquent writer was the swiftness with which time passes away & the brevity of human life. – Was it <u>chance</u> that caused me to preach that sermon on this day? --The coincidence at least is very striking. I certainly never thought of its instant application to myself with a reference to the nearest & dearest of all human beings. – I took it to church in common course – nor was it till sometime afterwards that I was struck with its full bearing & significance. The test, itself, is of general import – but the scope of the Apostle's argument & words which follow make it more particular. – Speaking of the troubles of that period of "<u>present distress</u>" – or persecution – when Christians were exposed to the utmost peril of their lives – St Paul gives his advice on some pointes with hesitation & reserve. – It was a matter of opinion & not of commandment. – But he adds – "This I say Brethren"! On this point there cannot be a doubt – "The time is short.—It remaineth that both they that have wives be as tho' they had none; & they that week as tho' they wept not; & they that rejoice as tho' they rejoiced not; & they that buy as tho' they possessed not - & they that use this world as not abusing it --- for the fashion of this world passeth away. ------ Caroline never forgot her duty to God. As I sat upon the bed in the evening talking to her, & the New Manual of Devotions lay beside her, she put it into my hand, & I read the thanksgiving for her safe deliverance.

Monday Oct 6th – Still every thing seemed to be going on well. I walked to the Town & returned a little before dinner – Mr. Chorley had paid a visit within the hour. -- Upon going into her room, I saw her face was flushed & I noticed it to her – She said "never mind my dear Love! it will soon go off—" & I thought no more of it. -- In the course of the afternoon she repeatedly asked for water & when I said "you are always drinking, you must be very feverish – the nurse said – "it is only the fever which attends the secretion of the milk – it always is so – everybody has it." – This was backed - & repeated over & over again – in so many ways & with such positiveness – that poor Caroline herself was persuaded of it - & my own ignorance on the subject made me acquiesce -- It is surely a little remarkable that I was the only one who all along apprehended things were not going on right – was earnest & anxious on the subject t- & yet gave way to the opinions & persuasions of those – whose experience entitled them to confidence. – So blind & feeble are our best powers when left to depend upon themselves. -- -- As her sweet Baby lay in her bosom – she pointed to it with extreme pleasure. – Her wish to be able to nurse had always been strong. – It was a satisfaction she had ever contemplated with delight. ---- She was now reaping it. – The little stranger was nestling at her breast. ---- In the evening the following letter came from Mr. Wainman.

My dear Sir,

I cannot express what I felt when I learnt that Dear Dear Caroline had suffered so much more than usual on such occasions. – Give my best love to her, & say that I hope that by this time, she & little William are as well as ought to be expected, & that he will ever be to you and herself a great comfort & blessing.

    Carhead   I am

    Monday Oct 6   yours most affec^{ly}

    1817--   Wm Wainman

As I sat upon the bed & read it to her, her countenance was lighted up with pleasure, & when I had concluded it she said with great animation – "How elegant! How delightful! What an elegant letter! This over pays me for all my sufferings!" -- Some conversation arose upon the name of "William" – mentioned in the letter when Mrs. Wainman suggested that "Henry" should be added to it – in which we both acquiesced. –.

-- We afterwards repeated the Thanksgiving Prayer which we had used the evening before. – At 10 O Clock when I went to wish her good night – she was suckling the dear Child of our Hopes - & looking up to me with a smiling & delighted face – said with greatest sweetness of expression – "See! I have got him here again!" – I told her – "I have scarcely noticed him – for my whole heart has been absorbed about yourself" – To which she answered in a playful manner "I shall be quite angry with you:-- -- Kiss him." -- -- It was now – that going to leave her for some hours – I felt anxious about her feverish state - & I questioned the nurse upon it – She assured me more strongly than ever that it was the ordinary milk fever – common to all - & that there was not any cause for alarm or uneasiness. -- -- Under this fatal impression I left her & went to bed. –.

7th Tuesday ---- Very early in the morning the nurse came to me & said Mrs Wray wished me to go to her. – I went immediately – She complained of being restless – hot & unable to sleep –I told her I would lay down by her, & she should compose herself to rest. – Whilst lying by her side I said – "I fear this nurse is an ignorant woman & knows nothing about you" - & some conversation passed about her feverish state & the singularity of such symptoms attending the ordinary secretion of the milk. – My beloved Caroline began to be apprehensive that all was not right – But the crisis was coming on – Her breathing grew short, quick & labored & at 4 O'Clock she exclaimed in the greatest alarm ----- describing her sensations. – I was panic struck -- -- & calling the nurse said to her with some warmth – "Must I <u>now</u> send for Mr Chorley?" – To which she answered – "Aye to be sure – send immediately." -- -- Having ordered every thing around to be kept quiet -- & begged my dear wife to be still, & compose herself till Mr. Chorley arrived, I left the room & sent off for him. – The state of my mind cannot be well described. – I suspected at once the nature of the malady – It flashed instantaneously on my mind – Its fatality was no secret to me – for I had myself been witness to it. Alarmed for the result & vexed at having been for hours the dupe of ignorance – I waited with tremendous impatience for Mr. C—'s arrival – My dear Caroline's last words as I left her room – entreating her to be composed – deserve to be for ever recorded – they were so like herself – "I will, love! – but don't be angry then." – They were not lost upon me.

At 5 O Clock Mr. C arrived – I told him all I knew. – he visited his patient - & brought me this account – "Mrs Wray has a considerable degree of fever & seems rather confused. I find upon enquiring that she had a shivering fit at 10 O Clock last night – Her pulse is high about 164. It will be proper to take some blood from her, & she must be kept as quiet as possible. – Let no one go near but the nurse – Talking will agitate her & increase her fever - & in this case quietness is every thing." – I directly asked him – "Is it the Puerperal Fever"? – He answered, "I can't say but it partakes of the nature of that disorder – but at present it is difficult to determine what it will prove." – He then left me – bled her in both arms - & lowered her pulse to 120. – Upon my observing what an ignorant woman the nurse was! – he said – "What can you expect from a monthly nurse! They are all alike ignorant – they know nothing of diseases." -- -- -- -- It afterwards appeared upon enquiring that she had never seen a similar case before.[13] ---- Mr. C—came again twice in the course of the day - & at my request brought Dr. Thorp with him in the Evening. – Mr. C—staid the night with us.

---

[13] Note in Original Text:

It is a remarkable circumstance that a young lady whom this nurse attended immediately after my dear wifes confinement, & who then laid lay in of her first child, died in childbirth early in this year, 1821. When brought to bed of her third child, & her death occurred in the same way but under circumstances much more rapidly fatal, than my dear wifes, whilst this very woman was again in attendance as nurse. And Mr. Chorley, whose patient she was, blamed the stupidity of the nurse, in some striking & analogous particulars which he mentioned to me.

8 Wednesday ----- Mr. Chorley came to my room at 4 O Clock & said – "I have been called up to Mrs Wray – the fever has returned with great strength - & I have told her I must cut off her hair & open the jugular vein. – She says she is very willing – if you will have no objection – but I must mention it to you." –My answer was – "Do whatever you think right Mr Chorley – you know best – you are the proper judge." – He accordingly returned to her & as he told me afterwards – "Her pulse was running so high that I had not the patience to count it, but cut off her hair as quick as possible & plunged her head in cold water – The effect was surprising but the palpitation of the heart was such that I do not remember ever meeting with a similar case. I heard a beating noise & was going to ask what it was when to my great surprise I found it proceeded from her heart." ----- -- By copious bleeding & the application of cold water for hours the fever [sic] went down to 120 & remained there. – It had risen far above the periodical attack of the preceding morning. – When Dr Thorp came he approved of what Mr. Chorley had done. From this time both the medical men attended each morning & evening - & Mr. C—always once or twice besides in the course of the day.

9 Thursday – Mr. Chorley had been called up to her in the night & relieved her. – This day passed over much the same as the preceding – the intermitting fits of fever being frequent – which as they rose – were subdued by a course of cold water applications from wrung flannels. ----- - It is the nature of this distressing disease to occasion the greatest anxiety of mind & depression of spirits. The rapidity with which the hot fit advances excites immediate alarm, & in the present deplorable case, by the fever flying to the head – this agitation was increased till confusion or temporary delirium ensured – amid all the trials of this eventful period, that was not the least which spring from her repeated messages & earnest importunities to see me – all of which I was constrained to resist – in conformity to the rule laid down. – This rule, as a general one, might be excellent & indeed it appears from Mr. Wm Heys treatise on this disorder that one of his patients who appeared to be recovering – relapsed & lost her life from the intrusion of her Friends. – But the present care did not require it. -- -- Hard as the trial was it had been & will be my consolation. That I did my duty against my feelings – Had I prevailed with the Faculty to wave the order - & the final result have remained – as it must have done – the same; - I might have reproached myself – or been open to reproach – for voluntarily contributing to the fatal consequence. -- -- To mark how essential quietness is in a fever of this description – the pulse generally rose ten strokes in a minute when the medical men were making their enquiries of her. Yet she was either so conscious of this or so willing to comply with their advice, that whenever she had occasion to speak with the nurses, she

commonly ended any little question with – "But Nurse! I must not talk." -- ---
Mr. Chorley who again staid the night – said to me before going to bed – "as nearly as we can determine Mrs Wray's case it is Phrenitis" – by which I understood fever on the brain.[14]

10th Friday. – Between 4 & 5 O Clock in the morning (the hour of the fever's periodical return in its greatest strength) M^r C- came to my room & said – "I am sorry to say that a new cause of distress has arisen. – The fever has left the head and seems to have gone to the bowels – Let your servant go to my house for the things I want & he may as well at the same time call up Dr Thorp." ---- This was immediately done. Dr Thorp came & by proper applications the inflammation as removed. – But whilst the disorder began to move about – the great weakness to which this ever dear sufferer was reduced caused a considerable accumulation of wind upon the stomach which irritated her complaint. – Still however the general symptoms began to wear a more favorable object – the pulse varied from 100 to 120 – the hot fits were of shorter continuance - & the case was far from desperate. – To a question which she put to Dr. Thorp – whether he considered her in danger – his answer was – "No! nothing like so much as on Wednesday." – Indeed he was always full of sanguine expectations -- -- She sent her love to me by him. – Mr. Chorley being exhausted & indisposed – the Doctor took his place at night -- & staid with us.

11th Saturday. -- -- The D^r was called up to his patient early in the morning. He went & sat by her till he had soothed her to rest. – She slept about two hours -- & this was the first sleep of any continuance since her confinement. – The day passed over much the same as the last – Her fever varied & she sent me many messages when it rose – but on the whole she was decidedly better & her pulse fell to 94. --- -- It was one of the many occasions on which she wished to see me – that she feelingly said – "I am sure I can bear it – if he can." ----- Dr Thorp resumed his bed at night.

12. Sunday – The Doctor made a most favorable report. – Every symptom was good & augured well – and this flattering prospect continued through the day: - but it was the calm which precedes a terrible storm. – At 8 O Clock in the Evening the Nurse came hurrying to me & said "nothing would pacify her Lady but seeing me" – It was evident the fever was rising - & it rose

---

[14] Oct 9. 1823 ---- Mr. Chorley informed me a few days ago that the fever, which has again made its appearance in the neighborhood, & is epidemical, results from a peculiar state of atmosphere, - a humid, foggy, & unwholesome state, the consequence of immediate rain, that it is not peculiar to lying in females, though they, from their condition, are extremely liable to it, & that it is an inflammatory contagion purely. – He farther said, that it is prevailing quietly at this very time in Edinbro & that he was now confidently in the opinion which he had always held of it. – Puerperal fever it certainly was not, as he had been satisfied, by his inspection of a peron who had died under it.

indeed with all its strength. – a scene of distress followed that cannot be conceived -- -- -- Let a veil be drawn over it for humanity's sake. – The medical men were sent for & Dr Thorp presently arrived – A word from him restored all to right – "you shall see Mr Wray as soon as you are composed." ----- ----- In a very little time I was allowed to visit her. – It was our first interview since Tuesday morning when Mr. Chorley was called in. – She was sat up in bed with the crimson shawl[15] thrown over her shoulders – her countenance not much altered – but her eyes emitting a glazy lustre, that indicated the strength & influence of her fever. – The attendants all left the room: ---- Such a meeting will not bear description. --- -- When the first moments were passed - & as I sat by her upon the bed. – she said with a look & tone so expressive & so tender that I never can forget them – "Take care of Baby! I feel this will be too much for me" --- I said "I hope not – Dr Thorpe has a good opinion of your case – I hope it will please God to restore you" – She replied – "If I might have seen you, I think I could have recovered" – but &c &c – I answered – "I have always longed to see you but the Doctors feared it would have a bad effect & this alone has prevented it." – "Yes" she said – "but they did not know me when they thought so." ----- Among other things I told her – "Baby is a very fine Child & I often kiss it for you" – She exclaimed with animation – "That's delightful – that's delightful" – Let me look at you – bring the candle here – let me see you" – desirous as I thought to observe what effect her illness had produced upon me. – I accordingly brought her a candle - & she looked me very earnestly in the face. ---- After some further conversation – I told her "I dare not trespass on my leave – but now, Caroline, that I have free access to you, send whenever you with to see me & I will immediately come to you." --- She put her arms round my neck & drew me to her lips so passionately – saying "God bless you" – that she might have known, as it really proved – that this was nature's last & fondest effort. --- I left her with a conviction that neither of us had cause for any great hope - & neither of us entertained such – yet between Hope & Despair there is an immense difference. – Had I been made acquainted at the time with what was said & what was done between her message to me - & Dr Thorp's arrival – I should have better understood her affecting charge "To take care of Baby." ----- I told Dr Thorp who again passed the night with us – "you will never persuade me that she can be restored. Those eyes tell a fatal truth." – He said with great confidence – that his opinion was otherwise – that he had great hopes - & that the lustre of the eyes would soon be taken away. – He also added – "whenever Mrs Wray wishes to see you, we agree in thinking you may go to her but don't talk much

---

[15] This shawl which was a gift of Mr. [unreadable] I afterwards gave to Mrs. [unreadable].

to her – nor worry her by staying too long." – Alas! This privilege came too late – the die was already cast. ----- -- Leeches were applied to her temples - & when I went to her again to wish her good night – she smiled & said "I am better." This seems to have been the crisis of the disorder.

13 Monday --- The night passed without any return of fever – but a deep & immoveable languor succeeded the last attacks. – From the frequent sound of her bell & a continual stir & bustle with the attending nurses – such a solemn stillness prevailed that the House might have been already possessed by death. – The change was awfully striking. – Tho' at full liberty to see me, she did not once send – nor speak much at all throughout the day. – Her dear little Baby she had never seen from the preceding Monday night when I left her cherishing & feeding it & most delighted with it; -- nor did she ever see it more: -- made many enquiries after it – rejoiced to hear its praises - & felt for the loss it was soon to have. – To some commendations of the fever – nurse in speaking of it – she said – "It's a pity"-- --- alluding as the nurse supposed to the prescience of her own mind – that it would soon be motherless. -- -- Indeed she was sensible beyond us all that her recovery was impossible.[16] – She felt <u>that</u> within her – which all human beings must feel once, & which sometimes eludes the sagacity of the best medical skill to penetrate & discover. – She commanded her Husband to the care of Heaven – "May God the Lord Almighty support my dear Husband as he has supported me." – These words - & words to this effect were frequently offered up by her. – They shew the feeling of her heart - & the conviction of her approaching end. -- --- -- But the sentiments of the medical men were encouraging. – Her great debility was in her favor - & no worse symptom appeared. ----- Hope ever lingers over life. – I pressed it to my bosom - & as no alteration had taken had taken place when Mr. Chorley came as usual, at noon – I could not part with it. --- Night drew on & still no amendment – anxiety & apprehension began to harass me – for no Doctors came. – It was midnight when Mr. Chorley arrived & he was along ---- Dr. Thorp had been thrown from his gig & was laid up in bed. – As the D^r had been always the most sanguine of the two – I received the account with a consternation which amounted to despair.

---

[16] The following particulars were communicated to me by the Head-Nurse in 1819 when she attended me in a dangerous illness. ----- On Monday, the day before she died – she said to this nurse & another steward who was attending her – "Do you think I can recover? – I have a most disagreeable smell in my nose – it is like the smell of death. – Don't you smell it?" – In the course of the day she again said – "I taste it in my mouth." ----- These observations which should have been communicated to the medical men, never were. They clearly prove, that a mortification, had taken place; -- that the freedom from pain & the great languor were the result of this fatal state of the bowels, & that all possibility of recovery was at an end. – They leave us doubt, but that the dreadful attach of the preceding night, produced such a degree of inflammation as destroyed the power of the vital organs. Oct 14. 1821.

----- After Mr Chorley had visited his patient, we sat together half an hour – in which the despair of my mind was so great & evident that he said to me with an openness, & earnestness he had never used before – "Indeed I do not think Mrs Wray's case by any means desperate – I would not say so, if it were otherwise – but I do not despair of her recovery." ---- Well might such words relieve a fond Husband's aching heart. – His experience – his reserve – his great caution & his sincerity – were unquestionable grounds of reliance – He thought what he said. – Comforted with this opinion – we separated & went to our respective rooms.

14 – Tuesday – The Last – The Fatal Day. ----- Upon enquiring of the nurse what sort a night her M^{rs} had passed – the answer was boding & concise – "very bad Sir." – "Any sleep?" "No Sir! – she said to me in the night – "Nurse I am very badly.—" ----- When Mr. C-- got up & visited his patient – he told me – there is a great languor about Mrs. Wray which we must remove – I will go & see Dr Thorp & make up what he prescribes – Her pulse rose ten strokes in the minute in merely speaking to me." --- His opinion seemed to be unchanged – nor did he apprehend any more immediate danger. – His manner was rather otherwise.

----- Soon after he was gone she desired to see her mother. – Mrs W. Went to her. – Her voice was so feeble that her mother could not hear her – but she put her arms around her neck & blessed her. -- --- She then sent for me. – I knew her motive but had better hopes - & trusted she was yet to be returned to me. – As I sat down upon the bed – she <u>looked at me</u> – she could not speak. – It was one of those looks which no pencil ever drew – so expressive – so full of meaning – so touching – so affective – To relieve her heart I mentioned little Baby - & spoke about his name – but as Mr. Chorley had observed – the effort of conversation was immediately perceptible in a rapid rise of fever – for her face became flushed & I was alarmed at the consequences. – I therefore said to her – "My talking only agitates you – I had better leave you a little." – She faintly answered – "yes perhaps it does." --- -- It did not occur to me at the moment – for my hopes buoyed me up – that her agitation arose from the anguish of her soul, at what she meant to be a parting interview.

----- Her feelings proved a truer guide than all the experience of her skillful advisers.

She often said in this last stage of her illness to those about her – "I have now no wish to live – there was a time when I should have thought it a hard struggle [17] – but now I have no tie to the world." -- -- -- Yet tho' for herself she had no wish to live -- -- the tenderest emotions of her heart were all awake to his sad sufferings & his wretched state, who with a helpless infant of a few days old – must remain to bemoan her death. – This was the subject of her dying thoughts – this the burden of her dying prayer. "O my dear Husband!! may the Lord his Savior support him under all his troubles."

It was now when her medicines came. – One was immediately given – but it produced no effect. – She slept for about ten minutes in the afternoon – and awaking with a heavenly smile – said – "I have been in heaven." ----- About 3 O Clock I was called to her. – She seemed to be dying – her eyes were thrown back - & a strong perspiration had broken out upon her face. – I instantly felt her pulse:- it was so faint as scarcely to be discernable – but I counted it at 120. – When she was told I was with her – she opened her languid eyes & knew me perfectly – for she was quite sensible. – I asked her some questions which she answered me. – Soon afterwards she said, "I'll take another draft & compose myself." – The draft had a momentary effect. She was evidently relieved & the clammy perspiration abated. – We changed the posture of her head a little - & as she lay more composed – she said with a most uncommon sweetness of tone & manner of compassion – "<u>My</u> Love! how beautiful! – Providence all around" – and in the same instant as she spoke, her whole countenance changed & became illuminated. – The light which overspread her face gave me an idea of glory. – It was momentary – but it surpassed any thing which the mind can conceive. – Every feature was affected by it. -- --- As I was going out to meet Mr. Chorley – who had just arrived – she said with considerable strength of voice ---- "It is the sleep of death! – Is it not the sleep of death?" – alluding as I thought to the notion of the soul sleeping between death & the resurrection – which led me to say – "O no! my Love! No! --- -- Meeting Mr C I said – "I do hope Mr Chorley it is only an increase of fever – she is rather better" – but he soon undeceived me – sending for me to another room – he said – "I am sorry to say that since I was here in the morning an unfavorable change has taken place. The medicine I sent was judged proper upon a consultation with Dr Thorp - & nothing more can be done." – I returned to her immediately - & laying down beside her on the bed supported her arm in my arms & performed the little offices for her which her care required – She was sinking fast – but thoroughly sensible. – It occurred to me that her mother & Brother Richard would wish to see her once more - & after

---

[17] - of sickness we may likewise remark, how wonderfully it reconciles us to the thoughts, the expectations, & the approach of death; & how this becomes in the hand of Providence, an example of one evil being made to correct another – Paley. 33 Sermon.

consulting with Mr. Chorley I called them up. – They took their last farewell – when complaining of tightness she said – "you won't keep me long Mr Chorley"! – We raised her up – altered her pillows - & did what we could to relieve any pressure from her posture – but she bore it with difficulty - & nature was evidently almost exhausted. --- --- M^r C put his hand upon her head - & I saw his countenance alter to surprise. – Soon, very soon, the cause was obvious – Her breathing grew short & the mental agonies appeared --- O! what a sight! tho' there was no pain – nor any distortion. --- In the first feeling of surprise & panic – I exclaimed "O! she is dying! – she is dying"! --- Mr. C– put up his hand - & in a low tone said, "Hush"! --- As I knelt by the bedside grasping her hand – & in an agony or distress – he came round to take me out of the room – but I could not bear to leave her. – My distress however became such – that he soon came up to me again – took me by the hand & kindly said – "you had <u>better</u> leave the room – this is not a proper scene for you – We must submit to these things – They are ordered by Providence." ----- I yielded to his advice & he led me away. -- -- a few a very very few moments must have a short interval closed this heart-rending scene.[18] --- When next I saw this richest Gift of God – this heavenly Treasure – my dear dear wife – she was laid out – bearing even in her dead countenance much of the expressive sweetness of her living features.

Thus died in the bloom of life & vigor of health & in the full enjoyment of that happiness – which humanly speaking knew neither change nor interruption one of the sweetest – gentlest – Dearest of God's Creatures – so amiable – so affectionate as to be beloved by all – so passionately fond of him who doated on her, that no words can tell it, & no heart can know it. – Kind to the poor – kind to her friends – kind to all around – she seemed a being of a finer mould than common mortals boast. – Warm in her feelings her heart was formed for love; & that love beat with rapture in her breast when it was given to play in real life. – Her piety was free from shew & full of ardor. – Her life displayed it & her death attested it. – Yet why she died so early – so suddenly & at such an eventful time - & under such distressing circumstances – her little child just expanding its feeble new-born powers – her afflicted Husband restricted from her company. – Why was she cut off from the fair promise of maternal joys - & increasing comforts – from all she loved - & all that is given to love – is known to Him alone who knoweth all things. ----- Vain are all reasonings on a death like this. A veil intercepts our view & makes

---

[18] Anxious to dedicate my Child to God – I baptized him by the names of William Henry – as soon as I could do it. The ceremony it seems took place – just as his mother expired. Perhaps it was a quarter of an hour after I had left the room. 1820.

speculations foolish. – The God who crowned her last & happiest year with one unclouded sunshine of delight – could – by his gracious providence have added many more of equal or even greater felicity. -- - That he did not leaves a latitude for faith & trust in him, which the knowledge of his goodness will supply – Be it our care – be it mine above all – to write the remembrance of her virtues on the fairest portion of my heart – to copy her bright example as it shines & glows – to dwell & feed on her endearing love and tenderness – to regard her as separated more by my imperfection than by space – to look forward to a reunion with her in heaven that shall be final & complete' & to render up to God the utmost gratitude of which the soul is capable – for bountifully allotting the last year of a life so incalculably precious to my unspeakable comfort.

Dark & inscrutable as are the ways of Providence Heaven - & vain & foolish as it is to track them – a light is sometimes thrown upon the path – faint it may be & very glimmering – but enough to regulate the mind & hand it up to the providence of God. -----

Had I been killed in the dreadful accident of our over-turn – poor Caroline would have been left a wretched widow without one hope or solace from our marriage. -- -- The affliction is reversed & she is gone – but she has bequeathed me a heavenly Treasure in her darling child, to be my comfort till we meet again – to form a connecting link in the great chain of being that unites us all together – to interest my tenderest affections & to engage & occupy my heart. --- -- That we shall meet again & be united [19] is my persuasion & my holy hope – It is conceivable that God has no other end in our attachments but the momentary interest they awaken here – that whilst he gives to one happy pair years upon years of conjugal felicity, he severs in a few short months – not to be reunited – the bond which binds another pair – not less happy – perhaps not less acceptable to him? – But how - & when, & under what altered circumstances - & with what untried feelings & affections - & with what kind of felicity – we shall meet – I neither know nor can conceive – This life – some-how or other – is to be the plan and groundwork – of our eternal happiness. – Every thing we say & every thing we do, has a reference to our final state. – The affections of the Soul will outlive the body [20] & form our character in heaven. - There will be purified, & exhausted, & carried to the highest

---

[19] Is there a great difference between the thought of losing those we love for ever – of taking at their death or at our own an eternal farewell, never to see them more; & the reflection that we are about to be separated for a few years at longest, to be united with them in a new & better state of mutual existence? – Paley 34 Serm.
[20] See Butter analogy – Life on probation.

pitch of excellence of which they are capable - & on them – thro' the merits of the Prevailing Intercessor, will rest our condition through endless ages. ----------

Periodical Coverage of Princess Charlotte's Death in Childbirth (1817–1818)

Introduction

On 6 November 1817, Princess Charlotte Augusta of Wales died in childbirth with her first child, which brought Britain into a period of great mourning for the wildly popular young princess. The Princess was third in the line of succession, following her grandfather George III and father George IV (then George, Prince of Wales). Many periodicals covered the nation's mourning through a series of memorials, with some sharing the details of her decline and death after the delivery of a stillborn son. Princess Charlotte endured a long and difficult birth, during which she was attended by physician and accoucheur Sir Richard Croft, her personal physician Matthew Baillie, and later obstetrician John Sims. Croft was especially distraught about her death, and just three months later killed himself, leading the situation to be called "the triple obstetrical tragedy." The excerpts here include two about the death of Princess Charlotte and one about Croft's death by suicide.

Excerpt from "A Memoir of the Life, Death, and Funeral, of Her Royal Highness the Princess Charlotte Augusta" (*The Ladies' Monthly Museum*, December 1817)

This marriage, concluded with so great a prospect of felicity to the happy pair, was hailed by the nation as a propitious occurrence, and ominous of future good; but, to exemplify by what a frail tenure all mortal possessions are held, and at once to check the pride, the vanity, and presumption of man; the hopes and expectations of the Royal Family and the Nation have been by one stroke of fate destroyed. This happy union promised a descendant in the first year; and the Princess, after a long and painful labour, (the particulars of which, are given as under.) brought into the world a still-born son, and in less than six hours after, expired herself; thus leaving the Prince, her father, with a barren sceptre in his hands; bereft of his only child, the heir-apparent of his crown, and the infant that should have succeeded her; and the nation deprived of their most anxious hope, of that object whose amiable character they almost idolized; and under whose future reign they promised felicity to themselves or their posterity! This melancholy event has crossed the line of succession; and, though it will fall to the next Royal Brother, the expectations of the country are greatly disappointed.

On Monday the, 3rd instant, her Royal Highness first showed the usual symptoms of indisposition. Dr. Baillie and Dr. Croft were the medical attendants.[21] During the whole of Tuesday, the labour advanced slowly, but without any appearance of danger. Towards evening, it was deemed advisable to send for Dr. Sims,[22] who arrived in the middle of the night. At six on Wednesday evening, the throes of child-birth had become more decisive; and the child was then, and, it is said, even up to a few minutes before its birth, ascertained to be living; and, on delivery, was found to be a perfect fine-formed male infant. During this trying scene, and throughout the whole of her tedious labour, the Princess maintained the utmost firmness and expressed the most pious resignation; and after the birth, her Royal Highness appeared so tranquil and composed, that, between twelve and one, the medical gentlemen retired to rest. The Cabinet Ministers also had left Claremont soon after eleven o'clock, but were afterwards recalled. The first symptom of approaching danger is said to have discovered itself on some gruel being presented to her, which she found a difficulty in swallowing; severe chills and spasms succeeded. The physicians were called up, but their assistance was vain. For the last half-hour, the spasms subsided; she sunk into calm composure, nearly speechless, but apparently not insensible; and at half past two o'clock, she was no more. His Serene Highness the Prince of Saxe-Coburg felt all the anxieties natural to an affectionate husband, during the whole labour. On the report, that the Princess was "doing well," he consoled himself for the loss of the child, and retired to rest in the adjoining chamber, and was among the first who attended the summons on the fresh appearances of indisposition. He remained by the bed-side the whole time, endeavouring, as much as possible, to disguise from his suffering consort the grief and agony he felt at the unexpected turn that had taken place. Her Royal Highness, it is said, scarcely ever moved her eyes from the face of her beloved partner, extending her hand frequently to meet his--that hand which was, in one short hour, to be cold, insensible, and lifeless. About five minutes before her death, the Princess said to the medical attendants, "Is there any danger?" they requested her Royal Highness to compose herself; and shortly after she breathed a gentle sigh, and expired.

---

[21] Dr. Matthew Baillie and Sir Richard Croft were both physicians to George III and his family and had trained under Dr. Thomas Denman, a preeminent obstetrician.
[22] Dr. John Sims was an obstetrician and member of the Royal College of Physicians.

Excerpt from "Brief Memoir of her Royal Highness the Princess Charlotte, with an Account of her last Illness, Death, and Funeral" (*The Literary Panorama and National Register*, December 1817)

In the sweet retirement of Claremont, the Prince and Princess passed their time in the full enjoyment of domestic bliss, far from the dissipations of a town life; and presenting the most beautiful instance of conjugal affection and human happiness that can be imagined. But this scene of joy was not to continue. When every one was waiting and listening for the signal that was to proclaim the birth of England's heir, an event which was to complete the happiness of the Prince and Princess- when all were prepared for gratulation and joy-suddenly.

> All things that were ordained festival
> Turned from their office to black funeral;
> Our instruments to melancholy bells;
> Our wedding cheer to a sad burial feast;
> Our solemn hymns to sullen dirges changed;
> Our bridal flowers served for a buried corpse,
> And all things changed them to the contrary!

From the moment it was generally known that her Royal Highness was likely to add one more member to the Royal House of Brunswick, the greatest interest was excited throughout the nation, and from the general state of her Royal Highness's health during her pregnancy, the most pleasing hopes were entertained.

The more early stages of the Princess Charlotte's labour were favourable to the moment when the bulletin announced that the child was still-born, and the mother "doing well." The date of that official paper was 10 o'clock on Wednesday night, the Princess having then been delivered about an hour. At six, the throes of childbirth had become more decisive; and the child was then, and, it is said, even up to a few minutes before its birth, ascertained to be living. At its birth it was found a perfect fine-formed male infant. After the birth, her Royal Highness appeared so tranquil and composed, that between twelve and one the medical gentlemen retired to rest. The Cabinet Ministers, also, having full reason to believe that all danger was over, had left Claremont soon after 11 o'clock, but were afterwards recalled. The first symptom of approaching danger is said to have been on some gruel being presented to her, which she found a difficulty in swallowing; cold and spasms succeeded. The physicians were called up, but their aid was vain. For the last half hour her spasms are said to have subsided; she sunk into calm composure, speechless, but apparently not insensible; and at half past 2 o'clock she was no more!

The following are official details of this melancholy event.

Claremont, Nov. 4.—Her Royal Highness was in good health till a late hour last night, when she found herself indisposed, which continued till three o'clock this morning, when Sir R. Croft, her *Accoucheur*, who has been in constant attendance for the last three weeks upon her Royal Highness, had no hesitation in pronouncing that the symptoms were those of her accouchement. In consequence, a number of servants, who have been for some time kept in close attendance in their riding dresses, and their horses in readiness for them to mount, were dispatched at a quarter past three o'clock, in various directions to summon the different Privy Counsellors, who it had been previously arranged were to attend according to court etiquette, and for Dr. Baillie—Directions were given to the Messengers to make all possible speed, which they strictly attended to.

It is scarely necessary to say Prince Leopold has passd the day in the greatest anxiety in the house, as well as all the royal attendants and domestics, with the State Officers and others.

From the neighbouring towns and villages the most earnest and solicitous enquiries have been constantly made during the day.

Claremont, 4 o'clock p.m.—The last report of Sir Richard Croft to the Privy Counsellors assembled here, was, "The progress of her Royal Highness, the Princess Charlotte's illness, is in every respect, as favourable as could be wished."

The following was the circular communication of Wednesday night, relative to the Princess Charlotte.

Claremont, Nov. 5.—Her Royal Highness made little progress yesterday. Communications were sent off to the Prince Regent and other branches of the Royal Family. At night, on the suggestion of Sir Richard Croft, Dr. Sims was sent for, that he might be in readiness to be consulted if necessary. At three o'clock this morning Dr. Sims arrived here from London. This morning, a little before eight o'clock, the Privy Counsellors, assembled here, had a consultation with the Medical gentlemen in attendance, when, in consequence of the protracted state of the illness of the Princess, the following official report or bulletin, was drawn up.

Claremont, Wednesday Morning, 8 o'clock.—
"The labour of her Royal Highness the Princess Charlotte is going on very slowly, but we trust favourably

(Signed) "M. BAILLIE.
"RICHARD CROFT.
"JOHN SIMS."

The following are the different official notices which have appeared, in addition to those already recited, upon the subject of the accouchement and death of the Princess Charlotte. The first relate to the period just preceding the delivery, and is as follows:

"Claremont, Nov. 5, half-past 5 p.m.
"The labour of Her Royal Highness the Princess Charlotte has within the last three or four hours considerably advanced, and will, it is hoped, within a few hours be happily completed.
"M. BAILLIE.
"RICHARD CROFT.
"JOHN SIMS."

But at a quarter past nine the hope thus encouraged was destroyed by the following annunciation:—

"Claremont, Nov 5, ¼ past 9 in the Evening.,
"At nine o'clock this evening Her Royal Highness the Princess Charlotte was safely delivered of a still-born male child, and her Royal Highness is going on favourably"
(Signed as before.)

At ten, another bulletin was issued, which at least seemed to remove all apprehension as to the personal danger of her Royal Highness. It is as follows:

"Claremont, Nov. 5, 10 o'clock, p m.
"At nine o'clock this evening Her Royal Highness the Princess Charlotte was delivered of a still-born male child. Her Royal Highness is extremely well."
(Signed as before.)

...

But the public disappointment was doomed to be unmixed, or rather to be merged in complete despair, for at half past six on Thursday morning the following mournful letter was dispatched by Lord Sidmouth to the Lord Mayor;—

"Whitehall, Nov. 6, 6 a.m.

"My Lord,—It is with the deepest sorrow that I inform your Lordship, that her Royal Highness the Princess Charlotte expired this morning at half past two o'clock.
"I have the honour to be, &c.
(Signed) "SIDMOUTH"
"The Right Hon. the Lord Mayor."

The following letters contain the painfully interesting details of these afflicting occurrences:

"Claremont, 6 o'clock this morning (Thursday.)
"I had hoped to have sent you very, very different tidings; and yesterday, when I dispatched my last letter to you, I felt confident that my next would have announced the consummation of our wishes, in the birth of a future heir or heiress. That next!—————— However, I will endeavour to write all I have heard, as well as the general grief and consternation will allow me. On Monday in the night, or about 3 on Tuesday morning, her Royal Highness was taken ill, and expresses were sent off to the great Officers of State, the Archbishop of Canterbury, and the Bishop of London, desiring their immediate attendance. Lord Chancellor, Mr. Vansittart, together with Earl Bathurst, Lord Sidmouth, the Archbishop and Bishop, immediately attended. Dr. Baillie, and Dr. Croft were the medical attendants. During the whole of Monday the labour advanced slowly, but without the least appearance of danger. The Princess Charlotte showed uncommon firmness and the utmost resignation. Towards evening, as the labour still lingered, it was deemed advisable to send for Dr. Sims, who arrived in the middle of the night. Nothing could be going on better, though too slowly: and the excellent constitution of the Princess gave every assurance that she would not be too much exhausted by the delay. No language, no panegyric can be too warm for the manner in which the Prince Leopold conducted himself. He was incessant in his attendance, and no countenance could more deeply express the anxiety he felt. Once or twice he exclaimed to the medical attendants, 'that the unrepining patient endurance of the Princess, whilst it gave him comfort, communicated also a deep affliction at her sufferings being so lengthened.'

About six o'clock yesterday the labour advanced more rapidly, and no apprehensions were entertained of any fatal result: and the child was ascertained to be still living. At nine o'clock her Royal Highness was delivered of a male child, but still-born. Throughout the whole of this long and painful labour, her Royal Highness evinced the greatest firmness, and received the communication of the child being born dead with much resignation. Prince Leopold exclaimed to the medical attendants, as soon as the intelligence was communicated to him—"Thank God! thank God! the Princess is safe." The child was perfect, and one of the finest infants ever brought into the world. The Princess was composed after her delivery, and though of course much exhausted, every hope was entertained of her doing well. This pleasing intelligence being communicated to the great Officers of State, and the Archbishop of Canterbury, and the Bishop of London, they left "The Right Hon. the Lord Mayor." Claremont about 11 o'clock; the medical attendants of course remaining. A little after 12, a change was observed in her Royal Highness—her quiet left her—she became restless and uneasy—and the medical attendants felt alarmed. Expresses were sent off, I believe, to the Officers of State, stating the change that had taken place. From half-past 12 restlessness and convulsions increased till nature and life were quite exhausted, and her Royal Highness expired at half-past 2 this morning. Prince Leopold was with her Royal Highness at this agonizing moment."

Another Letter from Claremont

> "Claremont, Thursday morning, 9 o'clock.
> "The most melancholy and distressing event has happened—Princess Charlotte is no more! All is dismay and grief, rejoicing turned into mourning, in the death of the most lovely and affectionate of Princesses. The scene at this time exceeds all attempt at description. The awful event was not known at Esher till eight o'clock, and now there is scarcely an eye free from tears. The amiable and affectionate Prince Leopold is distracted and inconsolable, and the whole of the Royal establishment is in a similar state. The approach of the departure of the conveyance compels us to be brief in relating the tragic particulars. Her Royal Highness, after her delivery, had expressed herself resigned to the child lying dead, most piously observing that it was the will of God. She continued remarkably well from nine o'clock (the time of her delivery) till past twelve o'clock, probably a quarter past, when the medical gentlemen, Drs. Baillie, Croft, and Sims, considering that she could not be doing better under the circumstances, retired to rest. Her Royal Highness took some gruel, and expressed herself inclined to sleep; however, on the gruel being given to her, she expressed herself to find a difficulty in swallowing it. The lovely Princess afterwards complained of being very chilly, and a pain at her stomach. The nurse, Mrs. Griffiths, considering her Royal Highness's complaints to require the advice of the medical gentlemen in attendance, the Doctors were all instantly called up. They lost no time in giving their attendance, but human assistance was of no avail. Her Royal Highness's attack continued unabated, and she expired about half-past two o'clock, in a severe attack of spasms."

"Death of Sir Richard Croft, Bart." (*Examiner*, 15 February 1818)

On Friday morning (says the *Chronicle*) it was made known that Sir Richard Croft, the celebrated Accoucheur, had died suddenly at the house of a lady in Wimpole-street (Mrs. Thackeray), whom he was attending in child-bed. The circumstance produced no ordinary sensation, as it was known that ever since the fatal termination of the accouchement of the amiable Princess Charlotte, Sir Richard has labored under the most severe mental affliction.—The unfortunate circumstance of not having previously introduced the experienced and able physician Dr. Sims to the Princess, so as to have the advantage of his assistance and counsel in the important duty he had to discharge, preyed upon his mind, and his friends have long observed symptoms of uneasiness that alarmed them, and which, probably, prepared them for the event that has happened. Various rumours were circulated and among others his name was implicated in a most delicate affair that has occupied the attention of the higher circles for some days past, and to which we cannot give the smallest credit. The utmost industry was also used to suppress all knowledge of the manner of Sir Richard's death; And certainly, if we could have saved the feelings of his afflicted relatives without a dereliction of our duty to the public, we should have yielded to the earnest solicitations that have been made to us. It is one of the most irksome parts of an Editor's task to make known cases, which may appear to belong only to private suffering, and not to concern the public; but surely a little reflection must convince our Readers that it is not true, and that an Editor cannot yield to the applications of friends on such events, without incurring the charge of corruption, even where he indulges only the kindest emotions of the heart.—Our Reporters were prevented from access to the Inquest; a prohibition which the Coroner was not justified in authorising, since the law of the Coroner was intended undoubtedly to operate as a preventive of the dreadful and abhorrent crime of suicide, a crime which is probably rendered more frequent by the concealment too often arranged, and by the lenity of the verdicts.—By this exclusion, we can only state the circumstances, as communicated to us by a witness. The Inquest was taken at the house, No. 86, in Wimpole-street, before Thomas Stirling. Esq. and a jury of neighbours.

The following circumstances were proved in evidence:—on Monday morning early the deceased was summoned to attend the Lady of Rev. Dr. Thackeray, of No. 86, Wimpole-street, Cavendish-square. He was in attendance until Tuesday morning at eleven o'clock, when finding his continued presence not necessary he went out for a time on his other engagements. An apartment in the floor above that occupied Mrs. Thackeray, was appointed for the residence of Sir Richard. In this chamber there were two pistols belonging to Dr. Thackeray, hanging within reach of Dr. Croft. Sir Richard retired to bed about half-past twelve o'clock on Thursday morning; About one o'clock Dr. Thackeray heard a noise, apparently proceeding from the room occupied by Dr. Croft, and sent a female servant to ascertain the cause; she returned saying she found the doctor in bed, and conceived him to be asleep. A short time after a similar noise was heard and the servant was again sent. She rapped at the door, but received no answer. This circumstance created alarm, in consequence of which the door of his apartment was broken open. Here a shocking spectacle presented itself:—the body of Sir Richard Croft was lying on the bed, shockingly mangled; his arms extended over his breast and a pistol in each hand. One of the pistols had been loaded with slugs, the other with ball. Both were discharged and the head of the unfortunate the gentleman was literally blown to pieces.

Drs. Latham and Baillie, and *Mr. Finch*, proved that the deceased had, since the death of the Princess Charlotte, laboured under mental distress. He had repeatedly been heard to say, that "this lamentable circumstance weighed heavy upon his mind, and he should never get over it."

Mr. Finch said he was well aware that the deceased was labouring under a derangement of intellect for a considerable time passed, and he should not have reposed trust in him on any occasion, since the lamented catastrophe alluded to.

The Jury, which was summoned at eight o'clock, having heard the whole of the evidence adduced, retired about ten, after the Coroner (Mr. Stirling) had summed up the evidence with suitable comments. About eleven o'clock the jury returned the following verdict:—"The deceased destroyed himself while in a fit of temporary derangement."

Mrs. Thackeray, we are happy to state, was safely delivered about eight o'clock on Friday morning by Mr. Herbert, an occasional Assistant of Sir Richard Croft. The Lady was kept ignorant of the fatal event, and is in a fair way of doing well.

About ten o'clock a hearse arrived, to convey the body to the house of the deceased in old Burlington-street. He was in his 57th year. Lady Croft, who survives him, has been for some time in a very delicate state of health. Her ladyship is a daughter of the late Dr. Denman, and sister of Mr. Denman, the Barrister who so greatly distinguished himself on the late State Trials at Derby. He has also left three sons and a daughter. One of the sons is in the army, in which he served with great *eclat* in the late war on the Continent.

"On Men-Midwives" (1819)

Introduction

This editorial explores the debates about the different kinds of practitioners caring for women during childbirth, including the traditional women as midwives, the accoucheurs or men-midwives, and other physicians or surgeons who did not specialize in obstetrics. The argument suggests that the high rates of maternal mortality are due, in part, to the impatience of man-midwives, who rush women through childbirth and use instruments like forceps.

"On Men-Midwives and Particularly on Those Who Practise Medicine as Well as Midwifery" (*The Literary Journal*, March 1819)

To the Editor of the Literary Journal.

Sir.—In my former communication upon Parish Registers, inserted in your last number, I promised to make some observations upon the employment of male practitioners in midwifery, I therefore hasten to perform my promise.

Upon the death of the Princess Charlotte of Wales, I happened to refer to the bills of mortality, with an intention of collecting evidence respects the diminution of mortality in childbed since the employment of men-midwives, from their superior skill. The result of my inquiries turned out contrary to my expectation. From a collection of the yearly bills of mortality, from 1657 to 1758, London. quarto, 1759, with appendixes; and the last appendix, called A Comparative View of the Diseases and Ages, &c. by J. P, Esq. F. R.S. I have extracted the following summary of thirty years, of a time, during which, the profession was almost entirely in female hands, the male practisioners being called in only in desperate cases.

From 1723 to 1732 in 152.913 burials, 1196 Are stated to have died in child bed, i.e. in the month.

[From] 1733 [to] 1737 in 154,237 [burials,] 1241[Are stated to have died in child bed, i.e. in the month.]

[From] 1738 [to] 1742 in 141,720 [burials,] 1207 [Are stated to have died in child bed, i.e. in the month.]

[From] 1743 [to] 1747 in 129,753 [burials,] 952 [Are stated to have died in child bed, i.e. in the month.]

[From] 1748 [to] 1752 in 114,625 [burials,] 940 [Are stated to have died in child bed, i.e. in the month.]

[From] 1753 [to] 1758 in 106,071 [burials,] 945 [Are stated to have died in child bed, i.e. in the month.]

Total of 30 years [in] 750,322 [burials,] 6481 [Are stated to have died in child bed, i.e. in the month.]

Average of 1 year [in] 25,010 [burials,] 206 [Are stated to have died in child bed, i.e. in the month.]

General average [in] 1000 [burials,] 8, or rather more.

Taking, then, a series of eight years, of the bills of mortality, as quoted in the Monthly Magazine, tor a period in which, on the contrary, the male practitioners had nearly the whole of the practice, I found that

In 1807 in 18,334 burials, 164 Are stated to have died in child bed, i.e. in the month.
In 1808 [in] 19,954 [burials,] 172 [Are stated to have died in child bed, i.e. in the month.]
In 1809 [in] 16,680 [burials,] 123 [Are stated to have died in child bed, i.e. in the month.]
In 1810 [in] 19,893 [burials,] 183 [Are stated to have died in child bed, i.e. in the month.]
In 1811 [in] 17,043 [burials,] 208 [Are stated to have died in child bed, i.e. in the month.]
In 1812 [in] 18,295 [burials,] 152 [Are stated to have died in child bed, i.e. in the month.]
In 1813 [in] 17,322 [burials,] 186 [Are stated to have died in child bed, i.e. in the month.]
In 1814 [in] 19,783 [burials,] 216 [Are stated to have died in child bed, i.e. in the month.]
Total of 8 years [in] 147,304 [burials,] 1404 [Are stated to have died in child bed, i.e. in the month.]
Average of 1 year [in] 18,413 [burials,] 175 [Are stated to have died in child bed, i.e. in the month.]
General average 1000 [burials,] 10, or rather less

Now, as no alteration in drawing up these bills took place during these periods, whatever errors they contain must affect both periods equally. Two things, then, are peculiarly striking in these extracts. The one, that notwithstanding the great increase of buildings which has taken place in every part of the bills, and which would seem to indicate a greater population in the latter, than in the former period; yet the annual average of the burials in the latter period is much smaller, being, indeed, one quarter less. As a native of London, I can recollect the small space in which my grandfather and his relations were cooped up, compared to that occupied by an equal number of my own family at present, although our relative station in society remains the same as his. We may therefore conclude, the population of London remains either stationary, or has decreased; and that the expansion of the buildings arises merely from the greater room we occupy than our ancestors; so that we need neither to be surprised at the malignant fevers or plagues that formerly ravaged London, nor a their disappearance in the present age.

But that which falls more immediately within the province of medical polity, is the increased mortality of child-bed, being in proportion of nearly one-forth. In endeavouring to discover the cause of this increased mortality, it would certainly be an injustice to science, to attribute it solely to the change from female to male practitioners in midwifry, although there is too great reason to suppose, that this increase of mortality has indirectly arisen from this circumstance, and been in a great measure occasioned by the practice of man-midwifry not having been made universally a separate branch of the profession, or at least conjoined only with pure surgery. Unfortunately, some of the apothecaries, and those surgeons who also practised medicine, took it up, and thus, almost necessitated the others, either to adopt the same course, or to take in a partner, who, generally, at the end of the term, or even before, got possession of the whole of their business, the employment by the mistress usually securing the attendance upon the whole family. Now, an apothecary must have several medical patients to visit every day, or he cannot live by his profession, and these require a regular attendance once, and, in some cases, twice a-day, which is incompatible with a sedulous attendance upon slow cases of midwifry. It is, therefore, but too probable, that an impatience of the confinement has led to a too frequent use of instruments, to hasten the delivery, and thus produced a greater mortality by child-bed, than when females only were employed, who, having no other calls to attend to, waited patiently for the natural termination—an opinion that receives confirmation from an apothecary having, lately, in one of the Medical Journals, deprecated the employment of females in midwifry, as not capable of using instruments, thus making the use of them the distinguishing point of male practice. Now, as surgeons, who do not practice medicine, are not tied to so strict an attendance upon their patients, so they can have little or no occasion to hurry the delivery; and therefore, it is probable, that if the practice of man-midwifry was a separate profession, or only conjoined with that of the surgeons, who do not practice medicine, this increased mortality would not take place. As Dr. Burrows is totally unmindful of the famous answer of the French merchants to the Prime Minister, Colbert, when he offered to issue regulations concerning their trade, even to their own desire, Laissez nous faire, and is well known to have a rage for legislating in respect to the profession, it were to be wished, that, if he cannot refrain from gratifying this penchant, among his other objects, he would endeavour to have the practice of medicine and man-midwifry made incompatible employments, like the professions of a butcher and a tanner; and in this, he would be less liable to incur obloquy than on a former occasion, as he would, on one hand, displease few or none, and on the other, please the very numerous class of apothecaries, who only practice midwifry to retain their medical practice, while, in their heart, they loath and abhor the other, still more those who linger in obscurity, because they cannot conquer their aversion to it; and above all, if such a consideration can have any weight with him, when mounted on his hobby-horse, would injure none, and probably save the lives of many mothers, to the great advantage of their young families, which lives are now sacrificed, and the children bereaved of their tenderest parents, by the impatience of the general practitioner, to visit the other persons under his care.

The population of the bills of mortality is usually taken as one eighth of that of the whole kingdom; therefore, the yearly burials will be 147,304, and the annual mortality in childbed, according to the present rate, now men-midwives are employed, will be 1404, but, according to the old proportion of eight in 1000 burials, as when women midwives only were employed, it would be only 1176, or rather more; hence the yearly increased mortality in childbed, is 228; and this increase, in fifty-six years, that is to say, from the year 1762, when our late Queen was delivered of the Prince Regent, and introduced the fashion of employing men midwives, although no absolute necessity existed for their interference, to the present, amounts to 12,768 females, who have been sacrificed to this fashion, or, at least, to the union of medical practice with that of midwifry.

Epicurus.

"Childbed: A Prose Poem" by Leigh Hunt (1837)

Introduction

This brief literary piece comes from the *Monthly Repository*, a middle-class miscellany formerly associated with the Unitarian Church. In it, essayist and poet Leigh Hunt romanticizes the general scene of childbirth, detailing the roles of the nurse, physician, mother and baby, and husband. He then turns to describe a specific birth and his care for his wife, Marianne (Kent) Hunt, who bore ten children between 1810 and 1829.

"Childbed: A Prose Poem" (*Monthly Repository*, November 1837)

And is childbed among the graces, with its close room, and its unwilling or idle visitors, and its jesting nurse (the old and indecent stranger), and its unmotherly, and unwifely, and unlovely lamentations? Is pain so unpleasant that love cannot reconcile it? and can pleasures be repeated without shame, which are regretted with hostile cries and resentment!

No. But childbed is among the graces, with the handsome quiet of its preparation, and the smooth pillow sustaining emotion, and the soft steps of love and respect, and the room in which the breath of the universe is gratefully permitted to enter, and mild and venerable aid, and the physician (the urbane security), and the living treasure containing treasure about to live, who looks in the eyes of him that caused it and seeks energy in the grappling of his hand, and hides her face in the pillow that she may save him a pain by stifling a greater. There is a tear for what may have been done wrong, ever; and for what may never be to be mutually pardoned again; but it is gone, for what needs it? Angelical are their whispers apart; and Pleasure meets Pain the seraph, and knows itself to be noble in the smiling testimony of his severity.

It was on a May evening, in a cottage flowering with the green-gage, in the time of hyacinths and new hopes, when the hand that wrote this, took the hand that had nine times lain thin and delicate on the bed of a mother's endurance and he kissed it, like a bride's.

L. H., 1827.

The Ladies' Medical Friend by William Hamilton Kittoe (1845)

Introduction

Dr. William Hamilton Kittoe's *The Ladies' Medical Friend* includes information on treating diseases specific to women, information on infant care for mothers, and an appendix of prescriptions. The opening of the book lists his qualifications with MD after his name, his role as surgeon and accoucheur, and the location of his home in London as well as the hours he is available to consult patients. In the preface, Kittoe suggests that women readers will find the guide particularly useful in an emergency, noting that "in all serious cases, the information given is only to be adopted till professional aid can be procured, and that in others, a medical man may be consulted effectually, with a due regard to that delicacy so indispensable with the female character." In the sections on pregnancy and childbirth, Kittoe provides specific guidance on health and conduct for women, reassures them of the relative safety of childbirth, suggests the attendance of an accoucheur, and details the possible complications.

Excerpt from Pregnancy

Some females experience immediately after conception a very peculiar sensation which is not easily described, but the first circumstance which renders the state probable, is the suppression of the periodical evacuation; with this there is generally fullness of the breast, head-ache, flushings of the face, heat in the palms of the hands, and giddiness; yet as each of these symptoms are the usual consequence of suppression, they can only be regarded as a criterion of pregnancy when they absolutely depend on that state. Suppression may take place from causes which have already been enumerated under that head, therefor it is not an infallible sign. In the commencement of pregnancy there is generally a very irritable state of the stomach, the woman experiences nausea, and in some cases she actually vomits; this in most instances takes place in the morning on first rising, when she experiences qualms or fits of langour more or less during the remainder of the day; there is heartburn, disturbed sleep, the countenance undergoes a marked change, the features acquire a peculiar sharpness, the eyes are encircled with a dusky or livid halo, the mouth appears elongated; in a word, there is a peculiar appearance not easy to be described, but with which women who have been pregnant are intimately acquainted: the temper is irritable, and the mind desponding: the pulse increases in frequency during pregnancy, and articular sympathies take place, producing salivation, tooth-ache, and jaundice, these "breeding symptoms," as they are quaintly termed, originate from irritation set up in the womb by impregnation. But as it is by no means impossible that other circumstances capable of exciting that organ may induce them, they are not always to be relied on; in fact in every instance where the female is not young, or has not a continued suppression for at least three periods, the excitement on parts contiguous to the womb are equally ambiguous; therefore these symptoms during the first four months are always to be considered as doubtful, unless every on enumerated be distinctly and unequivocally present; in fact the woman can never be assured of her true situation till the period of quickening ...

After the fourth month the symptoms become less ambiguous; in general the child is so much enlarged that its motions begin to be distinguished by the mother, hence that symptom is furnished called quickening. Females describe this sensation to resemble a slight tremulous motion, but it rarely if ever occurs at the same period in every instance; yet even here mistakes have occurred, wind has been so pent up in the bowels that the pulsation of the large blood-vessels have been mistaken for the motion of the child. As the term quickening may not be generally understood, I will give a short explanation of it. The ancient opinion, and on which the laws of some countries have been founded, was, that the foetus became animated at this period, but is now abandoned; the foetus is properly speaking, as much a living being immediately after conception as at any time before delivery; and its future progress is but the development and increase of those constituent principles which it then received. The next theory attached to the term is, that from the increase of size, its motions, which hitherto had been feeble and imperfect, are now of sufficient strength to communicate a sensible impulse to the adjacent parts of the mother; in this sense quickening implies the first sensation the mother has of her offspring. A far more natural and correct opinion is that which considers this symptom to be produced by the impregnated womb starting suddenly into the cavity of the belly, which explains several peculiarities attendant on this phenomenon; the variety in the period of its occurrence, the faintness which usually accompanies it, owing to the pressure being removed from the large vessels and the blood suddenly rushing into them: the distinctness of its character, as all mothers assert, so different from any subsequent motion of the child: its occasional absence in some females is also readily accounted for from the ascent of the womb being gradual and unobserved. The progressive increase in the size of the belly, together with the presence of milk in the breasts, which circumstance has invariably been considered of great importance by all medical men, are the best distinguishing characters of pregnancy that can be depended on (without resorting to examination, which is the province of the accoucheur alone). From this period the action of the child becomes more vigorous, though in some instances it is languid throughout the pregnancy, and in a few rare cases scarcely perceptible, notwithstanding which, the infant at birth has been large and lively.

…

Abortion, Or Miscarriage

The natural term of pregnancy is forty weeks, or nine calendar months; examples are, however, related of children being born after ten full months, but such instances are always doubtful, as it is very difficult to determine the exact period of conception. In France, the legislature has fixed the principle that child-birth may take place the 229th day of pregnancy. Miscarriage is a circumstance of frequent occurrence in the early months, particularly among females in the poorer classes of society, who are exposed to severe bodily fatigue and mental anxiety; it is also liable to occur in those of a full habit, or nervous temperament, or who may have been weakened by some previous malady. Besides these, there are other causes, as dancing, the use of warm baths, violent purgatives, emetics, diarrheas, piles, violent passions of the mind, excess in sexual intercourse, a generally relaxed state of the system, violent pressure of tight stays, sudden shocks, as falls, blows, fright, and lifting heavy weights; fainting will likewise often induce miscarriage, and when once this affection has been produced, the organs with great difficulty recover their tone; it is also extremely liable to occur from very slight causes. One writer gives an account of fourteen miscarriages taking place in succession in the same female, and another of eight in a single year. It is remarkable that women who are in the habit of miscarrying go on very promisingly up to a certain period, and then abort, not once or twice, but for a number of times in succession, notwithstanding every effort to prevent it. In such cases it is to be an incapability of the womb to expand is the chief cause.

Symptoms

Flying pains in the back and loins, with sudden appearance of a coloured discharge, great depression of strength and spirits, faintness, a sensation of shivering, palpitation of the heart, flabbiness of the breasts; the stomach and bowels are also frequently in a disturbed and disordered state. When the child is dead, it is often expelled in a very short time, with little pain and trifling loss of blood; in other cases the process is protracted, occupying many days, and, in some instances, even months. The infant may die before the expiration of the twelfth week, and yet not be expelled till the fourth or fifth month; and an infant of seven or eight months may lose its vitality, and yet be retained in the womb till the full period of regular pregnancy has expired. In twin cases, one may die, remain in the womb, and be born with the living child.

Treatment

In all cases of threatened miscarriage, the female should be kept perfectly tranquil in mind and body; be placed in a recumbent position; and, if the habit is plethoric, a gentle aperient administered. A full dose of some anodyne will also be necessary, and is to be combined with an astringent. By prompt and judicious management, it is sometimes possible to ward off an unfortunate termination; at all events, it may be materially retarded, and the symptoms alleviated. The diet should be light and nourishing, without being stimulating; and whenever exercise is taken (which at all times is better avoided), it must be by means of a carriage or swing. Cold bathing, more especially that of the sea, will be of great advantage; and when not to be procured, the hip or shower-bath, with salt dissolved in the water, will be a valuable substitute. If the discharge is only trifling, it may be in our power to restrain it by injections of cold water, to which may be added a few grains of fine-powdered alum or sulphate of zinc; for this purpose a female syringe of ivory or glass, as advised under the head of whites, is be employed. It is very frequently necessary to plug the orifice of the vagina with lint or sponge, steeped in vinegar, or in some instances to use ice for this purpose. When the habit is naturally robust and vigorous, a soft bed should be exchanged for a hard mattress; but in delicate constitutions this may be dispensed with; a little white wine and some vegetable tonic is to be administered daily. In every instance it will be absolutely necessary to refrain from connubial intercourse. It has, of late, been much the fashion, to confine women threatened with miscarriage (especially after they have suffered once or twice), to a horizontal position for weeks and months; it has frequently happened that such a system has been adopted from the earliest symptoms of conception, and continued throughout the entire period of pregnancy; in a few instances, or under some peculiar circumstances, such a system may be requisite and beneficial, but it has been far too indiscriminately employed. Wherever there is an indisposition in the womb to expand, it can never be of the slightest service; when such is the case, the tepid hip-bath resorted to about the period when the miscarriage may be anticipated, will be likely to prove far more beneficial; indeed, one of the most useful applications in cases of this description, is a broad flannel swathe, moistened with warm water, applied round the loins and lower part of the belly, every night on retiring to rest; this is to be surrounded, externally, by another dry bandage of folded calico, and both worn during the night. At all events, when the constitution is delicate and relaxed, the patient herself forming an objection to confinement, it is well worth consideration whether tonics, gentle exercise, as swinging, sailing, or driving out in an easy carriage at a moderate pace, a palanquin, sofa-bed, or Merlin chair, would not be much more efficacious means, and stand afar better chance of being crowned with success; at all events it would not be attended with the evil effects to the habit which a protracted confinement of months to a close bedroom would be likely to induce; such a method, instead of exhausting, would have the effect of invigorating and tranquillizing the circulation and nervous system, producing calm and refreshing sleep, and must be much more satisfactory than a life of perfect indolence, which would most assuredly tend to produce general debility, however much the position might be supposed to favour the womb. We have, however, so far supposed miscarriage has averted.

Should the pain therefore, instead of confining itself to a local action, become steady, extending round the back and belly, accompanied by violent forcing, bearing down, or expulsatory efforts, no time must be lost in obtaining medical assistance. If, however, on the contrary, the pain be only trifling, and the discharge small in quantity, letting things take their course, at the same time carefully watching the symptoms and administering a draught composed of thirty drops of tincture of opium, with twenty-five of sal-volatile in a wineglass of cold water, camphor, julep, or cinnamon water. Whenever the discharge is profuse, the patient feeling faint, sinking, and ready to expire, there is always some ground for apprehension, inasmuch as death has occasionally taken place; but generally speaking, the danger is of trifling import, the woman rallying very speedily; in event even of complete faint, the symptom ought to be regarded as favourable, for in such instances the flooding is almost invariably suspended. The agency of cold externally and internally is always of importance; the bed-curtains are to be withdrawn, the windows thrown open, nothing but a sheet covering the patient; the vinegar cloths round the loins and belly being renewed as often as they become warm. These remedies are to be discontinued the moment the flooding ceases; if it occurs in spring or summer, no fire is to be permitted in the room, and very little in the winter. It is worthy of remark, that females of a consumptive habit, and who have always a great aptitude to conceive, rarely or never miscarry; while those who marry late in life, are peculiarly liable to the occurrence. In regard to the effect of miscarriage on the constitution, it may be stated, as a general fact, that in a very large majority of instances, the injury sustained, comparatively speaking, is slight; it is a circumstance of every-day occurrence in all countries, and it is not usual for permanent or fatal injury to be sustained, except when it is frequently repeated, and in quick succession, or where improper treatment has been adopted.

Rules for the Management of Pregnancy

…

Young, healthy, well-formed women, who are pregnant for the first time, need never entertain any fears, as it rarely ever happens in the present day that a woman dies in labour, and never from the consequences, without imprudence on her own part or mismanagement on that of her attendants. Besides there is now no case of labour which can possibly occur but may be managed, and the life of the mother preserved. It is absolutely lamentable to listen to the groundless expression of the fears of young females in this state, and which are for the most part excited in their minds by ignorant nurses and midwives, also by silly mothers and acquaintances; this is indeed not much to be wondered at, as there is no work in our language for the instruction of the sex, on this, and other important and delicate subjects; al their information is derived from ignorant persons. That there are as able practitioners in England as in any other country in the world cannot be for a moment doubted, at the same time it must be acknowledged that the study of midwifery and other female complaints, never became an exclusive study before the year 1828 in England: prior to that period it was shamefully neglected; even now the injuries that are inflicted on females and children by ignorant practitioners are lamentably frightful, and it is an indelible: disgrace that such persons are still permitted to practice with impunity in so difficult, delicate, and dangerous a department of the healing art.

Effects of Tight Lacing in Pregnancy

The ancient Greeks and Athenians were so careful with respect to their progeny, that magistrates were appointed by special laws to inquire into the nature of vestments worn by women who were in a state of pregnancy. Such also was the case among the ancient Venetians. They were well aware that either abortion or malformed children, in mature age, would be the result of the opposite practice in youth. For this reason females in all lands wear their vestments larger and lighter than the other sex. Women, while pregnant, should wear nothing that can exert the slightest compressive power on any part of the body. If constriction of the chest dispose females to irritations of the lungs, and lead to consumption, such an effect will be much more certainly produced during pregnancy, when the organs of the abdomen being pressed against the lungs, diminish the expansion of the upper cavity, producing difficulty of breathing. The pressure of clothing over the chest induces either inflammation or wasting of the breast. It causes, also, imperfect secretion of milk, with all the train of evils which result to both parent and child. It may, likewise, give rise to the rupture of a blood-vessel in the lungs, or to apoplexy. Pressure of clothes upon the belly is not less injurious; it either forces the inferior organs to take an upright direction, and leads to the accidents before alluded to, or else it opposes the growth of the infant, and may thus cause miscarriage. Distortions of the infant, and club, or twisted feet, are frequently occasioned by tight lacing, which is had recourse to in order to conceal pregnancy. This brief notice will, we trust, prove a warning to our fair readers.

Rules and Cautions Necessary to Be Observed During Labour, and in the Lying-In Chamber

Fortunately for the fair daughters of the creation, the progress of travail, in the majority of instances, is safe, more especially when the woman lives according to the laws of nature; but among the higher and middle, (in fact, every class in civilized society in which her laws are infracted or forgotten, or where the system is impaired by the luxury and dissipation of modern times) the progress of child-bearing is attended with more or less danger at the time, and after its completion. These remarks are particularly applicable to the lower orders of society, whose custom, habits, pursuits, and lamentable intemperance render them liable to severe accidents during labour, and a vast number of diseases afterwards. My assertions will, I feel persuaded, be confirmed by the willing testimony of every experienced medical practitioner; fortunate it is, however, for suffering humanity that the progress of this state may, from the late discoveries and improvements in medicine and surgery, be greatly accelerated, and that most intense of all human sufferings relieved by the skilful exertions of the professional attendant, with perfect safety to the mother and offspring. It is a well established fact that even the presence of the accoucheur will frequently inspire confidence, afford relief, and expedite delivery, without the necessity of any manual operation whatever; the confidant assurance given to the patient of her safety leads to the feeling of hope, invariably tending to hasten the desired event far better than any other means; it is on this account that few intelligent females object to the attendance of a well-educated surgeon. Attempts, it is true, have, from time to time, been made to calumniate them, and deter husbands from permitting such persons to give aid at this painful and interesting period. Such contemptible endeavours have, however, proved futile, as every man of common understanding will, on a moment's reflection, be convinced that passion and pain can never for a moment coexist, and that the responsibility of the accoucheur, as well as his moral, social and domestic obligations, obliterate every impure sentiment: he is generally a husband and a father, and his professional reputation is at stake; it is therefore a most unfounded libel for a moment to suspect him of unworthy motives; in a word, it is utterly false, and the idea only of abandoned, profligate, wretched libertines, or debauchees, and not for a moment tolerated by respectable society, being as contrary to reason and common sense as it is to justice and honour. I never yet knew a solitary instance of a female in any rank of life, who had been attended by an educated (not an ignorant or pretended) medical man, who would ever after submit to (if she could avoid it) the care of a midwife. I believe one cause of the calamity before alluded to has arisen out of the objection started by some surgeons to the presence of the husband in the lying-in chamber, which certainly is a most injudicious prohibition. There can never be the slightest reason why the husband should be interdicted at this period; on the contrary, it may not only tend to calm the irritability of the patient, but will at once disabuse the former of any prejudice he might have before entertained on the subject.

...

Child Bed Fever

Has been instrumental in destroying more women than all other disorders incident to the child-bed state, or, perhaps, peculiar to the sex. There is not a doubt but in particular seasons contagion has prevailed, inducing this disease. In many instances it has proved fatal from mere exhaustion rather than any other cause.

Symptoms

This fever attacks generally on the second, sometimes the third day after delivery: it has been known to occur so late as a week after. The earlier it attacks, the greater the danger. Few women recover who have the belly much swollen. It is very insidious in its approaches, which, in many cases, are devoid of the shiverings generally indicative of a febrile malady. In most instances, however, a slight shiver is perceived, accompanied by nausea, retching, quick pulse, pain in the head, particularly over the eyebrows: the night is sleepless and wretched, with confusion of mind, and often delirium. Sometimes the temper is extremely irritable; at others, there is timidity, listlessness, or apathy: hysterical symptoms are not unfrequently present from the beginning, or very shortly afterwards. A pain is perceived in the belly, at first slight, but soon increasing: it is sometimes so tender, that even the weight of the bed-clothes produces distress. A general fullness of this part precedes or accompanies it from the first, often making the female as large as before delivery. The face is flushed, or the cheeks suffused, at the beginning, but afterwards pale and ghastly; the eyes without animation, and the lips blanched.

In the progress of the malady, the vomiting is often so severe, that nothing will remain on the stomach; and towards the conclusion of the attack, the fluid thrown up is dark and fœtid, always denoting a fatal termination. There is so much listlessness, that the patient lies chiefly on her back, making little or no complaint. The skin is not very hot, but clammy and relaxed; the tongue white, but afterwards brown; the mouth and throat covered with small ulcerous spots; the bowels confined at first, but after the third day the motions are frequent, dark, and offensive, seeming to afford relief; the urine is dark, high-coloured, with a brown sediment; the child-bed discharge and secretion of milk suspended; the thirst is not urgent. When hiccough supervenes, the patient usually dies by the expiration of the fifth day. In some cases, existence is protracted till the fourteenth, and a few fall victims in forty-eight hours, death not unfrequently being preceded by stupor and low delirium; but often the mind continues unimpaired till within a few minutes of dissolution, and the woman is carried off in a convulsive fit.

Such are the prominent features of this melancholy and fearful disorder. In regard to the Treatment, it will be only in my power.

Treatment,

It will be only in my power to offer a few general observations, as it is far too dangerous a complaint to be treated by any but an experienced professional man. No time, therefore, should be lost in calling in such the moment the nature of the malady is even suspected. I shall, however, give in the Appendix a few prescriptions which may be depended on, and used with safety, till more efficient aid can be procured. There is no remedy which appears to exercise so salutary an influence over this fever as the various preparations of opium; they may be administered both by the mouth and in clysters. Cloths wet with warm spirit of turpentine, applied over the belly, are often productive of a soothing and beneficial effect. In the advanced stage of the disease, wine, camphor, and quinine will be necessary, of course only under the direction of the physician, unless in situations where one is not to be procured. Bleeding is not advisable under any circumstance, and whenever it has been used, the results have invariably proved its mischievous effects.

"Etherization in Childbirth" (1848)

Introduction

This report on the uses of ether as an anesthetic for childbirth brings to the common reader in America current medical news, with both applications of the new treatment and statistics for its uses in Channing's study. The author quotes heavily from Channing, framing the quotations with questions and observations in plain language. This text shares this form of pain relief in childbirth less than two years after it was first reported by James Simpson for that purpose in Britain and a year after it was first publicly used for childbirth in America.

"Etherization in Childbirth" (*Saturday Evening Post*, 23 December 1848)

A work with the above title has recently been published by Walter Channing, M. D., Professor of Midwifery and Medical Jurisprudence in the University of Cambridge. The New York Tribune gives an interesting summary of its contents. If the learned Doctor is correct in his facts and assertions, one of the greatest blessings to women that it is possible to conceive, has dawned upon the world. That he is correct, we are disposed to believe, from the fact that we knew of two instances in this city, where ether was administered, with the happiest results. But to the Tribune's summary:

The book on Etherization in Child-birth, lately published by Dr. Walter Channing, deserves to be widely read by the Medical Profession, and by parents. It is illustrated by more than *five hundred cases*, enabling every reader to judge of the SAFETY and EXPEDIENCY of employing this wonderful pain-removing agent. We shall merely condense some of the facts and conclusions stated by the author, whose long and varied experience in this special branch of professional duty entitles him to the most respectful consideration.

1. SAFETY.—This is the great point to be established; let us hear what Dr. Channing has to offer in relation to it:

> In 516 cases of Natural Labor, embracing all varieties of circumstances incident to this process, accomplished during etherization, we have *not a case in which the mother did not do well!* (pp. 302, 322)

"In 51 cases of Instrumental, Preternatural and Complicated Labor, in which etherization was used, there were only 4 deaths; and these after convulsions so grave by cause and symptoms as to afford little reason to look for recovery. The balance in favor of etherization,"

in such extreme cases, may be understood from the following comparisons:

> IN REGARD TO STILL-BIRTHS.—In 18 cases, where etherization was *not* employed, there were 17 still-births,--or 37.26...per cent. In 51 cases where etherization *was* employed, there were 19 still-births,--or 37.26...per cent. Balance *in favor* of etherization 57.19...per cent.

IN REGARD TO MORTALITY.—Of 18 labors *without* etherization, 15 were fatal, or 83.33...per cent. Of 51 labors *with* etherization, 4 were fatal, or 7.85...per cent. Balance *in favor* of etherization, 75.48...per cent. (p. 315)

But may not etherization injure children born under its influence? Hear Dr. Channing:

I have not met with a *single* instance of either mental or physical peculiarity in children, thus born, they are fully equal in health, growth and mind, to those who have been born in the midst of pressure of severest pain. I repeat, there is not the smallest evidence of any injurious agency on children born during etherization; and so far from there being any cause of apprehension, it is notorious that children born during etherization are much more rarely still-born; and that they continue to do perfectly well. (pp. 157, 158)

In further corroboration of the entire safety of etherization let us quote the following remarks:

The success of etherization in midwifery has, I believe, been perfect. I do not remember a case in which it has been induced either by ether or chloroform, in which there has been the least reason to question its entirely useful agency, both in regard to mother and child. (p. 83)

May not puerperal convulsions be produced by etherization?

My attention has been particularly directed to this subject. I have not, however, met with a single instance at home or abroad. So far from this, I have seen cases of the most grave puerperal convulsions, in which ether has been used as a remedy and with excellent effects. (p. 101)

So far from uterine contractions being diminished or suspended by ether, it is notorious that they are very often increased in force or efficacy. * * In short, a state most favorable to easy, rapid and safe delivery is produced and sustained. (p. 108)

How is it with convalescence after child-birth, following etherization?

I have made this matter a subject of special regard and question. The answer has been, 'I have none of that weakness, weariness and pain which have been usual, and after-pains have been in comparison as nothing. It seems to me ridiculous to be lying here; I am conscious of a degree of health and strength which fits me for my whole duties in my family.' (p. 130)

A few words now as to

2. EXPEDIENCY. "Pain does not *necessarily* belong to labor, since painless, or nearly painless, cases of Labor are too common to allow of such a statement for a moment. Pain is the consequence of *resistance*. * * Now it is to relieve the *unnecessary* suffering which results from the conditions referred to, that etherization is employed; And it gives relief by increasing dilatability, diminishing or suspending sensibility, preventing exhaustion, enlarging secretions, taking away the disturbing action of the will."—p. 20.

> I can and do say that I have not met with an untoward result in any case of midwifery in which etherization has been induced by which any violence or ingenuity of explication can be ascribed to etherization as its cause. I have met with no record of such. (p. 25)

> I have never observed any loss of strength following its use. On the contrary, the absence of pain during labor, has been attended and followed by a remarkable preservation of strength. (p. 36)

> Etherization does just what sleep does. It is sleep, profound sleep; and though effort is made, and because an impediment to easy performance of functions exists, still there is no pain. * * * Etherization suspends sensibility. Labor goes on, but is not perceived. It is without pain. (p. 39)

> "Instead of determining," says Prof. Simpson, of Edinburgh, who has observed and gathered the results of etherization not only in hundreds, but thousands of cases, "whether we shall be *justified* in using this agent, under the circumstances named, it will become necessary to determine whether, on any ground, moral or medical, a professional man could deem himself *justified* in withholding any such safe means of assuaging the last stage of natural labor."—p. 48.

> A highly accomplished surgeon has suggested that the occasional dangers and fatal results of etherization in slight operations, as tooth-drawing, for instance, may be the result of the suddenness with which the operation is done * * whereas, in midwifery practice more time is taken, less suddenness in the lesion, greater loss of blood. (p. 100)

Doubtless, in some cases, where bad or fatal effects have been attributed to *etherization*, persons have actually been *poisoned* or *suffocated*. The article should be *pure*; and sufficient atmospheric air should be admitted to the lungs. Dr. Channing gives full directions and cautions as to the preparation and use of ether and chloroform.

We close our extracts from this profoundly interesting and instructive book with the following words of its benevolent author:

> This book treats of a noble subject: the *remedy of pain*. After ages of suffering, and of frequently intermitted pursuit of such a remedy, one has been found. It remains with the medical profession to say whether it shall take its place among the permanent and most important agents; Or whether it shall pass away till a truer age so revive it and give it a wider sphere of usefulness and a sure perpetuity.

Periodical Coverage of Queen Victoria and Anesthesia (1848–1859)

Introduction

Throughout Queen Victoria's reign, periodicals reported on every detail of her political and personal life, including her births of nine children between 1840 and 1857. Between the births of fifth child in 1846 and sixth in 1848, anesthesia in the form of ether and chloroform became available to ease the pain of childbirth. As the periodicals report, the Queen consulted with James Simpson and may have contemplated using anesthesia in her 1848 birth but did not use it then or in her 1850 birth. However, in her eighth birth in 1853, Queen Victoria was given chloroform. This section includes coverage of the rumors about her use of anesthesia from periodicals in Britain (*The Satirist, The Standard, Blackburn Standard, The Englishwoman's Review*) and America (*The Nineteenth Century, Trumpet*).

"Paradise Regained!" (*The Satirist; or Censor of the Times,* 23 January 1848)

"They rest from their labours, and their works do follow them."

The sage obstetric trio[23] mean,
According to court whisper,
Next time our kind, prolific QUEEN
Brings forth a little *lisper*,
To "chloroform" Her HAJESTY,
From pains and pangs to keep her free!

To lapse into a state *so* still,
Like some *ethereal* dreamer,—
Nor know you are mother—'till
You hear the little screamer;
This is a marvellous transition,
Making your "labours" quite elysian!

We wish our SOVEREIGN LADY joy,
And all the sex inclusive,
To think that science can employ
An agent so conducive
(We utter it with perfect reverence)
To their relief and "good deliverance!"

One grateful song they all should chaunt;
But who should lead the chorus?
No one's so proper-all must grant—
As SHE who now reigns o'er us!
Oh! what a moving sight to see 'em—
Millions of Matrons sing *Te Deum*:
While maidens following, scatter posies—
"Now, marriage-beds are beds of roses!"

Excerpt from "Ether and Chloroform" (*The Nineteenth Century: A Quarterly Miscellany*, January 1848)

Death is sleep. The progress to it in the act of dying ought, in the true natural order, to be without pain, a going to sleep. In a pure, true life, without the corruptions of medicine, it would be a going to sleep. Birth is a purely natural function, the creation of man continued; and no more pain would be in it, in the true natural order, than belongs to it to make it birth, and give

---

[23] Original Text: Messrs. Locock, Ferguson, and Clarke. Only think of this, Master Brooke—it is a fact that several Scotch practitioners have peremptorily refused to relieve patients from the agonies of childbirth, on the ground that it is "uncanonical and irreligious" thus to abrogate or mitigate the primal curse on woman! "The force of folly—can it further go?" —Ed.

signification to a mother's love, and sacred devotion to a mother's office. In a pure, true life, without the corruptions of medicine, in a healthy frame, birth is tolerable, birth is easy. Deliverance it always must be, for that is its essence, and the crown of its rejoicing.

Shame upon the philosophy of medicine, which would thus filch from maternity its sacred meaning, and drug into unconsciousness the deepest capacity for experience in earthly life. How can we abide the philosophy of a practice, which presumes that a child can be a right child, thus chemically deposited from Lethe, not born of a mother? Shall we renew, in the daily habits of the nineteenth century of the Christian era, the fabulous witchery of Circe, and call it medical science? Let the philosophy of medicine apply itself to the regeneration of these organized bodies by purity, by simplicity of diet, by healthy conditions of active life, and then it need not meddle with birth and death. Let it lead us back to vital power in the frame and constitution, and then let birth and death be left to us, facts too near the unseen world to be tampered with. Let medical science affirm the grave fact, let it warn us personally of the dreadful truth, that there are frames and conditions of men and women in civilization, to whom the offices of father and mother are not suited. Let it terrify such of us from paternity and maternity, by the thought of pain to ourselves, and a life of pain and abridgment of the due functions of life to offspring. Let it authoritatively pronounce, in the name of the whole race, and with that sanction, that to be father and mother in such case is criminal, if the relation be knowingly taken; and let the knowledge of these matters be so much a habit of learning, and life, and conversation with us, that ignorance herein shall be impossible. What a noble gossip that would be! Let not medical science help on these unsuitable generations by promises of insensibility to pain. Let not drug science in ether and chloroform entice thus to degeneration of the species, by offering a bounty on acts of wrong.

To what a point of perversion habits of life may come, with the sanction of medical science, we see now in a conspicuous example. A steamer, last winter, brought this paragraph for our newspapers across the deep:

> Queen Victoria, according to the late London papers, has summoned Dr. Simpson, of Edinburgh, the first who employed chloroform in obstetrics, to London. If she gives it the benefit of her example, it will probably be introduced into general practice.

The steamer which brought us the news of the French revolution, brought us also the account of the delivery of the Queen of England.

Ever since her marriage, Queen Victoria bas been accustomed to bear her yearly tribute of offspring, for the breasts of the wet nurses, and the appropriations of the civil list. At the head of the most civilized nation on the globe; with a popular influence passing down from the throne into all the homes of her subjects, like the sun in his sphere, her accouchements announced to the four winds, she has hitherto performed no function of a mother, except the absolutely inevitable bearing of her children, not only unrebuked by, but with the authority of the highest medical science in the kingdom. All physical connection of mother and child has ceased with birth. Without the rebuke, and with the sanction of the best medical science of her kingdom, she is set conspicuously to be, not a woman, in the sacred completeness of that function, but a matrix. And the nobility is to follow the exemplary queen, and all the mothers of Great Britain are to receive the boon of chloroform at the couch of birth, Lethe for Latona, down to the cellars of the manufacturing cities, where the animal functions of labor and reproduction of species (*de*-generation, for it cannot be called generation) is all that the highest civilization of cultured Christendom has left to humanity.

The Edinburgh Doctors of Divinity fought against Dr. Simpson's use of chloroform in obstetrics, with the Bible, and the Doctor of Medicine fought against them with the Bible. They quoted against him the denunciation of sorrow in childbirth for the woman in the third chapter of Genesis; and he quoted against them "the deep sleep which the Lord God caused to fall upon Adam," preparatory to the surgical operation of removing the rib, recorded in the second chapter of Genesis. They give a poor reason against him, and he as poor against them. They both show how readily men may prove from the letter of texts of scripture whatever they mean to believe and practice. While both parties are settling between them their foolish theological argument *in re obstetrica*, a simple man may take the liberty of asking them both to consider how it is, that while the Scriptures of the second and third chapters of Genesis remain just as they are, a strong, well-formed, healthy woman, who lives a life of temperate activity, brings forth children without sorrow, and is not under the curse? And while they are considering this, a simple man may affirm the Scripture of the whole creation; namely this: that it lies in the free will of the human race, in a few generations of purity and temperance, in healthy conditions of life, to deliver all mothers from the present sorrow of birth, supposed to come of the perpetual theological curse in the third chapter of Genesis. Chloroform will not avoid, but confirm the sorrow, in some other and worse result, and form, to mother and offspring, as all kindred treatment of disorder has confirmed pain upon us. Alas for us, with theology for religion in the regeneration of the life of the soul, and physic and surgery for regeneration in the life of the body. What shall we do to escape Scylla and Charybdis, waiting for us on either side of this strait of life which we must all pass through? How long shall not the curse stand for us, thus, in the written scripture of a carnal religion, and the confirmatory and illustrative habit of a carnal life?

"Secrets from the Palace by a Royal Page" (*The Satirist; or Censor of the Times*, 13 February 1848)

There was a report, a little while ago, that the use of chloroform would be had recourse to at Her Majesty's approaching accouchement, and that a Scotch professor had been engaged to come all the way from Edinburgh to administer it. This report was soon after contradicted; as everything is in connection with Court movements, if a secret, or what is intended to be kept a secret, happens to ooze out before its time. I can only assure you, and the dowager lady governess is no mean authority, that had it not been for the very recent fatal result, in the case of a female to whom chloroform was administered, and which was read *to* the Queen (for Her Majesty never reads a paper herself, or looks at one, if I except the picture papers) by Miss Skirrett, the aid of chloroform would most assuredly have been resorted to. That, however, is now entirely out of the question. In fact, neither Dr. Locock nor Sir James Clark will venture to run the risk of administering it, however much the relatives of the Queen might be anxious for the experiment to be tried. I think they are quite right.

"The Latest Absurdity" (*Trumpet and Universalist Magazine*, 4 March 1848)

Of all the difficulties and annoyances that men of genius have to encounter and overcome, that engendered by religious bigotry and superstition is the most vexatious.— This reflection has been suggested by the most intolerant officiousness of certain ministers in Edinburgh, who have taken it into their heads to object to the use of chloroform by medical men in obstetric cases. Our readers may laugh, but the fact is certain, that the mitigation of pain during the time of childbirth is objected to by these men, on the ground that God, in consequence of the fall, ordained man to be brought forth in sorrow, &c, Dr. Simpson, the successful discoverer of the inestimable qualities of chloroform in deadening the nervous system, and rendering the body incapable of feeling during surgical operations, has been at pains to combat this clerical anathema; and well has he done it. He has quoted from the original text the accounts of the first surgical operation recorded in holy writ—we say it with all reverence—that performed by God himself. 'The Lord caused a deep sleep,' &c. As no one will call in question the object to be gained by the deep sleep, we are satisfied we shall have no more appeals to Scripture or clerical anathemas against the use of chloroform, in surgical cases at any rate.— *Abroath Guide.*

"Multiple News Items" (*The Standard*, 22 April 1853)

The *Gazette des Hôpitaux* states a circumstance which we consider in the highest degree improbable, namely that in the recent accouchement of the Queen of England, chloroform was administered to her Majesty by Dr. Snow, with the approbation of Sir James Clark, Dr. Locock, and Dr. Ferguson. The effect, it is added, was very advantageous, and the Queen expressed her satisfaction at it.

"Court and High Life" (*Blackburn Standard*, 27 April 1853)

The Queen is convalescent and the infant Prince continues well. On Saturday, it is said the Court will leave Buckingham Palace for Osborne.

HER MAJESTY CHLOROFORMED. — On the occurrence of the recent interesting event, Dr. Snow, with the sanction of Sir James Clark and Dr. Locock, administered chloroform to the royal patient during the latter part of the labour. — *Magnet.*

"Chloroform at the Royal Accouchement" (*The Englishwoman's Review*, 8 January 1859)

From a memoir of the late Dr. Snow, in the "Medical Times," we learn that on April the 7th, 1853, he administered chloroform to Her Majesty at the birth of the Prince Leopold. A note in his diary records the event.

The inhalation lasted fifty-three minutes. The chloroform was given on a handkerchief, in fifteen minim doses, and the Queen expressed herself as greatly relieved by the administration. He had previously been consulted on the occasion of the birth of Prince Arthur, in 1850, but had not been called to render his services. Previous to the birth of Prince Leopold, he had been honoured with an interview with His Royal Highness the Prince Albert, and returned much over-joyed with the Prince's kindness and great intelligence on the scientific points which had formed the subject of the conversation. On the 14th of April, 1857, another note in the diary records the fact of the second administration of chloroform to Her Majesty at the birth of the Princess Beatrice. The chloroform again exerted its beneficent influence; and Her Majesty once more expressed herself as much satisfied with the result. Inquisitive folk often overburdened Snow, after these events, with a multitude of questions of an unmeaning kind. He answered them all with goodnatured reserve. "Her Majesty is a model patient," was his, usual reply—a reply which, he once said, seemed to answer every purpose, and was very true. One lady of an inquiring mind, to whom he was administering chloroform, got very loquacious during the period of excitement, and declared she would inhale no more of the vapour until she were told what the Queen said, word for word, when she was taking it. "Her Majesty," replied the dry doctor, "asked no questions until she had breathed very much longer than you have; and if you will only go on in loyal imitation, I will tell you everything." The patient could not but follow the example held out to her. In a few seconds she forgot all about the Queen, Lords, and Commons; and when the time came for a renewal of hostilities, found, that her clever witness had gone home to his dinner, leaving her with the thirst for knowledge still on her tongue.

A Popular Manual of Female Diseases by Robert Hall Bakewell (1859)

Introduction

The title page of this volume lists Dr. Robert Hall Bakewell's medical qualifications through the Royal College of Surgeons in midwifery and his past positions as a surgeon at several hospitals in London and during the Crimean War. In the preface, Bakewell explains his purpose of "supplying a want in medical literature" and preventing "quacks and quackeries of every description" by educating "the public respecting the principles and practice of legitimate medicine." He insists that the conditions listed are mostly preventable with care and knowledge, and that women should understand "the physiology of their own bodies and of the diseases to which they are peculiarly liable." In the section on pregnancy and childbirth excerpted here, Bakewell quotes directly from the standard nineteenth-century manual for midwives by Dr. Fleetwood Churchill, bringing specialized medical knowledge to his women readers. He is also unique in mentioning mental health in a brief section on "puerperal mania."

Excerpts from Chapter IX: Pregnancy and Its Diseases

The period of pregnancy, and the first few weeks after delivery, are naturally times of much anxiety, even to those who have frequently endured the pains and cares of maternity before. By those who experience them for the first time, an undefined sense of fear and dread is felt, which adds doubly to the weight of their anxieties. It is not to be wondered at that, under such circumstances, the mother, and especially the young mother, should trust confidingly to those whose age and experience give them a title to be heard. Hence we find that nowhere do the traditions of the past retain so firm a hold on the mind as in the lying-in room. Maxims that have been handed down from generation to generation, though too often originating in the grossest ignorance of physiology and pathology, are received with the profoundest respect and implicitly obeyed.

To state, as clearly and simply as possible, what are the duties of the mother and the nurse during the period of pregnancy and parturition, is the object of this Chapter.

During pregnancy a female is liable to many disorders, most of which, though troublesome and annoying, are not dangerous. These may be very much lessened by careful attention to the general health, without any treatment directed to the particular complaint. If a pregnant woman takes plenty of active exercise in the open air, has her bed and sitting rooms well ventilated, is regular and simple in her diet, and attends carefully to the state of the bowels, most of the common diseases of pregnancy will be either altogether prevented, or very much mitigated.

...

It is not my purpose to describe the rarer diseases of pregnancy, nor such as, from their importance, necessitate medical treatment. The frequency and danger of miscarriage require that some allusion should be made to it.

A female may miscarry at any period of pregnancy, that is to say, the child may be expelled from the womb at any time previous to the completion of the forty weeks which constitute the full term. The symptoms vary greatly at different periods, but it would occupy too much space, and be attended with no useful result, were I to give an account of them all. My purpose is only to impress upon those mothers who do me the honour to read this little work, the importance of obtaining proper medical advice in every case of miscarriage. Now there are two classes of miscarriages; those which arise from some accidental cause, such as a fall, a blow, severe fright, a strain, or the occurrence of some acute disease like small pox, and those which are habitual. The former are attended with much more suffering, as a rule, than the latter. Some women, who have frequently miscarried, have remarkably little pain, while others may have pain almost as severe as labour for a week or more. The essential symptoms of miscarriage are pains resembling more or less labour-pains, according to the period of pregnancy, and flooding. A slight degree of both may occur without miscarriage coming on, and the person may go her full time, but whenever the flooding is considerable, and the pain severe, the miscarriage is sure to occur. At the commencement, these symptoms may frequently be stopped, unless the child is dead, in which case, of course, the sooner it is expelled the better; but in every case when the two symptoms before mentioned occur, proper medical advice ought at once to be obtained. It is useless to wait in the hope that matters may improve, for the probability, almost the certainty, is, that without prompt and efficient medical treatment, they will go on from bad to worse. When miscarriage has frequently happened, it becomes an exceedingly difficult matter to prevent it. A case is related where a woman, in spite of everything that could be done, miscarried twenty-three times at the third month.

It is an undoubted fact, that although the severe flooding which often attends miscarriage is generally recovered from, yet that the patient is quite as liable to puerperal fever as after an ordinary confinement. The same regimen ought therefore to be pursued in the one case as the other, and a female who has just miscarried ought to take even more care of herself than one who has been delivered at the full time.

Dr. Churchill, one of the greatest authorities on the subject, in his work on Midwifery, says:

> The popular belief is, that abortion is more dangerous than labour, and I am not sure that it is far wrong. No doubt exists that women are as liable to puerperal diseases after abortion, or premature labour, as after delivery at the full time, and they require a more careful management than is generally adopted by them.
>
> The patient should rest in bed the usual time, and then return gradually to her usual occupations. Attention should be paid to the lochia that they be not checked, and to the bowels. The diet for some days should be bland and unstimulating.[24]

Excerpts from Chapter X: Labour

It is hardly needful to mention, that everything in the shape of baby - linen, or that is necessary for the mother during her confinement, should be quite

---

[24] Original Text: Churchill on Midwifery, p. 169, 170.

ready some weeks before the expected time, in case of a premature birth. It is not needful for me to say anything about these articles, with one exception — the binder. This is so important to the comfort and safety of the patient after delivery, that I cannot pass it by without stating how it ought to be made. It should be of some stout, strong material, that will not yield too much. It should be just long enough to go once round the patient's body, and overlap four or five inches; if it is longer, the portion overlapping is in the way. And, above all, it should be sufficiently broad to reach from an inch below the projections of the hip bones to the waist just below the breasts. Put on in this way with strong pins, it is surprising how comfortable the patient feels. It makes an even and gentle pressure on the womb, and thereby ensures its contraction, and it forms a support for the abdominal walls, which, after being so much stretched and distended, require something of the kind. I look upon the proper application of the bandage after delivery as one of the most important parts of the accoucheur's duty, and make a point of always performing it myself.

The bed upon which delivery is to take place should be made up in a particular way. The patient ought to lie on the mattress, and not on a feather or flock bed.

A piece of India-rubber sheeting or oil-cloth, should be placed over the mattress, and over this a sheet, folded several times, so as to soak up the discharge. As will be more particularly described hereafter, this sheet and the oil cloth will be drawn away after delivery, and the patient thus left on the clean mattress. The inconvenience of lying on the bed is, that, during the labour, the woman is sure to get into the middle of the bed, out of the accoucheur's reach. It is, besides, extremely difficult to keep the bed free from the discharge that always takes place during and after labour.

It may appear that these details are too minute and insignificant to require notice; but it is not so. On such trifles the patient's comfort very greatly depends; and nothing that promotes, ever so slightly, her quick and safe recovery, is unworthy of attention.

...

I cannot allow this opportunity to escape, without protesting in the strongest possible terms, against the employment of midwives. I do this not from any professional jealousy, or because they may be supposed to interfere with the profits of medical men, because this is not the case—every one who can pay a medical man will have one but because I believe that even the poorest ought to have a properly qualified attendant at this time of trouble and danger. The best educated and instructed midwives are not qualified. They are never acquainted with even the rudiments of medicine, they know nothing of anatomy or physiology, and they are always more impatient and use more force than medical men do. It is a remarkable fact, but it is one of which I have frequently been assured by patients who have been attended by midwives, that the latter seem to lose all the gentleness of their sex, and in their examinations and manipulations use far more force than is ever used by a skilful accoucheur. With all the rashness of ignorance, they will, if there is the slightest delay, or even if the labour though advancing does not progress quite so rapidly as they wish, use means for forcing it on, utterly regardless of the state of the patient or the cause of the delay. I have seen some most horrible instances of the practice of midwives.

Still, cases may occur, when from an unusually rapid labour, the absence of the medical attendant from home, or the distance from which he has to come, the child is born before his arrival. In this case the nurse's duties are very simple. Tie the navel-string firmly about an inch from the belly with a stout piece of twine, or half-a-dozen threads twisted together; then tie it about an inch and a half further on, and divide it with scissors half way between the two ligatures. Care must be taken that the first ligature is applied firmly and tightly, so that no bleeding shall occur from the cut end of the navel-string; a child may soon bleed to death if this is not attended to. Then if the after-birth comes away, nothing more need be done, except to fasten on the binder. But if after a quarter of an hour or twenty minutes' time no pain has occurred, and the after-birth has not come away, no pulling at the navel-string must be used on any account, but the nurse may gently rub the lower part of the patient's body with her hand. A little gentle pressure on the womb used at the same time will cause a slight pain, by which, in most cases, the after-birth will be expelled. If, however, this should not be the case, the nurse must make no further attempts to extract it; but wait the arrival of the medical man. All attempts to extract it by pulling at the cord are highly dangerous, and may be attended, if force is used, by the most frightful consequences.[25] There may, however, on such an occasion be flooding, and that to a serious extent. If the patient should become pale and faint, or sick, and the flooding continues, the nurse should dip her hand in cold water and apply it suddenly to the lower part of the abdomen. This is a powerful stimulus to the womb to contract; if this does not succeed, a cloth dipped in the coldest water may be slapped suddenly and repeatedly on the same part. This hardly ever fails to produce contraction of the womb, and stoppage of the flooding, unless the after-birth

---

[25] Original Text: Many instances are known in which the womb has been literally turned inside out, by ignorant midwives. I have several times known parts of the after-birth left in the womb by them, producing most dangerous flooding, and subsequent inflammation.

adheres to the inside of the womb. In these cases, which are fortunately very rare, it is impossible for any one but a properly educated accoucheur to be of service.

Brandy and water, or even neat brandy, may be given, and ought to be given, without hesitation, in cases where faintness occurs. In all other cases of bleeding fainting is salutary, as it tends to stop the hæmorrhage. But the reverse of this is the case after labour; nothing but the thorough contraction of the womb will cause the bleeding to stop, and as fainting has a tendency to prevent the contraction of the womb, it ought to be avoided by every means.

I have had occasion to give as much as a pint of pure brandy to a woman in the course of a few hours, and with the effect of only just sustaining life. In such cases not the slightest intoxication is produced, and a quantity which would make a woman in a state of health dead drunk, has only the effect of just keeping the pulse perceptible. These bad cases of hæmorrhage are the most frightful an accoucheur ever has to deal with-the attack is so sudden, the remedies must be prompt, and the treatment vigorous, or the patient will die. Fortunately such cases are rare; but as no one can tell when they may occur, who would neglect to engage a properly qualified medical man?

Before I quit this part of the subject, it is right to mention some of the faults frequently committed by nurses and patients in their estimate of the conduct of the medical attendant. They are impatient. They forget that if a labour is going on slowly, provided it is going on, there is no need to interfere, nor indeed is it wise or judicious to do so. It may be very annoying that a labour should be going on for eighteen or twenty hours, instead of being over in two or three, but, provided all is well, this is no reason for forcing the labour on. And as the medical man is after all the greatest sufferer (the patient excepted), it may be supposed that he will neglect no proper means of hastening the labour, if the case admits of, or requires any.

Another great mistake (very commonly made) is in supposing that the accoucheur can help the woman in the early part of labour. The accoucheur can do nothing until the last, and so far from his interference being of any service before this period, it does harm, and hinders rather than forwards the labour. A judicious accoucheur never meddles with the processes of Nature when he can possibly avoid it.

Nurses and friends of the patient are too apt to relate their experiences of difficult or fatal cases one leads to another until the poor patient may think that everybody, herself included, has to run the most dreadful risk of her life. She naturally feels anxious enough, and her spirits should rather be sustained by cheerful conversation and kind encouragement, than depressed by the silly tales alluded to.

During the early part of the labour, while the pains are of the kind denominated "grinding," the mouth of the womb is in process of dilatation. It is evident that, until this is fully accomplished, the head of the child cannot pass. Any voluntary efforts made during this period by the woman are, therefore, utterly useless, and can have no other effect than to fatigue and disappoint her. It is much better that she should sit up and walk about during this stage than that she should be in bed. Especially is this desirable in first labours, for as this is generally by far the longest part of any labour, and is always, from the little apparent progress made, the most trying, if the patient lie in bed she is led to expect the speedy termination of the labour. This expectation being disappointed, the time seems longer than it would otherwise do, and the patient becomes anxious and depressed in spirits. Let her walk about, or sit down, leaning on the back of a chair when a pain comes on; during the intervals let the conversation be directed to any subject but that of child-birth; let the woman have, at suitable intervals, a little light refreshment, such as a cup of tea and toast, or bread and butter, or a basin of warm broth. The practice of keeping a woman almost without food during a labour of any duration I highly disapprove of. It weakens her and weakens the pains, and thus retards delivery. On the other hand, except in some rare cases, stimulants should never be given. They almost invariably do harm.

During this stage a judicious accoucheur will not remain in the room with the patient. Nor will she or her friends expect him to do so. He can be of no service, he is, indeed, only in the way, and his continued presence is only likely to make the patient anxious and fidgety. He can tell, by merely listening to the patient's cry during the pain, how the labour is going on, and as soon as ever the expulsive pains commence, when only he can be of use, he will remain in the room.

The second stage of labour, when the forcing or bearing down pains commence, is frequently marked by a shivering fit, and by the breaking of the waters, as it is called. This occurs generally when the mouth of the womb is fully dilated and the head is passing through. When this takes place the woman should undress and go to bed. The practice pursued by some of the lower classes of keeping on their clothes until after delivery is most objectionable — the undressing and dressing after delivery disturbs the patient to a most dangerous extent. At this period of labour, the woman's own efforts in bearing down are very useful. The pains are very severe, sometimes almost excruciating, but if she will abstain as much as possible from loud cries, and keep in her breath, she will advance the labour. It is during this stage that severe cramps in the legs and thighs occur, and the pain in the back is described as dreadful, the bones feeling as if they were being forced asunder. Nothing but Chloroform, or delivery, effectually relieves these pains. If Chloroform is not given, the patient must bear them as well as she can, remembering that every pain brings her nearer to the last.

With respect to the use of Chloroform in labour, it may be expected that I should say a few words. It may be given to such an extent as to deaden the acuteness of the pains, and render them quite endurable, without in the least affecting their frequency, or, I believe, lessening their powers. This may be done without approaching insensibility; indeed, I have seen a patient who had had Chloroform previously administered, give directions when the handkerchief was to be taken away, or applied to the nose, when it needed a fresh charge of Chloroform, when the pain went off or was coming on, etc. And yet, after delivery, she said that all the severity of the pains was removed. In cases of natural labour, when all is going well, and no unnecessary suffering is felt, I would say, do not take Chloroform, although, even in such a case, if the patient expressed a strong wish for it, I would not refuse it. In some cases, as where women, who have previously borne children, have had very rapid and almost painless labours, its use would be decidedly wrong; but in those numerous cases where delicate women suffer much and long, where the pains are extremely severe, and yet the labour makes but little progress, in such cases Chloroform is invaluable. It causes a relaxation and softening of rigid parts, and, I firmly believe, hastens delivery. In all cases of instrumental labour I should give Chloroform to its full extent.

Excerpts from Chapter XI: Diseases of Childbed

It is not my intention to do more than briefly mention the most common of the diseases to which lying-in women are subject, inasmuch as the accoucheur being in attendance, he will discover and treat the earliest symptoms, and the patient's ignorance of these diseases is not likely to occasion any bad results. The natural anxiety women feel at this time induces them invariably to obtain medical assistance as soon as the slightest bad symptom arises; and it is well that it is so, for no diseases require more prompt and vigorous treatment, or are more entirely beyond the reach of domestic remedies than those which attack lying in women.

Puerperal Fever.—It has long been known that lying-in women are subject to a disease of remarkable fatality, characterized by symptoms of general fever and inflammation of some one or more of the organs of generation, in which the febrile symptoms are very rapidly followed by sinking. This disease is peculiarly fatal in lying-in hospitals, and in them has occurred epidemically;

thus years may pass without a case being seen, and then an epidemic like cholera breaks out, and case after case occurs and proves fatal. It is fearfully contagious. A practitioner attending one case will, in spite of the utmost precaution, convey the disease to other lying-in women he may be attending at the same time. The following instance, quoted by the late Dr. Gooch, shows this:

A practitioner in large midwifery practice lost so many cases from puerperal fever, that be determined to deliver no more for some time, but that his partner should attend in his place. He did so for a month, during which not a case of the disease occurred in their practice. The elder practitioner being then sufficiently recovered, returned to his practice, but the first patient he attended, being attacked by the disease, died. Again, a practitioner attended a post mortem examination of a case at two, P.M. He took care not to touch the body. At nine, P.M., he attended a woman, who was so nearly delivered that he had scarcely anything to do. The next morning she had shivering fits, and in forty-eight hours she died. The great practical point to be attended to by patients and nurses is this: whenever a lying-in woman complains of cold, shivering, or thirst, head ache, and general feverishness, with pain in the abdomen, or is attacked, without any evident cause, with vomiting, or complains of continuous pain in the abdomen (not like the after-pains, coming on and then going off again, but continuous pain), especially if the abdomen when pressed on feels tender or sore; when any of these symptoms occur the medical attendant should be sent for without a moment's delay. Prompt treatment, and that alone, can save the patient. It is true that there is a slight fever which attacks lying-in women, which passes off in a few days, and the commencement of which may, to a non-professional person, appear to resemble the more serious disease; but sending for the accoucheur will do no harm. The milk-fever is attended with thirst, hot skin, slight shiverings sometimes, and headache, but the pain and distension of the breasts and the absence of the proper flow of milk will show the difference. Nevertheless it is better that even the milk-fever should be properly attended to; but for further remarks on this point see the Chapter on Diseases of the Breast.

I have not room for many cases, but the following will show the advantages of prompt treatment. Several years ago I attended a lady with her fourth child. She had a tedious labour, followed by a good deal of hæmorrhage. Two days after her confinement, having previously gone on very well, I was sent for in great haste. I found that in the night she had had shivering, followed by heat, thirst, etc., and severe pain in the abdomen. She was lying with her thighs drawn up, in great suffering, breathing short and hurried, every breath giving pain, and unable to bear even the weight of the bed clothes-so tender was the abdomen. Her pulse was small, hard, and a hundred and twenty a minute. I immediately had a dozen leeches put on, and encouraged them to bleed freely, by fomentations, gave her calomel and opium every two hours, and ordered that she should have as little as possible to eat or drink. In the evening she was very much better, pulse fuller and slower, pain much less, could bear gentle pressure, etc. In a day or two she was nearly well. Now, in twelve hours, or even in less time, the above case would have been almost hopeless.

Puerperal Mania, a very distressing complaint, to which lying-in women are liable, is a species of insanity. It is rarely, if ever, permanent, but disappears under proper treatment: A very troublesome symptom, and one that re quires especial care on the part of the attendants, is a desire to murder the infant. This has frequently been accomplished during the paroxysm. The earliest symptoms are wakefulness, great excitability of the nervous system, attended with rapid and vehement talking, sometimes headache, with a wild look about the eye.

Surgical Affections.—Various injuries may be done to the organs of generation during labour, either by the body of the child, or by instruments used to accelerate delivery. Thus the interior of the vagina may be bruised and torn, or both, the vulva may be injured, the perinæum (or space between the orifice of the vagina and anus), may be torn through, even to such an extent as to cause the two canals to form but one opening; the bladder or uterus may be injured. These injuries will always be followed by more or less inflammation, perhaps by mortification and death. It would be obviously out of place to describe their treatment here, as they will invariably require the attendance of a skilful surgeon.

Incidents in the Life of a Slave Girl by Harriet Jacobs (1861)

Introduction

In this autobiography, Harriet Jacobs uses the pseudonym Linda Brent to detail her experiences while enslaved and then in her journey to freedom for herself and her children. In it, she represents some of the challenges specific to enslaved women, including sexual harassment and assault by enslavers and maternal efforts to protect her children. After a childhood of harassment by her enslaver under the pseudonym of Dr. Flint, Linda fears the completion of a cottage he is building as a space to assault her. She begins a consensual sexual relationship with Mr. Sands and hopes that he will help her gain freedom. In the excerpts provided here, Linda becomes pregnant by Mr. Sands and bears two children.

Excerpt from Chapter X: A Perilous Passage in the Slave Girl's Life

…

    When I found that my master had actually begun to build the lonely cottage, other feelings mixed with those I have described. Revenge, and calculations of interest, were added to flattered vanity and sincere gratitude for kindness. I knew nothing would enrage Dr. Flint so much as to know that I favored another, and it was something to triumph over my tyrant even in that small way. I thought he would revenge himself by selling me, and I was sure my friend, Mr. Sands, would buy me. He was a man of more generosity and feeling than my master, and I thought my freedom could be easily obtained from him. The crisis of my fate now came so near that I was desperate. I shuddered to think of being the mother of children that should be owned by my old tyrant. I knew that as soon as a new fancy took him, his victims were sold far off to get rid of them; especially if they had children. I had seen several women sold, with babies at the breast. He never allowed his offspring by slaves to remain long in sight of himself and his wife. Of a man who was not my master I could ask to have my children well supported; and in this case, I felt confident I should obtain the boon. I also felt quite sure that they would be made free. With all these thoughts revolving in my mind, and seeing no other way of escaping the doom I so much dreaded, I made a headlong plunge. Pity me, and pardon me, O virtuous reader! You never knew what it is to be a slave; to be entirely unprotected by law or custom; to have the laws reduce you to the condition of a chattel, entirely subject to the will of another. You never exhausted your ingenuity in avoiding the snares, and eluding the power of a hated tyrant; you never shuddered at the sound of his footsteps, and trembled within hearing of his voice. I know I did wrong. No one can feel it more sensibly than I do. The painful and humiliating memory will haunt me to my dying day. Still, in looking back, calmly, on the events of my life, I feel that the slave woman ought not to be judged by the same standard as others.

    The months passed on. I had many unhappy hours. I secretly mourned over the sorrow I was bringing on my grandmother, who had so tried to shield me from harm. I knew that I was the greatest comfort of her old age, and that it was a source of pride to her that I had not degraded myself, like most of the slaves. I wanted to confess to her that I was no longer worthy of her love; but I could not utter the dreaded words.

    As for Dr. Flint, I had a feeling of satisfaction and triumph in the thought of telling *him*. From time to time he told me of his intended arrangements, and I was silent. At last, he came and told me the cottage was completed, and ordered me to go to it. I told him I would never enter it. He said, "I have heard enough of such talk as that. You shall go, if you are carried by force; and you shall remain there."

I replied, "I will never go there. In a few months I shall be a mother."

He stood and looked at me in dumb amazement, and left the house without a word. I thought I should be happy in my triumph over him. But now that the truth was out, and my relatives would hear of it, I felt wretched. Humble as were their circumstances, they had pride in my good character. Now, how could I look at them in the face? My self-respect was gone! I had resolved that I would be virtuous, though I was a slave. I had said, "Let the storm beat! I will brave it till I die." And now, how humiliated I felt!

…

Excerpts from Chapter XI: The New Tie to Life

…

My uncle's stay was short, and I was not sorry for it. I was too ill in mind and body to enjoy my friends as I had done. For some weeks I was unable to leave my bed. I could not have any doctor but my master, and I would not have him sent for. At last, alarmed by my increasing illness, they sent for him. I was very weak and nervous; and as soon as he entered the room, I began to scream. They told him my state was very critical. He had no wish to hasten me out of the world, and he withdrew.

When my babe was born, they said it was premature. It weighed only four pounds; but God let it live. I heard the doctor say I could not survive till morning. I had often prayed for death; but now I did not want to die, unless my child could die too. Many weeks passed before I was able to leave my bed. I was a mere wreck of my former self. For a year there was scarcely a day when I was free from chills and fever. My babe also was sickly. His little limbs were often racked with pain. Dr. Flint continued his visits, to look after my health; and he did not fail to remind me that my child was an addition to his stock of slaves.

…

As the months passed on, my boy improved in health. When he was a year old, they called him beautiful. The little vine was taking deep root in my existence, though its clinging fondness excited a mixture of love and pain. When I was most sorely oppressed I found a solace in his smiles. I loved to watch his infant slumbers; but always there was a dark cloud over my enjoyment. I could never forget that he was a slave. Sometimes I wished that he might die in infancy. God tried me. My darling became very ill. The bright eyes grew dull, and the little feet and hands were so icy cold that I thought death had already touched them. I had prayed for his death, but never so earnestly as I now prayed for his life; and my prayer was heard. Alas, what mockery it is for a slave mother to try to pray back her dying child to life! Death is better than slavery. It was a sad thought that I had no name to give my child. His father caressed him and treated him kindly, whenever he had a chance to see him. He was not unwilling that he should bear his name; but he had no legal claim to it; and if I had bestowed it upon him, my master would have regarded it as a new crime, a new piece of insolence, and would, perhaps, revenge it on the boy. O, the serpent of Slavery has many and poisonous fangs!

Excerpts from Chapter XIV: Another Link to Life

I had not returned to my master's house since the birth of my child. The old man raved to have me thus removed from his immediate power; but his wife vowed, by all that was good and great, she would kill me if I came back; and he did not doubt her word. Sometimes he would stay away for a season. Then he would come and renew the old threadbare discourse about his forbearance and my ingratitude. He labored, most unnecessarily, to convince me that I had lowered myself. The venomous old reprobate had no need of descanting on that theme. I felt humiliated enough. My unconscious babe was the ever-present witness of my shame. I listened with silent contempt when he talked about my having forfeited *his* good opinion; but I shed bitter tears that I was no longer worthy of being respected by the good and pure. Alas! slavery still held me in its poisonous grasp. There was no chance for me to be respectable. There was no prospect of being able to lead a better life.

Sometimes, when my master found that I still refused to accept what he called his kind offers, he would threaten to sell my child. "Perhaps that will humble you," said he.

Humble *me*! Was I not already in the dust? But his threat lacerated my heart. I knew the law gave him power to fulfil it; for slaveholders have been cunning enough to enact that "the child shall follow the condition of the *mother*," not of the *father*, thus taking care that licentiousness shall not interfere with avarice. This reflection made me clasp my innocent babe all the more firmly to my heart. Horrid visions passed through my mind when I thought of his liability to fall into the slave-trader's hands. I wept over him, and said, "O my child! perhaps they will leave you in some cold cabin to die, and then throw you into a hole, as if you were a dog."

When Dr. Flint learned that I was again to be a mother, he was exasperated beyond measure. He rushed from the house, and returned with a pair of shears. I had a fine head of hair; and he often railed about my pride of arranging it nicely. He cut every hair close to my head, storming and swearing all the time. I replied to some of his abuse, and he struck me. Some months before, he had pitched me down stairs in a fit of passion; and the injury I received was so serious that I was unable to turn myself in bed for many days. He then said, "Linda, I swear by God I will never raise my hand against you again;" but I knew that he would forget his promise.

After he discovered my situation, he was like a restless spirit from the pit. He came every day; and I was subjected to such insults as no pen can describe. I would not describe them if I could; they were too low, too revolting. I tried to keep them from my grandmother's knowledge as much as I could. I knew she had enough to sadden her life, without having my troubles to bear. When she saw the doctor treat me with violence, and heard him utter oaths terrible enough to palsy a man's tongue, she could not always hold her peace. It was natural and motherlike that she should try to defend me; but it only made matters worse.

When they told me my new-born babe was a girl, my heart was heavier than it had ever been before. Slavery is terrible for men; but it is far more terrible for women. Superadded to the burden common to all, *they* have wrongs, and sufferings, and mortifications peculiarly their own.

Dr. Flint had sworn that he would make me suffer, to my last day, for this new crime against *him*, as he called it; and as long as he had me in his power he kept his word. On the fourth day after the birth of my babe, he entered my room suddenly, and commanded me to rise and bring my baby to him. The nurse who took care of me had gone out of the room to prepare some nourishment, and I was alone. There was no alternative. I rose, took up my babe, and crossed the room to where he sat. "Now stand there," said he, "till I tell you to go back!" My child bore a strong resemblance to her father, and to the deceased Mrs. Sands, her grandmother. He noticed this; and while I stood before him, trembling with weakness, he heaped upon me and my little one every vile epithet he could think of. Even the grandmother in her grave did not escape his curses. In the midst of his vituperations I fainted at his feet. This recalled him to his senses. He took the baby from my arms, laid it on the bed, dashed cold water in my face, took me up, and shook me violently, to restore my consciousness before any one entered the room. Just then my grandmother came in, and he hurried out of the house. I suffered in consequence of this treatment; but I begged my friends to let me die, rather than send for the doctor. There was nothing I dreaded so much as his presence. My life was spared; and I was glad for the sake of my little ones. Had it not been for these ties to life, I should have been glad to be released by death, though I had lived only nineteen years.

Always it gave me a pang that my children had no lawful claim to a name. Their father offered his; but, if I had wished to accept the offer, I dared not while my master lived. Moreover, I knew it would not be accepted at their baptism. A Christian name they were at least entitled to; and we resolved to call my boy for our dear good Benjamin, who had gone far away from us.

"The New Order of Medical Students" (1871)

Introduction

Though this essay is ostensibly about newly educated women physicians, it focuses primarily on the effects of traditional midwives and trained medical practitioners on maternal mortality. While explaining the differences in care, the essay details the causes of puerperal fever and recognizes the value of trained women physicians in obstetrics. Published by Samuel and Isabella Beeton, *The Englishwoman's Domestic Magazine* was a monthly periodical targeting an audience of middle-class women readers, offering them a mix of information and entertainment.

"The New Order of Medical Students" (*The Englishwoman's Domestic Magazine*, June 1871)

It is beyond a doubt that the Female Medical College is raising up an entirely new order in society. Students of that school of medicine, and more especially the certified practitioners, together with their friends and advocates, take their stand upon the proposition that when women become mothers it is more fitting that they should be attended by persons of their own sex. All history is conclusive upon the point, so far as it relates to the ancients, amongst whom there is abundant evidence that what are now called man-midwives were unknown. Later on, in the obscure haze at the expiring end of what are called the "Dark Ages," there is some evidence that men did occasionally intrude upon the office of attending lying-in women, for it is stated, as negative evidence of the fact, that it was considered disreputable for men to engage in that kind of practice, and the disrepute continued until the time of Charles I. It would be superfluous to adduce evidence in particular that there lived about the court of that "Merrie Monarch" a number of disreputable women, and when one of the most notorious of them needed a midwife, there was not a female practitioner to be found who would accept the office. In this extremity a medical man was called in, and as the case was got through safely and the attendant was well paid, and as other ladies of the court had some cause to fear the enmity of the midwives for similar reasons, the practice of regularly employing medical men on such occasions took firm root; gaining encouragement on the one hand from the patronage and example of the court, and stimulated by the extravagant fees for which the first emergency of the kind had created a precedent. The change not to be *entirely* deplored. Previously to that time midwifery and medical science had never been associated together. The latter remained for ages in the keeping of monks, and, as the science thraldom, there was nothing dogmas of the unlearned ancients who desired the advancement to guide the men of their profession. On the other hand, there is good reason to conclude that the best midwives of that time were entirely deficient in medical science, and were unable to call to their aid any kind of knowledge except that which was derived from the comparatively meagre personal experience of each practitioner. To this state of things was added a vast cloud of incongruous superstition which effectually prevented any progress towards additional light. Therefore, amongst the medical men of the time of Charles II, it is quite likely that some were actuated by a true nobility of purpose, which, in braving the odium of practising midwifery, sought to make it a matter of scientific study. The result has been that monopolising that branch of attendance amongst all sorts of people who can afford to employ them. Every year since has tended to make the gulf wider between qualified medical men and the old class of midwives. While the former have been slowly but certainly progressing, the latter have remained stationary, or, worse still, have retrograded in character—being, as a class, a national opprobrium.

Long since this evil has been rampant, and those who have pointed it out with the most assiduity have succeeded in establishing lying-in hospitals and maternity charities. The former seem to be gradually decaying in favour of institutions of the latter kind, which is scarcely surprising. The generality of women have a decided repugnance to transferring themselves to a public building, and therefore the maternity charities, especially in London and Birmingham, are gradually superseding the old form of relief. The reason is that attendance is given at the homes of the poor women, which course is so much in favour that several of the hospitals are entirely closed, and those which are open are by no means full. Considering that both plans have their relative merits, let us hope that emulation may enlarge the scope and tend eventually to the prosperity of each. Be that as it may, it is certain that the maternity charities are raising up a better class of midwives. Nothing is spared to give them intelligent training, a useful probation, and practical experience; and the results are beginning to form an important element in medical records. The statistics which have arisen appeal with unanswerable force to every mother in England who has a married daughter; to every husband whose regard for the true interests of his wife is greater than his respect for conventional prejudices; to every wife who looks forward to becoming the healthy mother of a healthy family. It must be borne in mind that the patients of the maternity charities dwell in the worst districts, and belong exclusively to very poor families. Notwithstanding this disadvantage, the cases are so successful that the number of deaths is recorded as only 133 in 47,600, or an average of 1 in 358; and at one period there were 3297 consecutive births, only 2 of which were fatal to the mothers. The deaths recorded include those which take place from the immediate consequences of parturition, and also those which take place from causes arising in the after-stages previously to recovery. Of these, the most usual come under the head of "puerperal causes," including the dreaded "puerperal fever," which is peculiar to such times. It is in this particular connection that we draw special attention to the comparison. The maternity cases in London, under the disadvantageous circumstances above alluded to, disclose an average of deaths from "puerperal causes" of 1 in 556, while the average of all the rest of London is 1 in 204; maternity deaths from "puerperal fever" 1 in 1567; deaths from that disease in all the rest of London, 1 in 492. Thus "puerperal causes" are about three times as fatal throughout London as they are in connection with the maternity charity. But the most striking feature of the inquiry is the fact that "puerperal fever" is prevalent among the higher ranks. The most remarkable case on record appears to have been that of the Princess Charlotte, who died of the fever after being attended by Sir Richard Croft. A Mrs. Thackeray, who was also under his care, soon afterwards died in like manner, and he blew out his brains in her house. A medical man in Edinburgh wrote a book against him, but within three months afterwards twenty-five women of rank, patients of the writer, died under his care. Forty cases occurred in rapid succession under the care of one surgeon and his assistant at Sunderland. These are but a few notices of events which are occurring around us daily, and it will be observed that the occurrence of "puerperal causes" is clearly traceable to the medical attendants, one of whom, as at Sunderland, may sometimes create a complete epidemic.

In seeking for an explanation, we turn our steps to the hospitals, where the beginning of the evil may be perceived. The practice of the hospitals sanctions the performance of surgical operations upon living subjects by gentlemen who are also engaged from day to day, and even five minutes previously, in dissection upon dead bodies. The combination of the two offices in the person of one man implies a degree of professional enthusiasm on his part which is in itself admirable. Engaged in the grim necessities of dissection performed upon half-putrid flesh, he is summoned at a moment's notice to the operating theatre, where, in the presence of a company of observers who cannot admire sufficiently the accuracy and rapidity with which he plies his terrible instruments, he manipulates, as he proceeds, the freshly-cut wounds of the unhappy patients. Such exhibitions tend to impress observers with the beneficence of such institutions, and they may well feel proud of the minute attention and ample comfort which surround and restore the more fortunate of the sufferers, who are thus indebted to the benevolent and the affluent for mitigations of their misery. But if such cases are followed up; if you would pour out oil and wine to hasten convalescence, and seek the individual patients for the purpose, you will discover how large a proportion of those who bore the operations with courage and without apparent harm, are carried off into the grave, not because the amputation hurt them so much, but because of the infection from the dissection-room, conveyed into their open wounds by the hands of the too enthusiastic practitioner. The disease they die of is known as hospital gangrene; and it is the very same thing in another form which is called "puerperal fever," the cause of most of the deaths which are falsely attributed to child-bearing. When you see that your family doctor has been engaged upon a *post-mortem* examination; and has given evidence theron to a jury, who have been dumb with astonishment at his profound acquirements, and before a coroner, who has complimented him; then, if a "little stranger" is immediately expected in your house, avoid that indiscreet doctor as if he were a pestilence, as indeed he is for the time being, The sanction of his hospital will keep him in countenance, but it is not safe to allow him under your roof. Scarcely less is the danger when a doctor, after leaving a case of ordinary fever, even when of a slight character, attends a mother, who at such times is sensitive beyond measure to all kinds of contagion.

This raises the whole question at issue between the medical profession and the patrons of the Female Medical College, who allege that the only really safe arrangement is for midwifery to be kept distinct from all other medical practice whatever, and that the only practicable solution of the difficulty is the one which they have adopted—the training of a new order of medical students, who, having a certificate of ability and experience, may be resorted to with confidence and satisfaction. This is, in fact, carrying the organisation of the maternity charities one step further, so that ladies of wealth and position may avail themselves of the advantages which have hitherto been restricted to the poor. Past students of the college are now practising as certified accoucheuses in London, especially at Hackney, Mildmay Park, Kentish Town, Newman-street, Oxford-street, Bolsover-street, Camberwell, Rotherhithe, and Deptford. Others are engaged in the provinces, notably at Birmingham, Newport, Isle of Wight, Bangor, Dublin, &c. Some of them have gone abroad. Miss Thompson, formerly in practice at York, is gone to Norway; Miss Curling, to Melbourne, Victoria; and Miss Ross is just gone or going to California. That these ladies are worthy of their vocation may be gathered from the fact that several cases which have come into their hands have obtained voluntary fees of ten guineas each; and handsome considerations, quite superior to those conceded by Dr. Bennet, are sufficiently frequent to be encouraging. Possibly yet better things may be in store for these worthy pilgrims. We may take some hints from days of old of which we have record. The register of the private purse of King Charles IX. informs us that, in 1572, Isabel Beaudonoir received 1250 livres (about £52) for attending the Queen Elizabeth of Austria as accoucheuse. In the year 1493–1494 Queen Anne de Bretagne made a handsome present to Pierre Bay, on the occasion of his marriage with the daughter of Thomina Baudeville, accoucheuse to the queen. On November 1st, 1648, a thousand livres were appropriated for the funeral of the deceased Madame Peronne du Montier, accoucheuse to the Queen and Princesses of France. These records not only suggest considerable rewards, but also personal distinction.

Meanwhile, there is no imperative rule to prevent ladies who have passed the college from proceeding to other walks of the profession; always bearing in mind that if they do they must restrict their practice so as to avoid contagion, or else abandon midwifery altogether. There is a gratifying instance of that conviction having been acted upon. Previously to the resolution arrived at by Mrs. Thorne to aim at becoming a physician, she was for some time in successful practice in London as an accoucheuse, bearing the certificate of the college. Some time after she had adopted the resolution she was requested to attend a lady under very gratifying circumstances, but she respectfully declined because she had recently been engaged upon dissection. It is also gratifying to learn that, since our last, the ladies studying at Edinburgh have competed in anatomy and surgery in a mixed class examination of the Royal College of surgeons, and that they took *first-class* honours.

Far from the Madding Crowd by Thomas Hardy (1874)

Introduction

In this novel by Thomas Hardy originally serialized in *Cornhill Magazine*, Fanny Robin and Sergeant Francis Troy planned to marry. However, Fanny mistakenly went to the wrong church, and Troy called off the wedding not aware that Fanny was pregnant with his child. After he marries another woman, Troy and his wife Bathsheba encounter the pregnant Fanny walking to a workhouse to deliver her baby. Troy gives her all of his money and promises to meet her there in a few days. This excerpt begins with the weakening Fanny's continued walk toward the Casterbridge workhouse.

Chapter XL: On Casterbridge Highway

For a considerable time the woman[26] walked on. Her steps became feebler, and she strained her eyes to look afar upon the naked road, now indistinct amid the penumbræ of night. At length her onward walk dwindled to the merest totter, and she opened a gate within which was a haystack. Underneath this she sat down and presently slept.

When the woman awoke it was to find herself in the depths of a moonless and starless night. A heavy unbroken crust of cloud stretched across the sky, shutting out every speck of heaven; and a distant halo which hung over the town of Casterbridge was visible against the black concave, the luminosity appearing the brighter by its great contrast with the circumscribing darkness. Towards this weak, soft glow the woman turned her eyes.

"If I could only get there!" she said. "Meet him the day after to-morrow: God help me! Perhaps I shall be in my grave before then."

A manor-house clock from the far depths of shadow struck the hour, one, in a small, attenuated tone. After midnight the voice of a clock seems to lose in breadth as much as in length, and to diminish its sonorousness to a thin falsetto.

Afterwards a light—two lights—arose from the remote shade, and grew larger. A carriage rolled along the road, and passed the gate. It probably contained some late diners-out. The beams from one lamp shone for a moment upon the crouching woman, and threw her face into vivid relief. The face was

---

[26] Fanny Robin

young in the groundwork, old in the finish; the general contours were flexuous and childlike, but the finer lineaments had begun to be sharp and thin.

The pedestrian stood up, apparently with revived determination, and looked around. The road appeared to be familiar to her, and she carefully scanned the fence as she slowly walked along. Presently there became visible a dim white shape; it was another milestone. She drew her fingers across its face to feel the marks.

"Two more!" she said.

She leant against the stone as a means of rest for a short interval, then bestirred herself, and again pursued her way. For a slight distance she bore up bravely, afterwards flagging as before. This was beside a lone copsewood, wherein heaps of white chips strewn upon the leafy ground showed that woodmen had been faggoting and making hurdles during the day. Now there was not a rustle, not a breeze, not the faintest clash of twigs to keep her company. The woman looked over the gate, opened it, and went in. Close to the entrance stood a row of faggots, bound and unbound, together with stakes of all sizes.

For a few seconds the wayfarer stood with that tense stillness which signifies itself to be not the end, but merely the suspension, of a previous motion. Her attitude was that of a person who listens, either to the external world of sound, or to the imagined discourse of thought. A close criticism might have detected signs proving that she was intent on the latter alternative. Moreover, as was shown by what followed, she was oddly exercising the faculty of invention upon the speciality of the clever Jacquet Droz, the designer of automatic substitutes for human limbs.

By the aid of the Casterbridge aurora, and by feeling with her hands, the woman selected two sticks from the heaps. These sticks were nearly straight to the height of three or four feet, where each branched into a fork like the letter Y. She sat down, snapped off the small upper twigs, and carried the remainder with her into the road. She placed one of these forks under each arm as a crutch, tested them, timidly threw her whole weight upon them—so little that it was—and swung herself forward. The girl had made for herself a material aid.

The crutches answered well. The pat of her feet, and the tap of her sticks upon the highway, were all the sounds that came from the traveller now. She had passed the last milestone by a good long distance, and began to look wistfully towards the bank as if calculating upon another milestone soon. The crutches, though so very useful, had their limits of power. Mechanism only transfers labour, being powerless to supersede it, and the original amount of exertion was not cleared away; it was thrown into the body and arms. She was exhausted, and each swing forward became fainter. At last she swayed sideways, and fell.

Here she lay, a shapeless heap, for ten minutes and more. The morning wind began to boom dully over the flats, and to move afresh dead leaves which had lain still since yesterday. The woman desperately turned round upon her knees, and next rose to her feet. Steadying herself by the help of one crutch, she essayed a step, then another, then a third, using the crutches now as walking-sticks only. Thus she progressed till descending Mellstock Hill another milestone appeared, and soon the beginning of an iron-railed fence came into view. She staggered across to the first post, clung to it, and looked around.

The Casterbridge lights were now individually visible. It was getting towards morning, and vehicles might be hoped for, if not expected soon. She listened. There was not a sound of life save that acme and sublimation of all dismal sounds, the bark of a fox, its three hollow notes being rendered at intervals of a minute with the precision of a funeral bell.

"Less than a mile!" the woman murmured. "No; more," she added, after a pause. "The mile is to the county hall, and my resting-place is on the other side Casterbridge. A little over a mile, and there I am!" After an interval she again spoke. "Five or six steps to a yard—six perhaps. I have to go seventeen hundred yards. A hundred times six, six hundred. Seventeen times that. O pity me, Lord!"

Holding to the rails, she advanced, thrusting one hand forward upon the rail, then the other, then leaning over it whilst she dragged her feet on beneath.

This woman was not given to soliloquy; but extremity of feeling lessens the individuality of the weak, as it increases that of the strong. She said again in the same tone, "I'll believe that the end lies five posts forward, and no further, and so get strength to pass them."

This was a practical application of the principle that a half-feigned and fictitious faith is better than no faith at all.

She passed five posts and held on to the fifth.

"I'll pass five more by believing my longed-for spot is at the next fifth. I can do it."

She passed five more.

"It lies only five further."

She passed five more.

"But it is five further."

She passed them.

"That stone bridge is the end of my journey," she said, when the bridge over the Froom was in view.

She crawled to the bridge. During the effort each breath of the woman went into the air as if never to return again.

"Now for the truth of the matter," she said, sitting down. "The truth is, that I have less than half a mile." Self-beguilement with what she had known all the time to be false had given her strength to come over half a mile that she would have been powerless to face in the lump. The artifice showed that the woman, by some mysterious intuition, had grasped the paradoxical truth that blindness may operate more vigorously than prescience, and the short-sighted effect more than the far-seeing; that limitation, and not comprehensiveness, is needed for striking a blow.

The half-mile stood now before the sick and weary woman like a stolid Juggernaut. It was an impassive King of her world. The road here ran across Durnover Moor, open to the road on either side. She surveyed the wide space, the lights, herself, sighed, and lay down against a guard-stone of the bridge.

Never was ingenuity exercised so sorely as the traveller here exercised hers. Every conceivable aid, method, stratagem, mechanism, by which these last desperate eight hundred yards could be overpassed by a human being unperceived, was revolved in her busy brain, and dismissed as impracticable. She thought of sticks, wheels, crawling—she even thought of rolling. But the exertion demanded by either of these latter two was greater than to walk erect. The faculty of contrivance was worn out. Hopelessness had come at last.

"No further!" she whispered, and closed her eyes.

From the stripe of shadow on the opposite side of the bridge a portion of shade seemed to detach itself and move into isolation upon the pale white of the road. It glided noiselessly towards the recumbent woman.

She became conscious of something touching her hand; it was softness and it was warmth. She opened her eyes, and the substance touched her face. A dog was licking her cheek.

He was a huge, heavy, and quiet creature, standing darkly against the low horizon, and at least two feet higher than the present position of her eyes. Whether Newfoundland, mastiff, bloodhound, or what not, it was impossible to say. He seemed to be of too strange and mysterious a nature to belong to any variety among those of popular nomenclature. Being thus assignable to no breed, he was the ideal embodiment of canine greatness—a generalization from what was common to all. Night, in its sad, solemn, and benevolent aspect, apart from its stealthy and cruel side, was personified in this form. Darkness endows the small and ordinary ones among mankind with poetical power, and even the suffering woman threw her idea into figure.

In her reclining position she looked up to him just as in earlier times she had, when standing, looked up to a man. The animal, who was as homeless as she, respectfully withdrew a step or two when the woman moved, and, seeing that she did not repulse him, he licked her hand again.

A thought moved within her like lightning. "Perhaps I can make use of him—I might do it then!"

She pointed in the direction of Casterbridge, and the dog seemed to misunderstand: he trotted on. Then, finding she could not follow, he came back and whined.

The ultimate and saddest singularity of woman's effort and invention was reached when, with a quickened breathing, she rose to a stooping posture, and, resting her two little arms upon the shoulders of the dog, leant firmly thereon, and murmured stimulating words. Whilst she sorrowed in her heart she cheered with her voice, and what was stranger than that the strong should need encouragement from the weak was that cheerfulness should be so well stimulated by such utter dejection. Her friend moved forward slowly, and she with small mincing steps moved forward beside him, half her weight being thrown upon the animal. Sometimes she sank as she had sunk from walking erect, from the crutches, from the rails. The dog, who now thoroughly understood her desire and her incapacity, was frantic in his distress on these occasions; he would tug at her dress and run forward. She always called him back, and it was now to be observed that the woman listened for human sounds only to avoid them. It was evident that she had an object in keeping her presence on the road and her forlorn state unknown.

Their progress was necessarily very slow. They reached the bottom of the town, and the Casterbridge lamps lay before them like fallen Pleiads as they turned to the left into the dense shade of a deserted avenue of chestnuts, and so skirted the borough. Thus the town was passed, and the goal was reached.

On this much-desired spot outside the town rose a picturesque building. Originally it had been a mere case to hold people. The shell had been so thin, so devoid of excrescence, and so closely drawn over the accommodation granted, that the grim character of what was beneath showed through it, as the shape of a body is visible under a winding-sheet.

Then Nature, as if offended, lent a hand. Masses of ivy grew up, completely covering the walls, till the place looked like an abbey; and it was discovered that the view from the front, over the Casterbridge chimneys, was one of the most magnificent in the county. A neighbouring earl once said that he would give up a year's rental to have at his own door the view enjoyed by the inmates from theirs—and very probably the inmates would have given up the view for his year's rental.

This stone edifice consisted of a central mass and two wings, whereon stood as sentinels a few slim chimneys, now gurgling sorrowfully to the slow wind.

In the wall was a gate, and by the gate a bellpull formed of a hanging wire. The woman raised herself as high as possible upon her knees, and could just reach the handle. She moved it and fell forwards in a bowed attitude, her face upon her bosom.

It was getting on towards six o'clock, and sounds of movement were to be heard inside the building which was the haven of rest to this wearied soul. A little door by the large one was opened, and a man appeared inside. He discerned the panting heap of clothes, went back for a light, and came again. He entered a second time, and returned with two women.

These lifted the prostrate figure and assisted her in through the doorway. The man then closed the door.

"How did she get here?" said one of the women.

"The Lord knows," said the other.

"There is a dog outside," murmured the overcome traveller. "Where is he gone? He helped me."

"I stoned him away," said the man.

The little procession then moved forward—the man in front bearing the light, the two bony women next, supporting between them the small and supple one. Thus they entered the house and disappeared.

Excerpt from Chapter XLI: Suspicion—Fanny Is Sent For

...

"Died of what? did you say, Joseph?"

"I don't know, ma'am."

"Are you quite sure?"

"Yes, ma'am, quite sure."

"Sure of what?"

"I'm sure that all I know is that she arrived in the morning and died in the evening without further parley. What Oak and Mr. Boldwood told me was only these few words. 'Little Fanny Robin is dead, Joseph,' Gabriel said, looking in my face in his steady old way. I was very sorry, and I said, 'Ah!—and how did she come to die?' 'Well, she's dead in Casterbridge Union,' he said, 'and perhaps 'tisn't much matter about how she came to die. She reached the Union early Sunday morning, and died in the afternoon—that's clear enough.' Then I asked what she'd been doing lately, and Mr. Boldwood turned round to me then, and left off spitting a thistle with the end of his stick. He told me about her having lived by seampstering in Melchester, as I mentioned to you, and that she walked therefrom at the end of last week, passing near here

Saturday night in the dusk. They then said I had better just name a hint of her death to you, and away they went. Her death might have been brought on by biding in the night wind, you know, ma'am; for people used to say she'd go off in a decline: she used to cough a good deal in winter time. However, 'tisn't much odds to us about that now, for 'tis all over."

"Have you heard a different story at all?" She looked at him so intently that Joseph's eyes quailed.

"Not a word, mistress, I assure 'ee!" he said. "Hardly anybody in the parish knows the news yet."

Excerpts from Chapter XLII: Joseph and His Burden—Buck's Head

It had gradually become rumoured in the village that the body to be brought and buried that day was all that was left of the unfortunate Fanny Robin who had followed the Eleventh from Casterbridge through Melchester and onwards. But, thanks to Boldwood's reticence and Oak's generosity, the lover she had followed had never been individualized as Troy. Gabriel hoped that the whole truth of the matter might not be published till at any rate the girl had been in her grave for a few days, when the interposing barriers of earth and time, and a sense that the events had been somewhat shut into oblivion, would deaden the sting that revelation and invidious remark would have for Bathsheba just now.

…

Every one except Gabriel Oak then left the room. He still indecisively lingered beside the body. He was deeply troubled at the wretchedly ironical aspect that circumstances were putting on with regard to Troy's wife, and at his own powerlessness to counteract them. In spite of his careful manœuvering all this day, the very worst event that could in any way have happened in connection with the burial had happened now. Oak imagined a terrible discovery resulting from this afternoon's work that might cast over Bathsheba's life a shade which the interposition of many lapsing years might but indifferently lighten, and which nothing at all might altogether remove.

Suddenly, as in a last attempt to save Bathsheba from, at any rate, immediate anguish, he looked again, as he had looked before, at the chalk writing upon the coffin-lid. The scrawl was this simple one, "*Fanny Robin and child.*" Gabriel took his handkerchief and carefully rubbed out the two latter words, leaving visible the inscription "*Fanny Robin*" only. He then left the room, and went out quietly by the front door.

Excerpts from XLIII: Fanny's Revenge

...

In five or ten minutes there was another tap at the door. Liddy reappeared, and coming in a little way stood hesitating, until at length she said, "Maryann has just heard something very strange, but I know it isn't true. And we shall be sure to know the rights of it in a day or two."

"What is it?"

"Oh, nothing connected with you or us, ma'am. It is about Fanny. That same thing you have heard."

"I have heard nothing."

"I mean that a wicked story is got to Weatherbury within this last hour—that—" Liddy came close to her mistress and whispered the remainder of the sentence slowly into her ear, inclining her head as she spoke in the direction of the room where Fanny lay.

Bathsheba trembled from head to foot.

"I don't believe it!" she said, excitedly. "And there's only one name written on the coffin-cover."

"Nor I, ma'am. And a good many others don't; for we should surely have been told more about it if it had been true—don't you think so, ma'am?"

"We might or we might not."

...

Bathsheba in after times could never gauge the mood which carried her through the actions following this murmured resolution on this memorable evening of her life. She went to the lumber-closet for a screw-driver. At the end of a short though undefined time she found herself in the small room, quivering with emotion, a mist before her eyes, and an excruciating pulsation in her brain, standing beside the uncovered coffin of the girl whose conjectured end had so entirely engrossed her, and saying to herself in a husky voice as she gazed within—

"It was best to know the worst, and I know it now!"

She was conscious of having brought about this situation by a series of actions done as by one in an extravagant dream; of following that idea as to method, which had burst upon her in the hall with glaring obviousness, by gliding to the top of the stairs, assuring herself by listening to the heavy breathing of her maids that they were asleep, gliding down again, turning the handle of the door within which the young girl lay, and deliberately setting herself to do what, if she had anticipated any such undertaking at night and alone, would have horrified her, but which, when done, was not so dreadful as was the conclusive proof of her husband's conduct which came with knowing beyond doubt the last chapter of Fanny's story.

Bathsheba's head sank upon her bosom, and the breath which had been bated in suspense, curiosity, and interest, was exhaled now in the form of a whispered wail: "Oh-h-h!" she said, and the silent room added length to her moan.

Her tears fell fast beside the unconscious pair in the coffin: tears of a complicated origin, of a nature indescribable, almost indefinable except as other than those of simple sorrow. Assuredly their wonted fires must have lived in Fanny's ashes when events were so shaped as to chariot her hither in this natural, unobtrusive, yet effectual manner. The one feat alone—that of dying—by which a mean condition could be resolved into a grand one, Fanny had achieved. And to that had destiny subjoined this reencounter to-night, which had, in Bathsheba's wild imagining, turned her companion's failure to success, her humiliation to triumph, her lucklessness to ascendency; it had thrown over herself a garish light of mockery, and set upon all things about her an ironical smile.

The Wife's Handbook by Henry Arthur Allbutt (1888)

Introduction

In this book, Dr. H. Arthur Allbutt follows many of the other guides to health for women in aiming "to save the lives and preserve the health of thousands of women, to rescue from death and disease children who may be born, to teach the young wife how to order her health during the most important period of her life, to remove from her mind the popular ignorance in which she may have been reared, and to enable her to learn truths concerning her duties as wife and mother." As this is not also a guide for women acting as midwives, he generally avoids technical details but includes recipes or specific brands for items women can use when facing mild symptoms in their pregnancy, birth, and postpartum period. He specifically includes miscarriage as a part of pregnancy. The *Handbook* includes a chapter on contraception, which was deemed indecent and cost him his medical license (see more in Chap. 3).

Excerpts from Chapter II: How to Keep the Health During Pregnancy

A woman who desires a good time when she is confined, and to get up well after her confinement, and who also wants to have a fine healthy baby, should be very careful of her health during the nine months of her pregnancy.

A few simple directions as to how she is to regulate her every-day life, and how she is to treat a few of the common ailments of the pregnant state, will not therefore come amiss in this chapter.

As soon as a woman believes herself to be pregnant, she should at once begin to look after her health, and should endeavor to keep in check the various disorders which are apt to arise. Any woman with ordinary common sense need feel no difficulty in doctoring herself for simple troubles. Of course, if anything takes place which alarms her, and which she finds she cannot with confidence attend to herself, then she should call in the doctor and get his advice. But as pregnancy is a perfectly natural condition, no woman of proper formation need fear anything going wrong if she only takes care of herself.

Diet, clothing, rest, fresh air and attention to the bowels are the things mostly to be attended to.

…

If a woman, before the beginning of the seventh month of pregnancy, has a discharge of blood and suffers from bearing-down pains, she is no doubt threatened with an abortion or miscarriage. If the same symptoms occur after the beginning of the seventh month, a premature labor will no doubt take place.

I may remark here that a child born before the beginning of the seventh month cannot live. If born after the beginning of the seventh month it may live with care.

A woman threatened with either a miscarriage or a premature labor should immediately send off for the doctor. She should go to bed and keep perfectly quiet till he arrives. She would do wisely to take about ten drops of laudanum in cold water. All her food and drink should be nearly cold. The lighter her diet is, the better. If flooding should be profuse, I would advise the application of cloths wrung out in cold water to the lower parts of the body. No brandy should betaken, as it usually makes flooding worse.

Some women look upon "a slight miscarriage" with contempt. This is foolish, because if a woman who has miscarried gets up too early she exposes herself to very many serious dangers, such as inflammation of the womb, and putting of the womb out of place. She may also incur the awful risk of blood-poisoning. Therefore, let every woman who has suffered a miscarriage put herself completely in the hands of her doctor, and follow out his instructions to the letter.

Other disorders of pregnancy no woman should try to treat herself, but should obtain medical advice as soon as possible. During pregnancy a woman should avoid, as far as possible, everything of a disagreeable nature, especially unpleasant sights. She should keep her mind free from all harass and care. This is important if she wishes to bear a healthy child.

Excerpts from Chapter IV: After Delivery

The doctor has now left, and the mother is attended to by the nurse or by some intelligent neighbor. Although the pains and perils of pregnancy and labor are past, still for another month great care will be required to keep well and to escape other dangers which accompany the lying-in state.

After the mother has laid quietly for half an hour or so, the nurse should put on her a clean night-dress previously warmed, should again wash the genitals with warm water and Condy's Fluid, should take away the napkins applied by the doctor, and put in their place clean warm ones. She should also arrange her comfortably in bed, drawing from under her any soiled linen, and putting clean sheets, nicely warmed, for her to lie upon. Whilst being made comfortable the mother must on no account sit up. To sit erect immediately after labor is very dangerous.

Whilst speaking of napkins, to apply to the genitals after labor, I would advise all women who can obtain them to use either Southall's "Sanitary Towels," sold by all chemists and ladies' outfitters atone shilling per dozen, or the "Sanitas Towels," which are washable, and which can be obtained at the same places at three shillings per dozen. These two kinds of "Towels" absorb all discharges, and are much more healthful and comfortable than the ordinary napkins. They must, however, never be allowed to remain on too long, so as to become offensive or uncomfortable. Women, during the ordinary monthly flows, will find these Towels far superior to the stiff and unpleasant ordinary napkins.

The mother being settled quietly in bed, and the baby having been washed, the nurse hands it to the mother, who should apply it to her breast for a few moments. The suction at the breast helps the womb to contract, and so keeps off flooding.

The husband may now pay a few minutes' visit to the lying-in room, but the mother must not talk or excite herself. She can have a basin of oatmeal gruel, made half of milk; and a little sleep, if she can afterwards obtain it, will do her good. The body bandage, if it becomes slack, must be tightened.

The room must be kept at a comfortable heat, neither too hot nor too cold. A shilling thermometer, hung on the wall near the bed, will show when the room gets chilly or over-heated. About 65 to 70 degrees is the proper heat at which to keep a lying-in room.

The above directions will, in most cases, suffice for the first few hours after delivery.

There are several things in connection with the lying-in state about which I wish to say a few words, and which it is necessary that the mother, as well as the nurse, should understand.

The management of the after-discharge is very important, and the health of the mother varies according to its condition and quantity. This discharge is called the lochia. As soon as delivery is over, the lochia sets in, and lasts for nearly three weeks. The first three or four days the discharge is almost pure blood. It then becomes thinner, and of a pale red color. In about a week it turns a greenish color, and is then sometimes called "green waters." It continues green till about the end of the third week. Now, it is well to let this discharge run off freely; and after the first two or three days the woman should be allowed to pass water kneeling. This position helps to drain off the discharges which collect in the vaginal passage. She should also sit up in bed several times daily after the first three days, so as to help a free discharge. If the lochia does not run off freely it decomposes in the passage and womb, and gives rise to blood-poisoning and fever. The napkins must be changed often during the day. If the discharge is offensive, or there is not much of it, a wine-glassful of Condy's Fluid must be mixed with half a pint of warm water, and the vagina must be syringed with the mixture night and morning. A Higginson's syringe is the best to use. If there is fever the doctor must be sent for.

After-pains need not cause any fear: they are necessary, and are produced by the womb contracting after labor. Some women have few pains, whilst others suffer sorely. As a rule, women in their first confinement have but few after-pains. It is the mother of many children who suffers. If the womb has contracted well directly after delivery, there will be but little after-pain, because all the clots of blood will have been driven out of the womb, and it is these clots of blood which excite the womb and cause pain.

By putting the baby to the breast within a couple of hours of delivery the womb will contract better, and after-pains will be usually avoided.

A woman should try and bear these pains, unless very excessive, because nature is acting to drive out some clot or other matter from the womb, which, if retained there, would set up fever and inflammation. At most she should do nothing more than take eight or ten drops of laudanum in a little water. It is best, if the pains are very severe, to consult the doctor.

In some first confinements the young mother is unable to pass her water for the first few days. The doctor or nurse may have to draw it away from the bladder through a catheter. This is an operation which gives no pain, and should never be objected to from a sense of false modesty. Many doctors can draw the water without uncovering the patient; and, even in those few cases where it is needful to uncover, there should be no foolish expostulation. The woman must assist her medical man to the best of her ability, and readily place herself in proper position at the edge of the bed, with her knees drawn up.

Suckling should be commenced as soon as possible after the mother is comfortable in bed. The baby applied to the breast within a couple of hours after delivery does a deal of good to the mother. Rarely will flooding take place if this is done, because the act of drawing the breast causes the womb to contract tighter, and so prevents excessive bleeding. If the baby is put to the breast soon, the flow of milk is promoted, and so the breast does not become too full. A long delay in suckling the baby causes the breasts to become full and hard, and then the nipple gets short, and is perhaps drawn in. I have seen many cases where, the baby being fed the first day or two before being put to suck, the breasts have become very full, and the nipples have been drawn quite in; the result being that the nipples could not be drawn out again, the baby was unable to get suck, and, the breasts being too full of milk, milk fever has set in, and an abscess resulted.

…

The mother must keep in bed at least eight or ten days. Getting up too early is apt to bring on "falling of the womb," and, in consequence, life-long discomfort and bad health. She must have no company the first week.

Even when the woman does rise from bed she must be very careful not to engage in household duties for two or three weeks. As much rest as possible for a whole month after the confinement is necessary. It takes the womb a full month to get to its proper size and condition again.

No woman should allow her husband to have sexual connection with her until after the end of the first month from her confinement. On this she must strongly insist. Connection, before the womb has resumed its original condition, is hurtful to the woman's health, and if she should conceive it will be at the cost of future suffering, as the womb would be weakened.

During suckling, husband and wife must not embrace too often, otherwise the milk will be spoilt in quality and the wife's health will suffer. On the other hand, sexual connection at this period, in moderation, is beneficial.

A woman should not let her husband smoke in the lying-in room, or when she is suckling. The tobacco-smoke taken into the blood acts on the milk and poisons the child. Her husband should smoke in another room or out of doors.

No beer or porter must be taken after delivery or during suckling. A woman should not listen to the recommendations of her neighbors on this subject. Wine, spirits, beer and porter all spoil the milk and injure the baby. Mothers who wish to have good milk and strong children must avoid alcohol. A good diet of fresh meat, eggs, milk, puddings and fish will do more to give good milk for nursing than all the stimulants in the world.

After the first month the woman should get out in the fresh air as much as possible.

In concluding this chapter it may be well to give a lying-in woman a few words of advice as to what she is to do if flooding should come on. The doctor must be sent for without a moment's delay. The woman must lie flat on her back with her head lower than her body; she must on no account sit up. She must try and keep from moving about, and must not excite herself. The nurse must put cloths wrung out of cold water to the bottom of the body and to the genitals, renewing them every two or three minutes; she must also press with her hand firmly on the bottom of the body till the doctor comes. Every woman should provide herself before confinement with a tube of Chanteaud's dosimetric granules (small pills) of sulphate of strychnine; and if flooding comes on the nurse must give her two granules every ten minutes till medical advice can be obtained. They act by contracting the womb. These granules can be got from W. J. Bendell, Chemist, 26, Great Bath Street, Clerkenwell; or from E. Yewdall, Leeds; or F. Earle, Hull. The price of a tube containing twenty granules or small pills is sixpence. Drinks of icy cold water may check the flooding. After flooding, nourishing diet will be necessary to restore the strength and make new blood.

Excerpt from Chapter VI: On Some Complaints of Child-Bearing, and Their Treatment

Hysterical Fits are very frequent in women whose blood has become poor, or whose nerves have been weakened. A woman affected with one of these fits will commence with a curious feeling of a ball rising in her throat. She will burst out laughing, sobbing, sighing, moaning, and talking wildly. If the fit is bad she may have convulsions, and to the bystanders may appear to be in a very dangerous condition. If these attacks are not checked, they may become an every-day occurrence, and lead to extreme family unhappiness, and even terminate in a kind of insanity.

Now a woman should try and control her mind, so as not to give way to these attacks. She should try and restore strength to the body and richness to the blood, by fresh air, good diet, and cheerful company. She should take one of the forms of iron mentioned for anaemia, should keep her bowels regular with an aloes and myrrh pill, and should be very careful to have only a moderate amount of sexual connection. If she feels an attack coming on, the best thing she can do is to sponge her face with a little cold water, and take thirty drops of tincture of Valerian in a little water.

Epileptic fits may sometimes be induced as a consequence of the irritations to which the nervous system has been exposed, and by the anaemic condition too frequent pregnancies produce. If once epileptic fits are set up, one never knows when a woman will be free from them. She may have occasional fits for years. Every fit, too, has a tendency to weaken the intellect. Women who suckle for eighteen months or two years often come on with various nervous disorders, and if they become pregnant while suckling, they are apt to sink into a very low state of both mind and body. A woman who has had one fit must put herself in the doctor's hands without delay. She must be careful to keep her bowels regular, and not to eat anything which may cause indigestion or promote the formation of wind in the stomach and bowels.

"The Yellow Wallpaper" and "Why I Wrote 'The Yellow Wallpaper'" by Charlotte Perkins Gilman (1892, 1913)

Introduction

In this short story, Charlotte Perkins Gilman writes from the first-person perspective of a woman who has recently given birth and is in the room of an old mansion her doctor husband has rented for the summer. This story is recognized as a response to physician Silas Weir Mitchell's "rest cure" as a treatment for hysteria. His treatment, which Gilman underwent in 1887, focused on isolating women, forcing rest from intellectual pursuits and physical activity and a strict diet. It relied on the patient becoming childlike in agreeing to the rules. Two decades after the story was published, Gilman described her motivations in writing "The Yellow Wallpaper" in an essay which is included after the story.

"The Yellow Wallpaper" (*The New England Magazine*, January 1892)

It is very seldom that mere ordinary people like John and myself secure ancestral halls for the summer.

A colonial mansion, a hereditary estate, I would say a haunted house, and reach the height of romantic felicity—but that would be asking too much of fate!

Still I will proudly declare that there is something queer about it.

Else, why should it be let so cheaply? And why have stood so long untenanted?

John laughs at me, of course, but one expects that in marriage.

John is practical in the extreme. He has no patience with faith, an intense horror of superstition, and he scoffs openly at any talk of things not to be felt and seen and put down in figures.

John is a physician, and perhaps—(I would not say it to a living soul, of course, but this is dead paper and a great relief to my mind)—perhaps that is one reason I do not get well faster.

You see, he does not believe I am sick!

And what can one do?

If a physician of high standing, and one's own husband, assures friends and relatives that there is really nothing the matter with one but temporary nervous depression—a slight hysterical tendency—what is one to do?

My brother is also a physician, and also of high standing, and he says the same thing.

So I take phosphates or phosphites—whichever it is, and tonics, and journeys, and air, and exercise, and am absolutely forbidden to "work" until I am well again.

Personally, I disagree with their ideas.

Personally, I believe that congenial work, with excitement and change, would do me good.

But what is one to do?

I did write for a while in spite of them; but it does exhaust me a good deal—having to be so sly about it, or else meet with heavy opposition.

I sometimes fancy that in my condition if I had less opposition and more society and stimulus—but John says the very worst thing I can do is to think about my condition, and I confess it always makes me feel bad.

So I will let it alone and talk about the house.

The most beautiful place! It is quite alone, standing well back from the road, quite three miles from the village. It makes me think of English places that you read about, for there are hedges and walls and gates that lock, and lots of separate little houses for the gardeners and people.

There is a delicious garden! I never saw such a garden—large and shady, full of box-bordered paths, and lined with long grape-covered arbors with seats under them.

There were greenhouses, too, but they are all broken now.

There was some legal trouble, I believe, something about the heirs and co-heirs; anyhow, the place has been empty for years.

That spoils my ghostliness, I am afraid; but I don't care—there is something strange about the house—I can feel it.

I even said so to John one moonlight evening, but he said what I felt was a draught, and shut the window.

I get unreasonably angry with John sometimes. I'm sure I never used to be so sensitive. I think it is due to this nervous condition.

But John says if I feel so I shall neglect proper self-control; so I take pains to control myself,—before him, at least,—and that makes me very tired.

I don't like our room a bit. I wanted one downstairs that opened on the piazza and had roses all over the window, and such pretty old-fashioned chintz hangings! but John would not hear of it.

He said there was only one window and not room for two beds, and no near room for him if he took another.

He is very careful and loving, and hardly lets me stir without special direction.

I have a schedule prescription for each hour in the day; he takes all care from me, and so I feel basely ungrateful not to value it more.

He said we came here solely on my account, that I was to have perfect rest and all the air I could get. "Your exercise depends on your strength, my dear," said he, "and your food somewhat on your appetite; but air you can absorb all the time." So we took the nursery, at the top of the house.

It is a big, airy room, the whole floor nearly, with windows that look all ways, and air and sunshine galore. It was nursery first and then playground and gymnasium, I should judge; for the windows are barred for little children, and there are rings and things in the walls.

The paint and paper look as if a boys' school had used it. It is stripped off— the paper—in great patches all around the head of my bed, about as far as I can reach, and in a great place on the other side of the room low down. I never saw a worse paper in my life.

One of those sprawling flamboyant patterns committing every artistic sin.

It is dull enough to confuse the eye in following, pronounced enough to constantly irritate, and provoke study, and when you follow the lame, uncertain curves for a little distance they suddenly commit suicide—plunge off at outrageous angles, destroy themselves in unheard-of contradictions.

The color is repellant, almost revolting; a smouldering, unclean yellow, strangely faded by the slow-turning sunlight.

It is a dull yet lurid orange in some places, a sickly sulphur tint in others.

No wonder the children hated it! I should hate it myself if I had to live in this room long.

There comes John, and I must put this away,—he hates to have me write a word.

We have been here two weeks, and I haven't felt like writing before, since that first day.

I am sitting by the window now, up in this atrocious nursery, and there is nothing to hinder my writing as much as I please, save lack of strength.

John is away all day, and even some nights when his cases are serious.

I am glad my case is not serious!

But these nervous troubles are dreadfully depressing.

John does not know how much I really suffer. He knows there is no reason to suffer, and that satisfies him.

Of course it is only nervousness. It does weigh on me so not to do my duty in any way!

I meant to be such a help to John, such a real rest and comfort, and here I am a comparative burden already!

Nobody would believe what an effort it is to do what little I am able—to dress and entertain, and order things.

It is fortunate Mary is so good with the baby. Such a dear baby!

And yet I cannot be with him, it makes me so nervous.

I suppose John never was nervous in his life. He laughs at me so about this wallpaper!

At first he meant to repaper the room, but afterwards he said that I was letting it get the better of me, and that nothing was worse for a nervous patient than to give way to such fancies.

He said that after the wallpaper was changed it would be the heavy bedstead, and then the barred windows, and then that gate at the head of the stairs, and so on.

"You know the place is doing you good," he said, "and really, dear, I don't care to renovate the house just for a three months' rental."

"Then do let us go downstairs," I said, "there are such pretty rooms there."

Then he took me in his arms and called me a blessed little goose, and said he would go down cellar if I wished, and have it whitewashed into the bargain.

But he is right enough about the beds and windows and things.

It is as airy and comfortable a room as any one need wish, and, of course, I would not be so silly as to make him uncomfortable just for a whim.

I'm really getting quite fond of the big room, all but that horrid paper.

Out of one window I can see the garden, those mysterious deep-shaded arbors, the riotous old-fashioned flowers, and bushes and gnarly trees.

Out of another I get a lovely view of the bay and a little private wharf belonging to the estate. There is a beautiful shaded lane that runs down there from the house. I always fancy I see people walking in these numerous paths and arbors, but John has cautioned me not to give way to fancy in the least. He says that with my imaginative power and habit of story-making a nervous weakness like mine is sure to lead to all manner of excited fancies, and that I ought to use my will and good sense to check the tendency. So I try.

I think sometimes that if I were only well enough to write a little it would relieve the press of ideas and rest me.

But I find I get pretty tired when I try.

It is so discouraging not to have any advice and companionship about my work. When I get really well John says we will ask Cousin Henry and Julia down for a long visit; but he says he would as soon put fire-works in my pillow-case as to let me have those stimulating people about now.

I wish I could get well faster.

But I must not think about that. This paper looks to me as if it knew what a vicious influence it had!

There is a recurrent spot where the pattern lolls like a broken neck and two bulbous eyes stare at you upside-down.

I get positively angry with the impertinence of it and the everlastingness. Up and down and sideways they crawl, and those absurd, unblinking eyes are everywhere. There is one place where two breadths didn't match, and the eyes go all up and down the line, one a little higher than the other.

I never saw so much expression in an inanimate thing before, and we all know how much expression they have! I used to lie awake as a child and get more entertainment and terror out of blank walls and plain furniture than most children could find in a toy-store.

I remember what a kindly wink the knobs of our big old bureau used to have, and there was one chair that always seemed like a strong friend.

I used to feel that if any of the other things looked too fierce I could always hop into that chair and be safe.

The furniture in this room is no worse than inharmonious, however, for we had to bring it all from downstairs. I suppose when this was used as a playroom they had to take the nursery things out, and no wonder! I never saw such ravages as the children have made here.

The wallpaper, as I said before, is torn off in spots, and it sticketh closer than a brother—they must have had perseverance as well as hatred.

Then the floor is scratched and gouged and splintered, the plaster itself is dug out here and there, and this great heavy bed, which is all we found in the room, looks as if it had been through the wars.

But I don't mind it a bit—only the paper.

There comes John's sister. Such a dear girl as she is, and so careful of me! I must not let her find me writing.

She is a perfect, and enthusiastic housekeeper, and hopes for no better profession. I verily believe she thinks it is the writing which made me sick!

But I can write when she is out, and see her a long way off from these windows.

There is one that commands the road, a lovely, shaded, winding road, and one that just looks off over the country. A lovely country, too, full of great elms and velvet meadows.

This wallpaper has a kind of sub-pattern in a different shade, a particularly irritating one, for you can only see it in certain lights, and not clearly then.

But in the places where it isn't faded, and where the sun is just so, I can see a strange, provoking, formless sort of figure, that seems to sulk about behind that silly and conspicuous front design.

There's sister on the stairs!

Well, the Fourth of July is over! The people are gone and I am tired out. John thought it might do me good to see a little company, so we just had mother and Nellie and the children down for a week.

Of course I didn't do a thing. Jennie sees to everything now.

But it tired me all the same.

John says if I don't pick up faster he shall send me to Weir Mitchell in the fall.

But I don't want to go there at all. I had a friend who was in his hands once, and she says he is just like John and my brother, only more so!

Besides, it is such an undertaking to go so far.

I don't feel as if it was worth while to turn my hand over for anything, and I'm getting dreadfully fretful and querulous.

I cry at nothing, and cry most of the time.

Of course I don't when John is here, or anybody else, but when I am alone.

And I am alone a good deal just now. John is kept in town very often by serious cases, and Jennie is good and lets me alone when I want her to.

So I walk a little in the garden or down that lovely lane, sit on the porch under the roses, and lie down up here a good deal.

I'm getting really fond of the room in spite of the wallpaper. Perhaps because of the wallpaper.

It dwells in my mind so!

I lie here on this great immovable bed—it is nailed down, I believe—and follow that pattern about by the hour. It is as good as gymnastics, I assure you. I start, we'll say, at the bottom, down in the corner over there where it has not been touched, and I determine for the thousandth time that I will follow that pointless pattern to some sort of a conclusion.

I know a little of the principle of design, and I know this thing was not arranged on any laws of radiation, or alternation, or repetition, or symmetry, or anything else that I ever heard of.

It is repeated, of course, by the breadths, but not otherwise.

Looked at in one way each breadth stands alone, the bloated curves and flourishes—a kind of "debased Romanesque" with delirium tremens—go waddling up and down in isolated columns of fatuity.

But, on the other hand, they connect diagonally, and the sprawling outlines run off in great slanting waves of optic horror, like a lot of wallowing seaweeds in full chase.

The whole thing goes horizontally, too, at least it seems so, and I exhaust myself in trying to distinguish the order of its going in that direction.

They have used a horizontal breadth for a frieze, and that adds wonderfully to the confusion.

There is one end of the room where it is almost intact, and there, when the cross-lights fade and the low sun shines directly upon it, I can almost fancy radiation after all,—the interminable grotesques seem to form around a common centre and rush off in headlong plunges of equal distraction.

It makes me tired to follow it. I will take a nap, I guess.

I don't know why I should write this.

I don't want to.

I don't feel able.

And I know John would think it absurd. But I must say what I feel and think in some way—it is such a relief!

But the effort is getting to be greater than the relief.

Half the time now I am awfully lazy, and lie down ever so much.

John says I musn't lose my strength, and has me take cod-liver oil and lots of tonics and things, to say nothing of ale and wine and rare meat.

Dear John! He loves me very dearly, and hates to have me sick. I tried to have a real earnest reasonable talk with him the other day, and tell him how I wish he would let me go and make a visit to Cousin Henry and Julia.

But he said I wasn't able to go, nor able to stand it after I got there; and I did not make out a very good case for myself, for I was crying before I had finished.

It is getting to be a great effort for me to think straight. Just this nervous weakness, I suppose.

And dear John gathered me up in his arms, and just carried me upstairs and laid me on the bed, and sat by me and read to me till it tired my head.

He said I was his darling and his comfort and all he had, and that I must take care of myself for his sake, and keep well.

He says no one but myself can help me out of it, that I must use my will and self-control and not let any silly fancies run away with me.

There's one comfort, the baby is well and happy, and does not have to occupy this nursery with the horrid wallpaper.

If we had not used it that blessed child would have! What a fortunate escape! Why, I wouldn't have a child of mine, an impressionable little thing, live in such a room for worlds.

I never thought of it before, but it is lucky that John kept me here after all. I can stand it so much easier than a baby, you see.

Of course I never mention it to them any more,—I am too wise,—but I keep watch of it all the same.

There are things in that paper that nobody knows but me, or ever will.

Behind that outside pattern the dim shapes get clearer every day.

It is always the same shape, only very numerous.

And it is like a woman stooping down and creeping about behind that pattern. I don't like it a bit. I wonder—I begin to think—I wish John would take me away from here!

It is so hard to talk with John about my case, because he is so wise, and because he loves me so.

But I tried it last night.

It was moonlight. The moon shines in all around, just as the sun does.

I hate to see it sometimes, it creeps so slowly, and always comes in by one window or another.

John was asleep and I hated to waken him, so I kept still and watched the moonlight on that undulating wallpaper till I felt creepy.

The faint figure behind seemed to shake the pattern, just as if she wanted to get out.

I got up softly and went to feel and see if the paper did move, and when I came back John was awake.

"What is it, little girl?" he said. "Don't go walking about like that—you'll get cold."

I thought it was a good time to talk, so I told him that I really was not gaining here, and that I wished he would take me away.

"Why darling!" said he, "our lease will be up in three weeks, and I can't see how to leave before.

> The repairs are not done at home, and I cannot possibly leave town just now. Of course if you were in any danger I could and would, but you really are better, dear, whether you can see it or not. I am a doctor, dear, and I know. You are gaining flesh and color, your appetite is better. I feel really much easier about you.

"I don't weigh a bit more," said I, "nor as much; and my appetite may be better in the evening, when you are here, but it is worse in the morning when you are away."

"Bless her little heart!" said he with a big hug; "she shall be as sick as she pleases! But now let's improve the shining hours by going to sleep, and talk about it in the morning!"

"And you won't go away?" I asked gloomily.

"Why, how can I, dear? It is only three weeks more and then we will take a nice little trip of a few days while Jennie is getting the house ready. Really, dear, you are better!"

"Better in body perhaps"—I began, and stopped short, for he sat up straight and looked at me with such a stern, reproachful look that I could not say another word.

"My darling," said he, "I beg of you, for my sake and for our child's sake, as well as for your own, that you will never for one instant let that idea enter your mind! There is nothing so dangerous, so fascinating, to a temperament like yours. It is a false and foolish fancy. Can you not trust me as a physician when I tell you so?"

So of course I said no more on that score, and we went to sleep before long. He thought I was asleep first, but I wasn't,—I lay there for hours trying to decide whether that front pattern and the back pattern really did move together or separately.

On a pattern like this, by daylight, there is a lack of sequence, a defiance of law, that is a constant irritant to a normal mind.

The color is hideous enough, and unreliable enough, and infuriating enough, but the pattern is torturing.

You think you have mastered it, but just as you get well under way in following, it turns a back somersault and there you are. It slaps you in the face, knocks you down, and tramples upon you. It is like a bad dream.

The outside pattern is a florid arabesque, reminding one of a fungus. If you can imagine a toadstool in joints, an interminable string of toadstools, budding and sprouting in endless convolutions,—why, that is something like it.

That is, sometimes!

There is one marked peculiarity about this paper, a thing nobody seems to notice but myself, and that is that it changes as the light changes.

When the sun shoots in through the east window—I always watch for that first long, straight ray—it changes so quickly that I never can quite believe it.

That is why I watch it always.

By moonlight—the moon shines in all night when there is a moon—I wouldn't know it was the same paper.

At night in any kind of light, in twilight, candlelight, lamplight, and worst of all by moonlight, it becomes bars! The outside pattern I mean, and the woman behind it is as plain as can be.

I didn't realize for a long time what the thing was that showed behind,—that dim sub-pattern,—but now I am quite sure it is a woman.

By daylight she is subdued, quiet. I fancy it is the pattern that keeps her so still. It is so puzzling. It keeps me quiet by the hour.

I lie down ever so much now. John says it is good for me, and to sleep all I can.

Indeed, he started the habit by making me lie down for an hour after each meal.

It is a very bad habit, I am convinced, for, you see, I don't sleep.

And that cultivates deceit, for I don't tell them I'm awake,—oh, no!

The fact is, I am getting a little afraid of John.

He seems very queer sometimes, and even Jennie has an inexplicable look.

It strikes me occasionally, just as a scientific hypothesis, that perhaps it is the paper!

I have watched John when he did not know I was looking, and come into the room suddenly on the most innocent excuses, and I've caught him several times looking at the paper! And Jennie too. I caught Jennie with her hand on it once.

She didn't know I was in the room, and when I asked her in a quiet, a very quiet voice, with the most restrained manner possible, what she was doing with the paper she turned around as if she had been caught stealing, and looked quite angry—asked me why I should frighten her so!

Then she said that the paper stained everything it touched, that she had found yellow smooches on all my clothes and John's, and she wished we would be more careful!

Did not that sound innocent? But I know she was studying that pattern, and I am determined that nobody shall find it out but myself!

Life is very much more exciting now than it used to be. You see I have something more to expect, to look forward to, to watch. I really do eat better, and am more quiet than I was.

John is so pleased to see me improve! He laughed a little the other day, and said I seemed to be flourishing in spite of my wallpaper.

I turned it off with a laugh. I had no intention of telling him it was because of the wallpaper—he would make fun of me. He might even want to take me away.

I don't want to leave now until I have found it out. There is a week more, and I think that will be enough.

I'm feeling ever so much better! I don't sleep much at night, for it is so interesting to watch developments; but I sleep a good deal in the daytime.

In the daytime it is tiresome and perplexing.

There are always new shoots on the fungus, and new shades of yellow all over it. I cannot keep count of them, though I have tried conscientiously.

It is the strangest yellow, that wallpaper! It makes me think of all the yellow things I ever saw—not beautiful ones like buttercups, but old foul, bad yellow things.

But there is something else about that paper—the smell! I noticed it the moment we came into the room, but with so much air and sun it was not bad. Now we have had a week of fog and rain, and whether the windows are open or not, the smell is here.

It creeps all over the house.

I find it hovering in the dining-room, skulking in the parlor, hiding in the hall, lying in wait for me on the stairs.

It gets into my hair.

Even when I go to ride, if I turn my head suddenly and surprise it—there is that smell!

Such a peculiar odor, too! I have spent hours in trying to analyze it, to find what it smelled like.

It is not bad—at first, and very gentle, but quite the subtlest, most enduring odor I ever met.

In this damp weather it is awful. I wake up in the night and find it hanging over me.

It used to disturb me at first. I thought seriously of burning the house—to reach the smell.

But now I am used to it. The only thing I can think of that it is like is the color of the paper! A yellow smell.

There is a very funny mark on this wall, low down, near the mopboard. A streak that runs round the room. It goes behind every piece of furniture, except the bed, a long, straight, even smooch, as if it had been rubbed over and over.

I wonder how it was done and who did it, and what they did it for. Round and round and round—round and round and round—it makes me dizzy!

I really have discovered something at last.

Through watching so much at night, when it changes so, I have finally found out.

The front pattern does move—and no wonder! The woman behind shakes it!

Sometimes I think there are a great many women behind, and sometimes only one, and she crawls around fast, and her crawling shakes it all over.

Then in the very bright spots she keeps still, and in the very shady spots she just takes hold of the bars and shakes them hard.

And she is all the time trying to climb through. But nobody could climb through that pattern—it strangles so; I think that is why it has so many heads.

They get through, and then the pattern strangles them off and turns them upside-down, and makes their eyes white!

If those heads were covered or taken off it would not be half so bad.

I think that woman gets out in the daytime!

And I'll tell you why—privately—I've seen her!

I can see her out of every one of my windows!

It is the same woman, I know, for she is always creeping, and most women do not creep by daylight.

I see her on that long shaded lane, creeping up and down. I see her in those dark grape arbors, creeping all around the garden.

I see her on that long road under the trees, creeping along, and when a carriage comes she hides under the blackberry vines.

I don't blame her a bit. It must be very humiliating to be caught creeping by daylight!

I always lock the door when I creep by daylight. I can't do it at night, for I know John would suspect something at once.

And John is so queer now, that I don't want to irritate him. I wish he would take another room! Besides, I don't want anybody to get that woman out at night but myself.

I often wonder if I could see her out of all the windows at once.

But, turn as fast as I can, I can only see out of one at one time.

And though I always see her she may be able to creep faster than I can turn!

I have watched her sometimes away off in the open country, creeping as fast as a cloud shadow in a high wind.

If only that top pattern could be gotten off from the under one! I mean to try it, little by little.

I have found out another funny thing, but I shan't tell it this time! It does not do to trust people too much.

There are only two more days to get this paper off, and I believe John is beginning to notice. I don't like the look in his eyes.

And I heard him ask Jennie a lot of professional questions about me. She had a very good report to give.

She said I slept a good deal in the daytime.

John knows I don't sleep very well at night, for all I'm so quiet!

He asked me all sorts of questions, too, and pretended to be very loving and kind.

As if I couldn't see through him!

Still, I don't wonder he acts so, sleeping under this paper for three months.

It only interests me, but I feel sure John and Jennie are secretly affected by it.

Hurrah! This is the last day, but it is enough. John is to stay in town over night, and won't be out until this evening.

Jennie wanted to sleep with me—the sly thing! but I told her I should undoubtedly rest better for a night all alone.

That was clever, for really I wasn't alone a bit! As soon as it was moonlight, and that poor thing began to crawl and shake the pattern, I got up and ran to help her.

I pulled and she shook, I shook and she pulled, and before morning we had peeled off yards of that paper.

A strip about as high as my head and half around the room.

And then when the sun came and that awful pattern began to laugh at me I declared I would finish it to-day!

We go away to-morrow, and they are moving all my furniture down again to leave things as they were before.

Jennie looked at the wall in amazement, but I told her merrily that I did it out of pure spite at the vicious thing.

She laughed and said she wouldn't mind doing it herself, but I must not get tired.

How she betrayed herself that time!

But I am here, and no person touches this paper but me—not alive!

She tried to get me out of the room—it was too patent! But I said it was so quiet and empty and clean now that I believed I would lie down again and sleep all I could; and not to wake me even for dinner—I would call when I woke.

So now she is gone, and the servants are gone, and the things are gone, and there is nothing left but that great bedstead nailed down, with the canvas mattress we found on it.

We shall sleep downstairs to-night, and take the boat home to-morrow.

I quite enjoy the room, now it is bare again.

How those children did tear about here!

This bedstead is fairly gnawed!

But I must get to work.

I have locked the door and thrown the key down into the front path.

I don't want to go out, and I don't want to have anybody come in, till John comes.

I want to astonish him.

I've got a rope up here that even Jennie did not find. If that woman does get out, and tries to get away, I can tie her!

But I forgot I could not reach far without anything to stand on!

This bed will not move!

I tried to lift and push it until I was lame, and then I got so angry I bit off a little piece at one corner—but it hurt my teeth.

Then I peeled off all the paper I could reach standing on the floor. It sticks horribly and the pattern just enjoys it! All those strangled heads and bulbous eyes and waddling fungus growths just shriek with derision!

I am getting angry enough to do something desperate. To jump out of the window would be admirable exercise, but the bars are too strong even to try.

Besides I wouldn't do it. Of course not. I know well enough that a step like that is improper and might be misconstrued.

I don't like to look out of the windows even—there are so many of those creeping women, and they creep so fast.

I wonder if they all come out of that wallpaper as I did?

But I am securely fastened now by my well-hidden rope—you don't get me out in the road there!

I suppose I shall have to get back behind the pattern when it comes night, and that is hard!

It is so pleasant to be out in this great room and creep around as I please!

I don't want to go outside. I won't, even if Jennie asks me to.

For outside you have to creep on the ground, and everything is green instead of yellow.

But here I can creep smoothly on the floor, and my shoulder just fits in that long smooch around the wall, so I cannot lose my way.

Why, there's John at the door!

It is no use, young man, you can't open it!

How he does call and pound!

Now he's crying for an axe.

It would be a shame to break down that beautiful door!

"John dear!" said I in the gentlest voice, "the key is down by the front steps, under a plantain leaf!"

That silenced him for a few moments.

Then he said—very quietly indeed, "Open the door, my darling!"

"I can't," said I. "The key is down by the front door under a plantain leaf!"

And then I said it again, several times, very gently and slowly, and said it so often that he had to go and see, and he got it, of course, and came in. He stopped short by the door.

"What is the matter?" he cried. "For God's sake, what are you doing!"

I kept on creeping just the same, but I looked at him over my shoulder.

"I've got out at last," said I, "in spite of you and Jane! And I've pulled off most of the paper, so you can't put me back!"

Now why should that man have fainted? But he did, and right across my path by the wall, so that I had to creep over him every time!

"Why I Wrote 'The Yellow Wallpaper'" (*The Forerunner*, October 1913)

Many and many a reader has asked that. When the story first came out, in the *New England Magazine* about 1891, a Boston physician made protest in *The Transcript*. Such a story ought not to be written, he said; it was enough to drive anyone mad to read it.

Another physician, in Kansas I think, wrote to say that it was the best description of incipient insanity he had ever seen, and–begging my pardon– had I been there?

Now the story of the story is this:

> For many years I suffered from a severe and continuous nervous breakdown tending to melancholia–and beyond. During about the third year of this trouble I went, in devout faith and some faint stir of hope, to a noted specialist in nervous diseases, the best known in the country. This wise man put me to bed and applied the rest cure, to which a still-good physique responded so promptly that

he concluded there was nothing much the matter with me, and sent me home with solemn advice to "live as domestic a life as far as possible," to "have but two hours' intellectual life a day," and "never to touch pen, brush, or pencil again" as long as I lived. This was in 1887.

I went home and obeyed those directions for some three months, and came so near the borderline of utter mental ruin that I could see over.

Then, using the remnants of intelligence that remained, and helped by a wise friend, I cast the noted specialist's advice to the winds and went to work again–work, the normal life of every human being; work, in which is joy and growth and service, without which one is a pauper and a parasite–ultimately recovering some measure of power.

Being naturally moved to rejoicing by this narrow escape, I wrote *The Yellow Wallpaper*, with its embellishments and additions, to carry out the ideal (I never had hallucinations or objections to my mural decorations) and sent a copy to the physician who so nearly drove me mad. He never acknowledged it.

The little book is valued by alienists and as a good specimen of one kind of literature. It has, to my knowledge, saved one woman from a similar fate–so terrifying her family that they let her out into normal activity and she recovered.

But the best result is this. Many years later I was told that the great specialist had admitted to friends of his that he had altered his treatment of neurasthenia since reading *The Yellow Wallpaper*.

It was not intended to drive people crazy, but to save people from being driven crazy, and it worked.

"La Belle Zoraïde" by Kate Chopin (1894)

Introduction

The story of Zoraïde is presented in the frame of a bedtime story that Manna Loulou is telling her mistress. In it, Zoraïde is a mixed-race enslaved woman who falls in love with an enslaved man, though Madame Delarivère wishes for her to marry a different man. The resulting pregnancy leads to manipulation by Madame Delarivère that has tragic consequences for Zoraïde.

"La Belle Zoraïde"

The summer night was hot and still; not a ripple of air swept over the marais. Yonder, across Bayou St. John, lights twinkled here and there in the darkness, and in the dark sky above a few stars were blinking. A lugger that had come out of the lake was moving with slow, lazy motion down the bayou. A man in the boat was singing a song.

The notes of the song came faintly to the ears of old Manna Loulou, herself as black as the night, who had gone out upon the gallery to open the shutters wide.

Something in the refrain reminded the woman of an old, half-forgotten Creole romance, and she began to sing it low to herself while she threw the shutters open:—

> "Lisett' to kité la plaine,
> Mo perdi bonhair à moué;
> Ziés à mouésemblé fontaine,
> Dépi mo pa miré toué."

And then this old song, a lover's lament for the loss of his mistress, floating into her memory, brought with it the story she would tell to Madame, who lay in her sumptuous mahogany bed, waiting to be fanned and put to sleep to the sound of one of Manna Loulou's stories. The old negress had already bathed her mistress's pretty white feet and kissed them lovingly, one, then the other. She had brushed her mistress's beautiful hair, that was as soft and shining as satin, and was the color of Madame's wedding-ring. Now, when she reentered the room, she moved softly toward the bed, and seating herself there began gently to fan Madame Delisle.

Manna Loulou was not always ready with her story, for Madame would hear none but those which were true. But to-night the story was all there in Manna Loulou's head—the story of la belle Zoraïde—and she told it to her mistress in the soft Creole patois, whose music and charm no English words can convey.

"La belle Zoraïde had eyes that were so dusky, so beautiful, that any man who gazed too long into their depths was sure to lose his head, and even his heart sometimes. Her soft, smooth skin was the color of café-au-lait. As for her elegant manners, her svelte and graceful figure, they were the envy of half the ladies who visited her mistress, Madame Delarivière.

"No wonder Zoraïde was as charming and as dainty as the finest lady of la rue Royale: from a toddling thing she had been brought up at her mistress's side; her fingers had never done rougher work than sewing a fine muslin seam;

and she even had her own little black servant to wait upon her. Madame, who was her godmother as well as her mistress, would often say to her: —

'Remember, Zoraïde, when you are ready to marry, it must be in a way to do honor to your bringing up. It will be at the Cathedral. Your wedding gown, your corbeille, all will be of the best; I shall see to that myself. You know, M'sieur Ambroise is ready whenever you say the word; and his master is willing to do as much for him as I shall do for you. It is a union that will please me in every way.'

"M'sieur Ambroise was then the body servant of Doctor Langlé. La belle Zoraïde detested the little mulatto,[27] with his shining whiskers like a white man's, and his small eyes, that were cruel and false as a snake's. She would cast down her own mischievous eyes, and say: —

"'Ah, nénaine,[28] I am so happy, so contented here at your side just as I am. I don't want to marry now; next year, perhaps, or the next.' And Madame would smile indulgently and remind Zoraïde that a woman's charms are not everlasting.

"But the truth of the matter was, Zoraïde had seen le beau Mézor dance the Bamboula in Congo Square. That was a sight to hold one rooted to the ground. Mézor was as straight as a cypress-tree and as proud looking as a king. His body, bare to the waist, was like a column of ebony and it glistened like oil.

"Poor Zoraïde's heart grew sick in her bosom with love for le beau Mézor from the moment she saw the fierce gleam of his eye, lighted by the inspiring strains of the Bamboula, and beheld the stately movements of his splendid body swaying and quivering through the figures of the dance.

"But when she knew him later, and he came near her to speak with her, all the fierceness was gone out of his eyes, and she saw only kindness in them and heard only gentleness in his voice; for love had taken possession of him also, and Zoraïde was more distracted than ever. When Mézor was not dancing Bamboula in Congo Square, he was hoeing sugar-cane, barefooted and half naked, in his master's field outside of the city. Doctor Langlé was his master as well as M'sieur Ambroise's.

"One day, when Zoraïde kneeled before her mistress, drawing on Madame's silken stockings, that were of the finest, she said:

"'Nénaine, you have spoken to me often of marrying. Now, at last, I have chosen a husband, but it is not M'sieur Ambroise; it is le beau Mézor that I want and no other.' And Zoraïde hid her face in her hands when she had said

---

[27] A term used to describe someone with one parent of European descent and one parent of African descent.
[28] Translates to "sister".

that, for she guessed, rightly enough, that her mistress would be very angry. And, indeed, Madame Delarivière was at first speechless with rage. When she finally spoke it was only to gasp out, exasperated: —

"'That negro! that negro! Bon Dieu Seigneur,[29] but this is too much!'

"'Am I white, nénaine?' pleaded Zoraïde.

"'You white! Malheureuse![30] You deserve to have the lash laid upon you like any other slave, you have proven yourself no better than the worst.'

"'I am not white,' persisted Zoraïde, respectfully and gently. 'Doctor Langlé gives me his slave to marry, but he would not give me his son. Then, since I am not white, let me have from out of my own race the one whom my heart has chosen.'

"However, you may well believe that Madame would not hear to that. Zoraïde was forbidden to speak to Mézor, and Mézor was cautioned against seeing Zoraïde again. But you know how the negroes are, Ma'zélle Titite," added Manna Loulou, smiling a little sadly. "There is no mistress, no master, no king nor priest who can hinder them from loving when they will. And these two found ways and means.

"When months had passed by, Zoraïde, who had grown unlike herself,— sober and preoccupied,—said again to her mistress:—

"Nénaine, you would not let me have Mézor for my husband; but I have disobeyed you, I have sinned. Kill me if you wish, nénaine: forgive me if you will; but when I heard le beau Mézor say to me, 'Zoraïde, mo l'aime toi,'[31] I could have died, but I could not have helped loving him."

"This time Madame Delarivière was so actually pained, so wounded at hearing Zoraïde's confession, that there was no place left in her heart for anger. She could utter only confused reproaches. But she was a woman of action rather than of words, and she acted promptly. Her first step was to induce Doctor Langlé to sell Mézor. Doctor Langlé, who was a widower, had long wanted to marry Madame Delarivière, and he would willingly have walked on all fours at noon through the Place d'Armes if she wanted him to. Naturally he lost no time in disposing of le beau Mézor, who was sold away into Georgia, or the Carolinas, or one of those distant countries far away, where he would no longer hear his Creole tongue spoken, nor dance Calinda, nor hold la belle Zoraïde in his arms.

---

[29] Translates to "Good god, lord!".
[30] Translates to "unfortunate".
[31] Translates to "I love you".

"The poor thing was heartbroken when Mézor was sent away from her, but she took comfort and hope in the thought of her baby that she would soon be able to clasp to her breast.

"La belle Zoraïde's sorrows had now begun in earnest. Not only sorrows but sufferings, and with the anguish of maternity came the shadow of death. But there is no agony that a mother will not forget when she holds her first-born to her heart, and presses her lips upon the baby flesh that is her own, yet far more precious than her own.

"So, instinctively, when Zoraïde came out of the awful shadow she gazed questioningly about her and felt with her trembling hands upon either side of her. 'Où li, mo piti a moin? where is my little one?' she asked imploringly. Madame who was there and the nurse who was there both told her in turn, 'To piti á toi, li mouri' ('Your little one is dead'), which was a wicked falsehood that must have caused the angels in heaven to weep. For the baby was living and well and strong. It had at once been removed from its mother's side, to be sent away to Madame's plantation, far up the coast. Zoraïde could only moan in reply, 'Li mouri, li mouri,'[32] and she turned her face to the wall.

"Madame had hoped, in thus depriving Zoraïde of her child, to have her young waiting-maid again at her side free, happy, and beautiful as of old. But there was a more powerful will than Madame's at work—the will of the good God, who had already designed that Zoraïde should grieve with a sorrow that was never more to be lifted in this world. La belle Zoraïde was no more. In her stead was a sad-eyed woman who mourned night and day for her baby. 'Li mouri, li mouri,' she would sigh over and over again to those about her, and to herself when others grew weary of her complaint.

"Yet, in spite of all, M'sieur Ambroise was still in the notion to marry her. A sad wife or a merry one was all the same to him so long as that wife was Zoraïde. And she seemed to consent, or rather submit, to the approaching marriage as though nothing mattered any longer in this world.

"One day, a black servant entered a little noisily the room in which Zoraïde sat sewing. With a look of strange and vacuous happiness upon her face, Zoraïde arose hastily. 'Hush, hush,' she whispered, lifting a warning finger, 'my little one is asleep; you must not awaken her.'

"Upon the bed was a senseless bundle of rags shaped like an infant in swaddling clothes. Over this dummy the woman had drawn the mosquito bar, and she was sitting contentedly beside it. It short, from that day Zoraïde was demented. Night nor day did she lose sight of the doll that lay in her bed or in her arms.

---

[32] Translates to "It died, it died".

"And now was Madame stung with sorrow and remorse at seeing this terrible affliction that had befallen her dear Zoraïde. Consulting with Doctor Langlé, they decided to bring back to the mother the real baby of flesh and blood that was now toddling about, and kicking its heels in the dust yonder upon the plantation.

"It was Madame herself who led the pretty, tiny little 'griffe'[33] girl to her mother. Zoraïde was sitting upon a stone bench in the courtyard, listening to the soft splashing of the fountain, and watching the fitful shadows of the palm leaves upon the broad, white flagging.

"'Here,' said Madame, approaching, 'here, my poor dear Zoraïde, is your own little child. Keep her; she is yours. No one will ever take her from you again.'

"Zoraïde looked with sullen suspicion upon her mistress and the child before her. Reaching out a hand she thrust the little one mistrustfully away from her. With the other hand she clasped the rag bundle fiercely to her breast; for she suspected a plot to deprive her of it.

"Nor could she ever be induced to let her own child approach her; and finally the little one was sent back to the plantation, where she was never to know the love of mother or father.

"And now this is the end of Zoraïde's story. She was never known again as la belle Zoraïde, but ever after as Zoraïde la folle (she is now called Zoraïde the Crazy instead of Zoraïde the Beautiful), whom no one ever wanted to marry—not even M'sieur Ambroise. She lived to be an old woman, whom some people pitied and others laughed at—always clasping her bundle of rags—her 'piti.'

"Are you asleep, Ma'zélle Titite?"

"No, I am not asleep; I was thinking. Ah, the poor little one, Man Loulou, the poor little one! better had she died!"

Butthisisthe wayMadameDelisleandMannaLoulou really talkedtoeachother:—

"Vou pré droumi, Ma'zélle Titite?"

"Non, pa pré droumi; mo yapré zongler. Ah, la pauv' piti, Man Loulou. La pauv' piti! Mieux li mouri!"[34]

---

[33] A term used to describe a person believed to be one-quarter European descent and three-quarters African descent.

[34] These two quotations repeat the last two lines of dialogue between Manna Loulou and her mistress in Creole.

"The Curse of Eve" by Arthur Conan Doyle (1894)

Introduction

This short story is from Arthur Conan Doyle's collection *Round the Red Lamp*, which brought together medical stories based on his own professional experience. The story follows a husband, Robert Johnson, on the evening his wife goes into labor with their first child in their home. Johnson seeks the doctor, a specialist, and a medication to be used for pain, encountering various challenges along the way. The story presents childbirth from the perspective of a Victorian husband, who is excluded from the birthing room and worries about the unknowns of the situation within it.

"The Curse of Eve"

Robert Johnson was an essentially commonplace man, with no feature to distinguish him from a million others. He was pale of face, ordinary in looks, neutral in opinions, thirty years of age, and a married man. By trade he was a gentleman's outfitter in the New North Road, and the competition of business squeezed out of him the little character that was left. In his hope of conciliating customers he had become cringing and pliable, until working ever in the same routine from day to day he seemed to have sunk into a soulless machine rather than a man. No great question had ever stirred him. At the end of this snug century, self-contained in his own narrow circle, it seemed impossible that any of the mighty, primitive passions of mankind could ever reach him. Yet birth, and lust, and illness, and death are changeless things, and when one of these harsh facts springs out upon a man at some sudden turn of the path of life, it dashes off for the moment his mask of civilisation and gives a glimpse of the stranger and stronger face below.

Johnson's wife was a quiet little woman, with brown hair and gentle ways. His affection for her was the one positive trait in his character. Together they would lay out the shop window every Monday morning, the spotless shirts in their green cardboard boxes below, the neckties above hung in rows over the brass rails, the cheap studs glistening from the white cards at either side, while in the background were the rows of cloth caps and the bank of boxes in which the more valuable hats were screened from the sunlight. She kept the books and sent out the bills. No one but she knew the joys and sorrows which crept into his small life. She had shared his exultations when the gentleman who was going to India had bought ten dozen shirts and an incredible number of collars, and she had been as stricken as he when, after the goods had gone, the bill was returned from the hotel address with the intimation that no such person had lodged there. For five years they had worked, building up the business, thrown together all the more closely because their marriage had been a childless one. Now, however, there were signs that a change was at hand, and that speedily. She was unable to come downstairs, and her mother, Mrs. Peyton, came over from Camberwell to nurse her and to welcome her grandchild.

Little qualms of anxiety came over Johnson as his wife's time approached. However, after all, it was a natural process. Other men's wives went through it unharmed, and why should not his? He was himself one of a family of fourteen, and yet his mother was alive and hearty. It was quite the exception for anything to go wrong. And yet in spite of his reasonings the remembrance of his wife's condition was always like a sombre background to all his other thoughts.

Dr. Miles of Bridport Place, the best man in the neighbourhood, was retained five months in advance, and, as time stole on, many little packets of absurdly small white garments with frill work and ribbons began to arrive among the big consignments of male necessities. And then one evening, as Johnson was ticketing the scarfs in the shop, he heard a bustle upstairs, and Mrs. Peyton came running down to say that Lucy was bad and that she thought the doctor ought to be there without delay.

It was not Robert Johnson's nature to hurry. He was prim and staid and liked to do things in an orderly fashion. It was a quarter of a mile from the corner of the New North Road where his shop stood to the doctor's house in Bridport Place. There were no cabs in sight so he set off upon foot, leaving the lad to mind the shop. At Bridport Place he was told that the doctor had just gone to Harman Street to attend a man in a fit. Johnson started off for Harman Street, losing a little of his primness as he became more anxious. Two full cabs but no empty ones passed him on the way. At Harman Street he learned that the doctor had gone on to a case of measles, fortunately he had left the address—69 Dunstan Road, at the other side of the Regent's Canal. Robert's primness had vanished now as he thought of the women waiting at home, and he began to run as hard as he could down the Kingsland Road. Some way along he sprang into a cab which stood by the curb and drove to Dunstan Road. The doctor had just left, and Robert Johnson felt inclined to sit down upon the steps in despair.

Fortunately he had not sent the cab away, and he was soon back at Bridport Place. Dr. Miles had not returned yet, but they were expecting him every instant. Johnson waited, drumming his fingers on his knees, in a high, dim lit room, the air of which was charged with a faint, sickly smell of ether. The furniture was massive, and the books in the shelves were sombre, and a squat black clock ticked mournfully on the mantelpiece. It told him that it was half-past seven, and that he had been gone an hour and a quarter. Whatever would the women think of him! Every time that a distant door slammed he sprang from his chair in a quiver of eagerness. His ears strained to catch the deep notes of the doctor's voice. And then, suddenly, with a gush of joy he heard a quick step outside, and the sharp click of the key in the lock. In an instant he was out in the hall, before the doctor's foot was over the threshold.

"If you please, doctor, I've come for you," he cried; "the wife was taken bad at six o'clock."

He hardly knew what he expected the doctor to do. Something very energetic, certainly—to seize some drugs, perhaps, and rush excitedly with him through the gaslit streets. Instead of that Dr. Miles threw his umbrella into the rack, jerked off his hat with a somewhat peevish gesture, and pushed Johnson back into the room.

"Let's see! You DID engage me, didn't you?" he asked in no very cordial voice.

"Oh, yes, doctor, last November. Johnson the outfitter, you know, in the New North Road."

"Yes, yes. It's a bit overdue," said the doctor, glancing at a list of names in a note-book with a very shiny cover. "Well, how is she?"

"I don't—"

"Ah, of course, it's your first. You'll know more about it next time."

"Mrs. Peyton said it was time you were there, sir."

"My dear sir, there can be no very pressing hurry in a first case. We shall have an all-night affair, I fancy. You can't get an engine to go without coals, Mr. Johnson, and I have had nothing but a light lunch."

"We could have something cooked for you—something hot and a cup of tea."

"Thank you, but I fancy my dinner is actually on the table. I can do no good in the earlier stages. Go home and say that I am coming, and I will be round immediately afterwards."

A sort of horror filled Robert Johnson as he gazed at this man who could think about his dinner at such a moment. He had not imagination enough to realise that the experience which seemed so appallingly important to him, was the merest everyday matter of business to the medical man who could not have lived for a year had he not, amid the rush of work, remembered what was due to his own health. To Johnson he seemed little better than a monster. His thoughts were bitter as he sped back to his shop.

"You've taken your time," said his mother-in-law reproachfully, looking down the stairs as he entered.

"I couldn't help it!" he gasped. "Is it over?"

"Over! She's got to be worse, poor dear, before she can be better. Where's Dr. Miles!"

"He's coming after he's had dinner." The old woman was about to make some reply, when, from the half-opened door behind a high whinnying voice cried out for her. She ran back and closed the door, while Johnson, sick at heart, turned into the shop. There he sent the lad home and busied himself frantically in putting up shutters and turning out boxes. When all was closed and finished he seated himself in the parlour behind the shop. But he could not sit still. He rose incessantly to walk a few paces and then fell back into a chair once more. Suddenly the clatter of china fell upon his ear, and he saw the maid pass the door with a cup on a tray and a smoking teapot.

"Who is that for, Jane?" he asked.

"For the mistress, Mr. Johnson. She says she would fancy it."

There was immeasurable consolation to him in that homely cup of tea. It wasn't so very bad after all if his wife could think of such things. So light-hearted was he that he asked for a cup also. He had just finished it when the doctor arrived, with a small black leather bag in his hand.

"Well, how is she?" he asked genially.

"Oh, she's very much better," said Johnson, with enthusiasm.

"Dear me, that's bad!" said the doctor. "Perhaps it will do if I look in on my morning round?"

"No, no," cried Johnson, clutching at his thick frieze overcoat. "We are so glad that you have come. And, doctor, please come down soon and let me know what you think about it."

The doctor passed upstairs, his firm, heavy steps resounding through the house. Johnson could hear his boots creaking as he walked about the floor above him, and the sound was a consolation to him. It was crisp and decided, the tread of a man who had plenty of self-confidence. Presently, still straining his ears to catch what was going on, he heard the scraping of a chair as it was drawn along the floor, and a moment later he heard the door fly open and someone come rushing downstairs. Johnson sprang up with his hair bristling, thinking that some dreadful thing had occurred, but it was only his mother- in- law, incoherent with excitement and searching for scissors and some tape. She vanished again and Jane passed up the stairs with a pile of newly aired linen. Then, after an interval of silence, Johnson heard the heavy, creaking tread and the doctor came down into the parlour.

"That's better," said he, pausing with his hand upon the door. "You look pale, Mr. Johnson."

"Oh no, sir, not at all," he answered deprecatingly, mopping his brow with his handkerchief.

"There is no immediate cause for alarm," said Dr. Miles. "The case is not all that we could wish it. Still we will hope for the best."

"Is there danger, sir?" gasped Johnson.

"Well, there is always danger, of course. It is not altogether a favourable case, but still it might be much worse. I have given her a draught. I saw as I passed that they have been doing a little building opposite to you. It's an improving quarter. The rents go higher and higher. You have a lease of your own little place, eh?"

"Yes, sir, yes!" cried Johnson, whose ears were straining for every sound from above, and who felt none the less that it was very soothing that the doctor should be able to chat so easily at such a time. "That's to say no, sir, I am a yearly tenant."

"Ah, I should get a lease if I were you. There's Marshall, the watchmaker, down the street. I attended his wife twice and saw him through the typhoid when they took up the drains in Prince Street. I assure you his landlord sprung his rent nearly forty a year and he had to pay or clear out."

"Did his wife get through it, doctor?"

"Oh yes, she did very well. Hullo! hullo!"

He slanted his ear to the ceiling with a questioning face, and then darted swiftly from the room.

It was March and the evenings were chill, so Jane had lit the fire, but the wind drove the smoke downwards and the air was full of its acrid taint. Johnson felt chilled to the bone, though rather by his apprehensions than by the weather. He crouched over the fire with his thin white hands held out to the blaze. At ten o'clock Jane brought in the joint of cold meat and laid his place for supper, but he could not bring himself to touch it. He drank a glass of the beer, however, and felt the better for it. The tension of his nerves seemed to have reacted upon his hearing, and he was able to follow the most trivial things in the room above. Once, when the beer was still heartening him, he nerved himself to creep on tiptoe up the stair and to listen to what was going on. The bedroom door was half an inch open, and through the slit he could catch a glimpse of the clean-shaven face of the doctor, looking wearier and more anxious than before. Then he rushed downstairs like a lunatic, and running to the door he tried to distract his thoughts by watching what; was going on in the street. The shops were all shut, and some rollicking boon companions came shouting along from the public-house. He stayed at the door until the stragglers had thinned down, and then came back to his seat by the fire. In his dim brain he was asking himself questions which had never intruded themselves before. Where was the justice of it? What had his sweet, innocent little wife done that she should be used so? Why was nature so cruel? He was frightened at his own thoughts, and yet wondered that they had never occurred to him before.

As the early morning drew in, Johnson, sick at heart and shivering in every limb, sat with his great coat huddled round him, staring at the grey ashes and waiting hopelessly for some relief. His face was white and clammy, and his nerves had been numbed into a half conscious state by the long monotony of misery. But suddenly all his feelings leapt into keen life again as he heard the bedroom door open and the doctor's steps upon the stair. Robert Johnson was precise and unemotional in everyday life, but he almost shrieked now as he rushed forward to know if it were over.

One glance at the stern, drawn face which met him showed that it was no pleasant news which had sent the doctor downstairs. His appearance had altered as much as Johnson's during the last few hours. His hair was on end, his face flushed, his forehead dotted with beads of perspiration. There was a peculiar fierceness in his eye, and about the lines of his mouth, a fighting look as befitted a man who for hours on end had been striving with the hungriest of foes for the most precious of prizes. But there was a sadness too, as though his grim opponent had been overmastering him. He sat down and leaned his head upon his hand like a man who is fagged out.

> I thought it my duty to see you, Mr. Johnson, and to tell you that it is a very nasty case. Your wife's heart is not strong, and she has some symptoms which I do not like. What I wanted to say is that if you would like to have a second opinion I shall be very glad to meet anyone whom you might suggest.

Johnson was so dazed by his want of sleep and the evil news that he could hardly grasp the doctor's meaning. The other, seeing him hesitate, thought that he was considering the expense.

"Smith or Hawley would come for two guineas," said he. "But I think Pritchard of the City Road is the best man."

"Oh, yes, bring the best man," cried Johnson.

"Pritchard would want three guineas. He is a senior man, you see."

"I'd give him all I have if he would pull her through. Shall I run for him?"

"Yes. Go to my house first and ask for the green baize bag. The assistant will give it to you. Tell him I want the A. C. E. mixture. Her heart is too weak for chloroform. Then go for Pritchard and bring him back with you."

It was heavenly for Johnson to have something to do and to feel that he was of some use to his wife. He ran swiftly to Bridport Place, his footfalls clattering through the silent streets and the big dark policemen turning their yellow funnels of light on him as he passed. Two tugs at the night-bell brought down a sleepy, half-clad assistant, who handed him a stoppered glass bottle and a cloth bag which contained something which clinked when you moved it. Johnson thrust the bottle into his pocket, seized the green bag, and pressing his hat firmly down ran as hard as he could set foot to ground until he was in the City Road and saw the name of Pritchard engraved in white upon a red ground. He bounded in triumph up the three steps which led to the door, and as he did so there was a crash behind him. His precious bottle was in fragments upon the pavement.

For a moment he felt as if it were his wife's body that was lying there. But the run had freshened his wits and he saw that the mischief might be repaired. He pulled vigorously at the night-bell.

"Well, what's the matter?" asked a gruff voice at his elbow. He started back and looked up at the windows, but there was no sign of life. He was approaching the bell again with the intention of pulling it, when a perfect roar burst from the wall.

"I can't stand shivering here all night," cried the voice. "Say who you are and what you want or I shut the tube."

Then for the first time Johnson saw that the end of a speaking-tube hung out of the wall just above the bell. He shouted up it,—

"I want you to come with me to meet Dr. Miles at a confinement at once."

"How far?" shrieked the irascible voice.

"The New North Road, Hoxton."

"My consultation fee is three guineas, payable at the time."

"All right," shouted Johnson. "You are to bring a bottle of A. C. E. mixture with you."

"All right! Wait a bit!"

Five minutes later an elderly, hard-faced man, with grizzled hair, flung open the door. As he emerged a voice from somewhere in the shadows cried, —

"Mind you take your cravat, John," and he impatiently growled something over his shoulder in reply.

The consultant was a man who had been hardened by a life of ceaseless labour, and who had been driven, as so many others have been, by the needs of his own increasing family to set the commercial before the philanthropic side of his profession. Yet beneath his rough crust he was a man with a kindly heart.

"We don't want to break a record," said he, pulling up and panting after attempting to keep up with Johnson for five minutes. "I would go quicker if I could, my dear sir, and I quite sympathise with your anxiety, but really I can't manage it."

So Johnson, on fire with impatience, had to slow down until they reached the New North Road, when he ran ahead and had the door open for the doctor when he came. He heard the two meet outside the bed-room, and caught scraps of their conversation. "Sorry to knock you up—nasty case— decent people." Then it sank into a mumble and the door closed behind them.

Johnson sat up in his chair now, listening keenly, for he knew that a crisis must be at hand. He heard the two doctors moving about, and was able to distinguish the step of Pritchard, which had a drag in it, from the clean, crisp sound of the other's footfall. There was silence for a few minutes and then a curious drunken, mumbling sing-song voice came quavering up, very unlike anything which be had heard hitherto. At the same time a sweetish, insidious scent, imperceptible perhaps to any nerves less strained than his, crept down the stairs and penetrated into the room. The voice dwindled into a mere drone and finally sank away into silence, and Johnson gave a long sigh of relief, for he knew that the drug had done its work and that, come what might, there should be no more pain for the sufferer.

But soon the silence became even more trying to him than the cries had been. He had no clue now as to what was going on, and his mind swarmed with horrible possibilities. He rose and went to the bottom of the stairs again. He heard the clink of metal against metal, and the subdued murmur of the doctors' voices. Then he heard Mrs. Peyton say something, in a tone as of fear or expostulation, and again the doctors murmured together. For twenty minutes he stood there leaning against the wall, listening to the occasional rumbles of talk without being able to catch a word of it. And then of a sudden there rose out of the silence the strangest little piping cry, and Mrs. Peyton screamed out in her delight and the man ran into the parlour and flung himself down upon the horse-hair sofa, drumming his heels on it in his ecstasy.

But often the great cat Fate lets us go only to clutch us again in a fiercer grip. As minute after minute passed and still no sound came from above save those thin, glutinous cries, Johnson cooled from his frenzy of joy, and lay breathless with his ears straining. They were moving slowly about. They were talking in subdued tones. Still minute after minute passing, and no word from the voice for which he listened. His nerves were dulled by his night of trouble, and he waited in limp wretchedness upon his sofa. There he still sat when the doctors came down to him—a bedraggled, miserable figure with his face grimy and his hair unkempt from his long vigil. He rose as they entered, bracing himself against the mantelpiece.

"Is she dead?" he asked.

"Doing well," answered the doctor.

And at the words that little conventional spirit which had never known until that night the capacity for fierce agony which lay within it, learned for the second time that there were springs of joy also which it had never tapped before. His impulse was to fall upon his knees, but he was shy before the doctors.

"Can I go up?"

"In a few minutes."

"I'm sure, doctor, I'm very—I'm very—"he grew inarticulate. "Here are your three guineas, Dr. Pritchard. I wish they were three hundred."

"So do I," said the senior man, and they laughed as they shook hands.

Johnson opened the shop door for them and heard their talk as they stood for an instant outside.

"Looked nasty at one time."

"Very glad to have your help."

"Delighted, I'm sure. Won't you step round and have a cup of coffee?"

"No, thanks. I'm expecting another case."

The firm step and the dragging one passed away to the right and the left. Johnson turned from the door still with that turmoil of joy in his heart. He seemed to be making a new start in life. He felt that he was a stronger and a deeper man. Perhaps all this suffering had an object then. It might prove to be a blessing both to his wife and to him. The very thought was one which he would have been incapable of conceiving twelve hours before. He was full of new emotions. If there had been a harrowing there had been a planting too.

"Can I come up?" he cried, and then, without waiting for an answer, he took the steps three at a time.

Mrs. Peyton was standing by a soapy bath with a bundle in her hands. From under the curve of a brown shawl there looked out at him the strangest little red face with crumpled features, moist, loose lips, and eyelids which quivered like a rabbit's nostrils. The weak neck had let the head topple over, and it rested upon the shoulder.

"Kiss it, Robert!" cried the grandmother. "Kiss your son!"

But he felt a resentment to the little, red, blinking creature. He could not forgive it yet for that long night of misery. He caught sight of a white face in the bed and he ran towards it with such love and pity as his speech could find no words for.

"Thank God it is over! Lucy, dear, it was dreadful!"

"But I'm so happy now. I never was so happy in my life."

Her eyes were fixed upon the brown bundle.

"You mustn't talk," said Mrs. Peyton.

"But don't leave me," whispered his wife.

So he sat in silence with his hand in hers. The lamp was burning dim and the first cold light of dawn was breaking through the window. The night had been long and dark but the day was the sweeter and the purer in consequence. London was waking up. The roar began to rise from the street. Lives had come and lives had gone, but the great machine was still working out its dim and tragic destiny.

"Progress Made in the Treatment of the Diseases of Women" by Charles Jewett (1895)

Introduction

The by-line to this essay describes Dr. Charles Jewett's position as Professor of Obstetrics and Diseases of Children at Long Island College Hospital in Brooklyn, New York. His position as a distinguished educator in the field offers a clear view of the changes in treatment and outcomes for women in childbirth over the preceding decades and leads to his pride in the work of Americans in women's health. This piece was published in *The Independent*, a weekly miscellany magazine that brought his medical perspective to a general audience.

"Progress Made in the Treatment of the Diseases of Women" (*The Independent*, 12 September 1895)

Great progress has been made in the treatment of feminine diseases during the past twenty-five years, especially from the surgical point of view. Marked improvements have made in surgery as related to obstetrics and gynecology. This statement is particularly true in reference to the treatment of what is called extra-uterine pregnancy and of the treatment of labor in contracted pelvis. Only twenty years ago hundreds of women bled to death from the rupture of extra-uterine pregnancy. At that time there were no surgeons who were bold enough to perform the necessary operation. At the present time, on the occurrence of such a rupture, the abdomen is opened and the bleeding is stopped; in this way a large proportion of lives have been saved. It may also be said that the operative methods for dealing with the different phases of extra-uterine pregnancy have undergone very important modifications within the last few years, and there is a corresponding gain in the number of lives saved.

In the case of contracted pelvis, what is called the operation of the Cesarean section, has been so perfected that the lives of more than ninety per cent. of women operated upon, can be saved under this operation, while, twenty years ago, the patients rarely survived. Another operation has been added to the methods of treating labor in contracted pelvis. This is called symphyseotomy, an operation which was practiced years ago, but has become obsolete. It has been revived and re-adopted by surgeons all over the world. This has only occurred within the last three years, and is an operation of great life-saving value. When first introduced it was practiced without the aid of the antiseptic methods, and the results were so bad that it had to be abandoned. Symphyseotomy performed according to the antiseptic methods of the present day, competes, in importance, with the Cesarean section, in properly selected cases.

One of the most important advances made in obstetric practice relates to the management of common, normal labor. Formerly the death rate after labor from child-bed fever was very great, sometimes reaching ten and twenty percent, in hospital epidemics, To-day the death rate from this cause in the well-managed hospitals and the best private practice is less than one-half of one per cent. This decrease has been brought about by the perfected antiseptic practice in modern obstetrics.

The late Professor Huxley, it is said, once stated that the civilized woman ought to be able to bear children as easily as the savage woman. It must be remembered that the civilized woman does not lead the same kind of life as her savage sister. While child bearing is a natural, physiological process, as a matter of fact, with most of our patients it is a process that borders very closely on the pathological; that is, it exhibits a dangerous condition because of the fact that women are not always well able to resist the dangers that confront them at such a time. It would hardly be expected that women in civilized, polite society could meet such a condition as readily as the savage woman; but it is not true that savage women are entirely free from suffering at such a time. The observations of intelligent travelers, who have studied this subject among the Eskimos and among savage races generally, go to show that a large proportion of childbirths among primitive people are painful. Among such women there are, as in civilized life, cases of contracted pelvis; and of course, such cases are not managed as well among them as they are in a community where educated physicians can be found. But I suppose, as a rule, in the case of simple labor the savage woman passes through the ordeal with less pain and trouble than her civilized sister.

In the special treatment of women the improvements along the medical line have been in the direction of a practice founded on a scientific basis. The activity of research, both in surgery and medicine, the cumulative progress that is belong made from year to year, is infinitely greater than it was twenty years ago.

…

It is pleasing to our national pride to know that the leading surgeons of the world in gynecology are Americans. They can stand against the world when it comes to the actual practice of the profession. The Germans are in the front rank as discoverers; but I think American surgeons are their superiors in practical skill. The teaching of gynecology and obstetrics to students and young physicians has made enormous strides during the last quarter of a century. One of the principal reasons for this has been, there has been a larger amount of bed-side instruction, In other words, the teaching of to-day results in producing practical obstetricians and gynecologists, while, in former times, the knowledge acquired by the college graduate was almost wholly theoretical.

Some idea can be formed of the improvement in medical teaching when it is remembered that twenty years ago it only required two courses of study of three months each to graduate physician, tho of course he was supposed to be engaged in the study of it three years in the intervals of his college attendance. To-day the requirement in our colleges is nine months of study annually for from three to four years.

The standard of general knowledge required of young men who desire to enter the profession is much higher than it was in former times. In New York State the young man who begins the study of medicine must have an educational preparation equivalent to that required for a college course.

The Awakening by Kate Chopin (1899)

Introduction

This novel by Kate Chopin is set in New Orleans and a resort in Grand Isle, Louisiana, focusing on the protagonist Edna Pontellier from a third-person perspective. Throughout the novel, Edna engages with her neighbor Madame Ratignolle, who is a doting mother and pregnant with another child. This is in direct contract with Edna's ambivalence about motherhood. In these scenes, from late in the novel, Madame Ratignolle goes into labor and requests Edna's presence at the birth.

Excerpt from Chapter XXXVI

There was a knock at the door. Old Celestine came in to say that Madame Ratignolle's servant had come around the back way with a message that Madame had been taken sick[35] and begged Mrs. Pontellier to go to her immediately.

"Yes, yes," said Edna, rising; "I promised. Tell her yes—to wait for me. I'll go back with her."

…

Excerpt from Chapter XXXVII

Edna looked in at the drug store. Monsieur Ratignolle was putting up a mixture himself, very carefully, dropping a red liquid into a tiny glass. He was grateful to Edna for having come; her presence would be a comfort to his wife. Madame Ratignolle's sister, who had always been with her at such trying times, had not been able to come up from the plantation, and Adèle had been inconsolable until Mrs. Pontellier so kindly promised to come to her. The nurse had been with them at night for the past week, as she lived a great distance away. And Dr. Mandelet had been coming and going all the afternoon. They were then looking for him any moment.

Edna hastened upstairs by a private stairway that led from the rear of the store to the apartments above. The children were all sleeping in a back room. Madame Ratignolle was in the salon, whither she had strayed in her suffering impatience. She sat on the sofa, clad in an ample white *peignoir*,[36] holding a handkerchief tight in her hand with a nervous clutch. Her face was drawn and pinched, her sweet blue eyes haggard and unnatural. All her beautiful hair had been drawn back and plaited. It lay in a long braid on the sofa pillow, coiled like a golden serpent. The nurse, a comfortable looking Griffe woman in white apron and cap, was urging her to return to her bedroom.

"There is no use, there is no use," she said at once to Edna. "We must get rid of Mandelet; he is getting too old and careless. He said he would be here at half-past seven; now it must be eight. See what time it is, Joséphine."

---

[35] Had gone into labor.
[36] Dressing gown.

The woman was possessed of a cheerful nature, and refused to take any situation too seriously, especially a situation with which she was so familiar. She urged Madame to have courage and patience. But Madame only set her teeth hard into her under lip, and Edna saw the sweat gather in beads on her white forehead. After a moment or two she uttered a profound sigh and wiped her face with the handkerchief rolled in a ball. She appeared exhausted. The nurse gave her a fresh handkerchief, sprinkled with cologne water.

"This is too much!" she cried. "Mandelet ought to be killed! Where is Alphonse? Is it possible I am to be abandoned like this—neglected by every one?"

"Neglected, indeed!" exclaimed the nurse. Wasn't she there? And here was Mrs. Pontellier leaving, no doubt, a pleasant evening at home to devote to her? And wasn't Monsieur Ratignolle coming that very instant through the hall? And Joséphine was quite sure she had heard Doctor Mandelet's coupé. Yes, there it was, down at the door.

Adèle consented to go back to her room. She sat on the edge of a little low couch next to her bed.

Doctor Mandelet paid no attention to Madame Ratignolle's upbraidings. He was accustomed to them at such times, and was too well convinced of her loyalty to doubt it.

He was glad to see Edna, and wanted her to go with him into the salon and entertain him. But Madame Ratignolle would not consent that Edna should leave her for an instant. Between agonizing moments, she chatted a little, and said it took her mind off her sufferings.

Edna began to feel uneasy. She was seized with a vague dread. Her own like experiences seemed far away, unreal, and only half remembered. She recalled faintly an ecstasy of pain, the heavy odor of chloroform, a stupor which had deadened sensation, and an awakening to find a little new life to which she had given being, added to the great unnumbered multitude of souls that come and go.

She began to wish she had not come; her presence was not necessary. She might have invented a pretext for staying away; she might even invent a pretext now for going. But Edna did not go. With an inward agony, with a flaming, outspoken revolt against the ways of Nature, she witnessed the scene of torture.

She was still stunned and speechless with emotion when later she leaned over her friend to kiss her and softly say good-by. Adèle, pressing her cheek, whispered in an exhausted voice: "Think of the children, Edna. Oh think of the children! Remember them!"

"Small vs. Large Families" by Ida Husted Harper (1901)

Introduction

In this essay for the weekly magazine *The Independent*, journalist and suffragist Ida Husted Harper describes the complicated issues facing women (and their husbands) who want few children. She specifically quotes from husbands on their reasons for limiting their family size, which mostly center on the suffering of women in childbirth. Harper's perspective on women's rights is clear throughout, with an interest in women's education and intellectual pursuits, though she also emphasizes the risk of illness or death that accompanies childbirth.

Excerpt from "Small vs. Large Families" (*The Independent*, 26 December 1901)

The point for consideration is simply this—that, in all this protest against the higher education, woman is not considered as an individual, but solely in relation to wifehood and motherhood. There is no recognition of the great pleasure and benefit she will derive from it, and no anxiety in regard to her health as it will affect her own comfort and happiness, but only as it may interfere with her becoming the wife of some man and the mother of his children. Woman never has attempted one advanced step which has not been blocked by these two words—wifehood and motherhood. In olden times the position of the "spinster" was so intolerable that she was glad to find refuge behind this barrier, but in the new freedom which has come to the unmarried woman she is ordering her own life according to her own ideas. When men would deprive her of a university education lest it should interfere with the functions of marriage, she says, "Very well; if I must choose I will take the education and remain single;" and in books, writing, art, music, travel, and, perhaps, a profession, she finds a very acceptable substitute. Marriage, nowadays, is by no means so necessary to women as men are apt to think; and while, if all the conditions were favorable, the average woman might prefer to be married, she may not consider it worth the sacrifices which are oftentimes required. The number of educated women who take this position is apt to increase so long as men continue to insist on a certain amount of ignorance and a strong constitution as the essentials of matrimony. After a while, when they become liberal enough and wise enough to make intellectual companionship, sympathy of thought and congeniality in tastes the prominent features, they may be able to convince such women of its great advantages.

There is another phase of this question which is being continually obtruded by men, viz.: The disinclination of women who do marry to have a number of children, or, in some cases, to have any, but in all of this one-sided discussion, for women themselves take no part in it in it, one indisputable fact is wholly ignored—that where there are one hundred wives who desire few or no children, there can be husbands of the same mind. There could be no greater injustice than to hold wives alone responsible for the failure to have a family. The mother instinct is much stronger in woman than is the father instinct in man, and, notwithstanding the far greater liabilities incurred by the wife, there is no hesitation in saying that as a rule she would be willing to assume them if there was a great desire for children on the part of the husband. But there is not. The average man does not want the burden of a large family, and there are many husbands who object for other reasons. With an apology for being personal the writer will mention several examples among her own acquaintances.

...

Another, the wealthy president of a corporation, also with one son, declared: "I would give half I am worth for a daughter, but when I saw what my wife endured before our boy was born, at the time and afterward, I thought, 'Not for ten times what I am worth would I ever allow this again.'"

A professional man of much refinement and sensibility said with emotion: "I would be willing to give my own life to save my wife from pain and sorrow and, much as I love children, I will do without them forever rather than permit her to pass through the necessary ordeal."

Still another, with a beautiful home and spacious grounds which would be paradise for children, said, when some one.suggested this: "My first wife died in childbirth. When I married the second I resolved that there should not be another sacrifice."

These instances might be multiplied. They will touch a responsive chord in the heart of more than one man who reads them, and admit that it is husbands as well as wives who are responsible for the small families of the present day.

When men criticise women so severely for avoiding maternity do they ever stop to consider what they themselves would do in her place? A man in New York, not long ago, sent the writer of this a letter regarding something which she had published, in which, in a burst of rage, he declared that all the "crimes against women," for which men are punished, are offset by the refusal of women to bear children, for which they are not punished. He would like a law to punish them.

It is only in recent years, since there has been a decrease in the number of children, that the life insurance companies will insure women. They refused on account of the terrible mortality in childbirth, which, as the ages go by, counts more victims than all the wars. Is it not asking a great deal of a woman to face death deliberately every few years from youth to middle age? We laud the soldier to the skies who risks his life in battle, but we take it as a matter of course that women should be continually putting their lives in peril, year after year, mother, daughter, granddaughter, from generation to generation, for all time.

Putting aside, however, the danger, the suffering, and all the intermediate inconveniences, think what it means for a woman to give the core of her life, the beautiful years between twenty and forty-five, the time when the mental powers are at their best, when enjoyment in the pleasant things of the world is keenest, to the exacting demands of the nursery. The society of little children has much in it that is sweet, but it is not mentally stimulating, and there is nothing that so wears on the nerves as to have their constant care. It would drive a man insane, and he would welcome a change to mining coal or excavating the New York tunnel. There never was a mother of a large family who was willing that her daughters should have a similar experience.

Women are encouraged with the assurance that motherhood is regarded as the most sacred office in the world. That is not true. Motherhood is only considered sacred when it is preceded by wifehood. Without this it is looked upon as a disgrace. The unmarried mother is repudiated by the whole world, including the father of her child. It is only when a woman has been consecrated to the one man and bears children who are to perpetuate his name and family that her "motherhood" becomes sacred either to the Church, the State, or the man himself. The most sacred thing about maternity is the divine love of the mother for her child, and in this she needs no instruction. There is no human being, however, who has the right to dictate to her the number of children she shall bear. The vast majority of, women gladly devote the years necessary to rearing two or three, but when there is a demand that they shall give up their entire life they object.

Woman in Girlhood, Wifehood, Motherhood by Myer Solis-Cohen (1906)

Introduction

In this popular guide, Dr. Myer Solis-Cohen addresses the health needs of women at all stages of life, though with more emphasis on beauty and wellness, which is the focus of the book's first section. Solis-Cohen opens with a preface that describes the purpose of explaining the components of health and wellness that a physician may not describe in detail, as he only attends a patient when she is sick or she forgets to ask the doctor during the visit. He seeks "to give all the information a woman requires for any of the emergencies that may occur during her own life and for the preservation of health and beauty," including her "childhood, maidenhood, wifehood and motherhood" and detailed coverage of childbirth and care for a baby. He distinguishes his volume by the fact that it is "accurate" and "has avoided generalities [to provide] directions [that are] pointed and definite."

Excerpts from Chapter XVI: The Symptoms of Pregnancy

As a rule, it is not a difficult matter to determine whether a woman is pregnant, although cases have occurred in which mistakes were made. Physicians have operated on a supposed abdominal tumor only to find a pregnant uterus.

There are certain symptoms, however, which are usually present in a woman who is with child. But they may occur in conditions other than pregnancy, and they may be absent, though the woman be "in a family way." The physician is the only person who is competent to decide.

The Commonest Symptoms of Pregnancy. — The most common symptoms of pregnancy experienced by the mother are (1) cessation of menstruation, (2) "morning sickness," (3) changes in the size, shape and appearance of the abdomen, (4) changes in the breasts, and (5) quickening.

...

The Occurrence of Quickening

A living fetus, or unborn child, moves about within the womb, but not until about midway between the fourth and fifth months are the movements powerful enough to be felt by the mother. The sensation the mother experiences when the fetus moves is called "quickening." It has been felt as early as the third month, but may not be noticed at all until the last month. During the advanced stages of pregnancy fetal movements can usually be felt by a person laying a cold hand suddenly upon the woman's abdomen. There are two kinds of sensations conveyed to the hand: a heaving and a sensation compared to that of a finger-tap under a blanket.

Necessarily, movements are never felt when the fetus is dead. They may be undetected even when it is living. There are many things, moreover, which may simulate these movements and thus lead one astray.

Alterations in the Nervous System

A pregnant woman usually exhibits some disorder of the nervous system, becoming more sensitive and irritable. Her disposition may change from placidity to vivacity, or from amiability to sullenness or moroseness. Sometimes the moral nature is affected, with impairment of the ability to distinguish between right and wrong. The appetite may become very fanciful and the most unusual articles of diet may be craved. Often a woman experiences a sense of dizziness or a feeling as if she were going to faint, or she may even lose consciousness. Neuralgia, especially of the face and teeth, is not uncommon.

Excerpts from Chapter XIX: Preparations for the Confinement

In preparing for the confinement, one should know what is best to do and, if possible, put that knowledge into practice. But, unfortunately, a woman is not always able to do as she wishes. The best is oftentimes unattainable, in which case the best under the circumstances must suffice. Whenever possible the directions given in this chapter should be implicitly followed; they are simple and necessary. However, persons who for any reason are unable to adopt the first and best suggestions made may be able to carry out the simpler methods also given, which, though less desirable, are yet serviceable and good.

The Lying-In Room

The room usually selected for the confinement is the prospective mother's own bed-room. It ought to be large and sunny, well lighted, well ventilated and properly heated. A communicating room for the nurse is a great convenience, leaving the mother the exclusive use of her own. Matters are also made easier if the bath-room be near. All unnecessary furniture, heavy curtains, and all bric-a-brac should be removed. If a carpet is on the floor it may be taken up, or the portion about the bed may be protected by a large rubber mackintosh, or oilcloth, or by several layers of newspaper. A rug should be removed. It is well to take out of the room anything that might collect dust, which often is a carrier of disease germs.

....

Engaging the Physician and Nurse

The Accoucheur. — As soon as pregnancy is suspected, the physician should be engaged. He should have general supervision over the life of the woman, her diet, clothing, exercise, and so forth, during the whole period between conception and labor.

Pregnancy, although usually a normal process, is subject to various complications, for whose recognition and treatment a physician is required. The kidneys, in particular, need constant watching, as they frequently become affected during this period. A four-ounce specimen of mixed night and morning urine should be sent to the physician for examination every two weeks until the last month, when it should be sent every week. A statement of the exact amount of urine passed, during the twenty-four hours should accompany the specimen.

When such symptoms as scanty urination, severe headache, dizziness, or swelling of the feet or face occur, they should be reported to the physician at once.

A *midwife*, in the opinion of the writer, is not desirable, except in those cases where it is impossible to secure the services of a physician or a medical student. The midwife rarely understands the meaning of surgical cleanliness, which is the most important factor in preventing infection or blood-poisoning. She, moreover, is unable to meet the various complications as they arise, but always must send out for a doctor, who often arrives too late. Promptness at such a time in recognizing and meeting a serious condition is all-important.

The Nurse. — A woman must choose between a trained nurse and the so-called monthly nurse.

A *trained nurse* or graduate nurse, one who has completed a course of training in a hospital, should be procured if she can be afforded. Such a person not only has the requisite knowledge as well as experience, but she has learned how to obey the orders of the physician.

The *monthly nurse*, on the other hand, has not had careful hospital training, being merely a woman who makes a practice of nursing maternity cases for thirty days. Nevertheless she often has acquired skill and experience with constant practice. Some monthly nurses, indeed, are very capable, and many are adaptable and able to carry out the doctor's orders in an intelligent manner. Frequently, however, they are filled with wrong ideas and queer, old-fashioned notions about the care both of mother and baby. Oftentimes they feel their experience to be of such great importance that they pay no attention to the advice or orders of the physician; they regard the care of the patients as their own particular business rather than the doctor's. In consequence, the monthly nurse is often directly responsible for much injury to mother and child. Still she is always a great help in the absence of any one better, and she is all the majority of women are able to afford.

The selection of a nurse should receive careful consideration. The woman must be known to be competent. It is not safe to employ a woman who is not known. Often the physician is able to recommend some one in whom he has confidence. In addition to ability, the nurse must have certain favorable personal qualities. She must be able to adapt herself to circumstances, to improvise when she cannot procure the object she requires. She also must possess tact, so as to get along with the family and the servants. Honesty and honor are two necessary traits: the first, because the nurse sometimes is almost in charge of the house and always has access to every part; the second, because there is no family secret kept from the nurse, no skeleton she does not see.

The duties of the nurse comprise everything that has to do with the care of both patients. She tends to the mother, washes her, arranges her meals, and so on, and at the same time takes charge of the baby, bathing it and caring for it in every way.

The nurse, ordinarily, does not perform any work outside of her own particular duties. She is not expected to wash the baby's clothes, with the exception of the diapers and flannels, nor wash her own garments, nor do the general cooking or sewing or cleaning. She may do all these, however, if she be so disposed, or if she be engaged with that understanding. The patient's meals, however, she is supposed to prepare. Where no servants are kept, the monthly nurse often prepares the meals for the family, and when not engaged in caring for her patients may tend to some of the other household duties.

The nurse must be properly cared for, in order that she maintain her own health as well as keep at the highest point of efficiency. Provision should be made for her obtaining sufficient sleep and getting some outdoor exercise every day. It is in relieving the nurse at such times that solicitous relatives can be of most service.

The nurse should be engaged several months before the expected confinement. At this time all arrangements about the work to be done and the compensation to be received should be definitely settled.

As the day for the confinement approaches, the nurse should be within reach, and a few days beforehand, especially if the patient has already borne children, she should go to the house and remain there until after the confinement. She should, of course, be able to recognize the signs of labor and to know when to send for the physician. As soon as the process has begun she should arrange the bed and prepare the patient.

Excerpts from Chapter XXI: The Management of Labor

It is not the author's purpose in this chapter to write a treatise on obstetrics. Nor is it his intention to so instruct a woman that she will be qualified to assume full charge of a labor. It must not be supposed that with a few minutes' reading a person can become proficient in what requires years of study and practice to acquire. The delivery of the child, known also as child-birth, labor, obstetrics, parturition, midwifery and tokology, is too serious a procedure to be entrusted to any but the most skillful hands. A physician should be engaged whenever possible; next in order of proficiency come the medical student and the midwife.

In assisting the physician, however, a woman can be of great service, especially if she is familiar with the work required of her. The present chapter will be devoted to instructing a woman in the requisite knowledge that will make her presence valuable in the lying-in room.

…

The Diagnosis of Labor

It is important for a woman to be able to recognize when she is in labor, in order, on the one hand, to summon the physician in time, and on the other to avoid ludicrous mistakes.

"Dropping." — A valuable premonitory sign is the "dropping" or sinking of the child's head in the pelvis, which is associated with a flattening of the upper part of the abdomen and a greater prominence of the lower portion. This may occur over night at the beginning of the last month of pregnancy in women who have never borne children, and two weeks or less before labor in a woman who is already a mother.

Labor Pains. — The sign that labor has actually begun is the occurrence of labor pains. These are of a characteristic duration, situation and nature. They last but a minute and are separated by intervals of from five minutes to half an hour, being usually about fifteen minutes apart. The pain is felt in the abdomen or in the back, or it may seem to pass from the navel to the spine.

The Show. — As the neck of the womb stretches, there is a slight oozing of blood which stains the large plug of mucus that fills the cervical canal. With the further dilation of the neck or cervix this blood-stained plug of mucus is expelled, when it is known as the "show."

…

Surgical Cleanliness the Guiding Factor Throughout Labor

A Talk on Germs. — Disease germs or bacteria are very minute; thousands could be present on the head of a pin without being seen with the naked eye. These microscopic organisms multiply with great rapidity; in the course of several hours two or three individuals can increase to billions. Whenever disease germs get inside the body they manufacture a poison which may produce disease and even cause death. While dangerous wherever found, they are especially so in certain localities, such as the interior of the womb and of the abdomen, in the latter place giving rise to peritonitis.

The introduction of a disease germ into the body is called infection. The presence of such a germ in the body is known as sepsis. Any article that has a germ on it is said to be infected or septic. By disinfecting or sterilizing an object we remove all germs from it and render it aseptic, sterile or surgically clean. There is consequently an important difference between ordinary cleanliness and surgical cleanliness. The former signifies that all dirt has been removed; the latter that all germs as well as dirt are absent.

How the Birth Canal Becomes Infected. — Disease germs are never normally present in any of a woman's organs of generation. They must come from without. When present in any part of the birth canal they have as a rule been introduced by the finger or hand, by an implement or instrument, or by the water. They can, however, themselves effect an entrance if deposited upon the external parts by one of the agents mentioned or by the bed linen, the body clothing, the mattress, the vulvar pads or by the material used to wash the vulva or external parts (rags, cloths, sponges, cotton, etc.). As soon as any germs have been introduced into the birth canal they are liable to multiply and cause both a local inflammation and a poisoning of the whole system. Such a condition occurring after labor is known to physicians as puerperal infection, puerperal sepsis or puerperal fever, and more popularly as child-bed fever or blood poisoning.

At any time other than during labor or shortly after it, the introduction of germs into the vagina is not attended with such serious results, because the cervix or neck of the womb is usually tightly closed and shuts off the germs from the parts above. But during the period from the beginning of labor, when the cervix begins to dilate, to the end of the puerperium, when it has firmly contracted again, a germ can easily travel through the open neck, then out the tube, and finally enter the abdominal cavity. In the womb the germ produces a septic inflammation; in the tube it may cause an inflammation, going on to the formation of an abscess known as a pus tube; in the abdomen it will set up a peritonitis. All these conditions give rise to blood poisoning.

Puerperal Infection Can Always be Prevented. — Knowing how child-bed fever is caused, it is possible to prevent it. If germs are never introduced into the birth canal they can do no damage there. The entrance of germs is prevented by not inserting into the vagina of a woman in labor, or even bringing in contact with the parts, anything that is not surgically clean. Some women indeed are lucky and may have germs introduced without suffering any evil consequences. But the majority are bound to pay the penalty. Most of the deaths that have occurred during or shortly after child-birth have been caused by puerperal infection, a preventable disease. If a woman should regard the precautions given in this chapter as being too troublesome and "fussy," let her reflect that they save human lives. Anything less is fraught with danger. No better picture of the result of carelessness and negligence can be given than the one presented by the physician and man of letters, Oliver Wendell Holmes:

"It is as a lesson," he says, "rather than as a reproach, that I call up the memory of the irreparable errors and wrongs. No tongue can tell the heart-breaking calamity they have caused. They have closed the eyes just opened upon a new world of love and happiness; they have bowed the strength of manhood into the dust; they have cast the helplessness of infancy into the stranger's arms, or bequeathed it, with less cruelty, the death of its dying parent. There is no tone deep enough for regret, and no voice loud enough for warning."

How to Prevent Puerperal Infection. — The only way to prevent puerperal infection is to keep disease germs out of the woman's vagina. This is accomplished by observing surgical cleanliness or asepsis. Nothing that is not sterile must enter the birth canal. In addition to this there must be ordinary cleanliness in everything concerning the woman. It is partly on account of their knowledge of asepsis that the physician is to be preferred to the midwife and the trained nurse to the monthly nurse.

All the directions given in Chapter XIX concerning the preparations for the confinement are to be rigorously followed: the room, the bed and the dressings should be made ready in the manner described. The rules laid down in this and the following chapter must be obeyed to the letter. Only water that has been boiled may be used about the patient, even when it is to be made up into a disinfectant solution. All articles that come in contact with the woman in labor should be boiled for at least five minutes, or if boiling would injure them they should be immersed for half an hour in a disinfectant solution, such as bichlorid of mercury 1 to 1000 or carbolic acid 1 to 20.

But it is not sufficient that everything employed about a woman in labor be rendered aseptic; it must be kept so. The moment a sterile object touches something that is not sterile the object is itself no longer sterile, but has become infected. An instrument that has been boiled remains aseptic or sterile if held in a hand that has been sterilized, but when touched by a hand that has not been rendered sterile it is no longer surgically clean. Consequently before they can touch any object or any part of the patient which is to remain sterile the hands themselves must first be sterilized.

A common and efficient method of sterilizing the hands is to scrub them for ten minutes with a nail brush, tincture of green soap and hot water, the latter being changed several times, and follow this by a thorough scrubbing with alcohol and then by an immersion for at least two minutes in a 1 to 1000 bichlorid of mercury solution. After this process the hands must not touch anything that is not sterile, for a hand that has been thoroughly sterilized becomes infected as soon as it touches the face or dress or any other object which has not been rendered aseptic. Consequently, should a person with sterile hands inadvertently touch something not surgically clean, should she for example scratch her face or brush her hand against her dress, she must immediately immerse her hands in the bichlorid solution or even scrub them again before so doing.

"Twilight Sleep in America" by Constance Leupp and Burton J. Hendrick (1915)

Introduction

This essay is representative of a movement toward new pain management options during childbirth. The concept of Dämmerschlaf, or twilight sleep, was developed in Germany to allow birthing women to forget the pain experienced. Interest in this method was incredibly popular among American women, who traveled to Germany to give birth before twilight sleep was available in the United States. *McClure's Magazine*, a periodical that pioneered investigative journalism, produced a series of essays on the topic that included journalists visiting Germany and researching the hospitals in New York that began using the method. Twilight sleep was controversial among doctors and needed precision to avoid negative results like overdose. Though its popularity waned in after 1916, it shaped twentieth-century approaches to medicalizing childbirth.

"Twilight Sleep in America" (*McClure's Magazine*, April 1915)

Ten months ago *McClure's Magazine* published the first account in this country of the Freiburg method of painless childbirth. The article met with an overwhelming response from every part of the United States. Hundreds of letters poured in from the women of the country, asking for further information regarding the method. At the same time, the article was vigorously attacked by medical journals and physicians, some of them of high standing, chiefly on the ground that the method had been tried in this country, had been found dangerous, and had been discarded.

Since last June, however, owing largely to the pressure of demand from the women themselves, numbers of American physicians have visited Freiburg, have studied the method at first hand, and have introduced it experimentally in hospitals in nearly all our large cities. The results are of extraordinary interest. The following article describes what American physicians have accomplished with Twilight Sleep, and what conclusions they have drawn regarding it.

In June, 1914, *McClure's Magazine* published an article describing, under the head of "Painless Childbirth," a new procedure developed in the women's clinic of the University Hospital in Freiburg, Germany. For many thousands, probably many millions, of years, the infant of the human species had entered the world only at the cost of unimagined agony to its mother; now we learned, for the first time, that there was at least a possibility that this suffering was to end. This announcement had an immediate interest for two classes in society. Inevitably it appealed strongly to all women, in themselves nearly half of human-kind. It also attracted the attention of that small minority of men, the doctors, whose business it is to assist women in the greatest ordeal of their lives.

Naturally, the women welcomed this announcement. In a few weeks the whole lay world was discussing the news. It was about the only subject not smothered by the European war. Soon, however, the first enthusiasm gave way to the keenest disappointment. The newspapers began to report, and the word was passed from mouth to mouth, that the whole thing a humbug. We were amazed to learn that the Freiburg method was nothing new—that wide-awake American physicians had tried it years before, and dismissed it in disgust; that not only did it not relieve pain, but that it frequently killed both the mother and the child. The entire performance, we were told, was an especially vulgar and criminal advertising dodge—a scheme of two German doctors, Krönig and Gauss, to entice American dollars out of the pockets of hysterical American women.

What had so suddenly changed American opinion? The explanation was simple: authority had spoken. Many important medical journals in the United States had denounced the Freiburg Twilight Sleep in almost vituperative terms.

Gradually, however, the situation changed again. Scattered pieces of information began to leak through to the public. Newspaper items announced that medical societies were discussing the Freiburg idea. Moreover, professional opinion did not now seem quite unanimous. Authoritative statements ranged all the way from utter scorning to suggestions that there "might be something in it" and reports that certain doctors were actually making progress with this method. Medical journals which had been most forward in their denunciations began to print articles describing the successful use of Twilight Sleep. Several of the very doctors who had tried the method years before, and discarded it, now declared that, after all, it seemed to work. The professional attitude was still deprecating and judicial. Only under exceptional circumstances, we were told, could painless childbirth be realized; the procedure was for only the most skilful operators, working under extremely favorable conditions; the method of its introduction was a shocking case of sensational journalism and an indecent violation of medical ethics. Still, Twilight Sleep was not a demonstrated fraud, and Krönig and Gauss were not a new edition of Dr. Friedman, of turtle-serum fame.

Has Twilight Sleep Made Good in America?

What, then, is the present situation? Has Twilight Sleep "made good" in the United States? What are its successes and its failures? What, according to American experience, are its limitations? What are the chances that, in the hands of trained physicians, it will supplant the family doctor, the midwife, the forceps, and the other traditions of the lying-in chamber?

It was, perhaps, not surprising that the scientific world received this announcement so unfavorably. As the medical journals said, the method was not new. In fact, its present appearance is the third in the last twelve years. Medical men first learned of it in 1902. Scopolamin-morphine had already been demonstrated to have a distinct value in general surgery. An injection preliminary to ether or chloroform robbed these established anesthetics of many of their terrors; it quieted the patient, removed the apprehension with which the average man or woman anticipates an operation, and abolished many of the unpleasant after effects. In 1902, however, von Steinbüchel of Gritz suggested a new and startling use for these drugs. He had tried them in twenty cases of parturient women, and found that they greatly diminished the agonies of childbirth.

Von Steinbüchel's work has little practical importance now, as he had developed no available technique. He sounded one warning, however, that still has particular value. He insisted that, because of the special knowledge required and the close attention demanded, scopolamin-morphine could not be used in general practice. Steinbüchel's method was not a twilight sleep: he was not attempting to destroy pain, but merely to diminish it; he had a wholesome respect for the dangers of the drugs, and so gave very small amounts. The obstetricians in Germany and Italy who tried Steinbüchel's procedure aimed at the same goal: while several obtained results more or less satisfactory to themselves, their reports inspired little general confidence and remained for many years in the dusty pigeonholes of scientific literature.

...

Gauss Technique the Secret of Success

In order to understand the situation, we must keep firmly in mind this fact: there is a system of scopolamin-morphine anesthesia, and a system known as Twilight Sleep. The former fails wherever it is tried; the latter, in all reports made since the Krönig and Gauss publication, has succeeded. Merely injecting scopolamin-morphine into the system of a parturient woman will not produce a painless childbirth. The Gauss technique, in nearly eight thousand cases, has, however, accomplished this result. In reality, Twilight Sleep is not a method of anesthesia at all. The word "anesthesia" was devised by Oliver Wendell Holmes to describe the physical and mental condition induced by the inhalation of sulphuric ether. It is derived from the Greek, and means "without feeling." An anesthetic person is unconscious, both mentally and physically; his ego receives no impressions; his muscles likewise are quiescent — temporarily paralyzed. An anesthetic woman could never give birth to a child, since the entire pelvic musculature must be actively at work. There is another physical condition, known as analgesia. In this the patient, although she may or may not be conscious or partly conscious, has no sensibility, or has a greatly reduced sensibility, to pain. There is still another condition, known as amnesia, in Which the woman, although she may receive certain reflex impressions of pain, does not consciously perceive them, and immediately forgets them.

This is the psychological state now so widely known as Twilight Sleep. It is apparently the only state in which anything approaching a painless childbirth can be attained. Scopolamin-morphine, used in these cases, is not an anesthetic: it is an analgesic and an amnesic. Recent writings, lay and professional, have insisted that this treatment does not actually abolish pain but merely makes the patient forget it. From the beginning, however, the German experts have described their method as both painlessness and forgetfulness. The title of Krönig's famous paper, "Painless Childbirth in Dämmerschlaf," clearly accentuates this claim. The twilight condition, indeed, does not represent the deep insensibility of anesthesia; in most cases, however, there is so great a diminution of pain that the birth process loses its distressing character.

Steinbüchel's original treatment failed because he gave such small doses that the patients received very little relief. Gauss' American successors, in 1907 and 1908, failed because they went to the other extreme and tried to secure absolute painlessness; hence their large doses and the consequent bad effects on mother and child. The Freiburg experimenters, however, discovered the half-way station—the condition that was neither complete consciousness nor complete unconsciousness; the state in which the mind received impressions, but made no particular note of them; in which it perceived particular objects, but made no mental associations; in which it felt, but in greatly diminished degree, the pangs of childbirth, but instantaneously forgot them. The process, so far as pain and other sensations are concerned, is a continuous realization and a continuous forgetting. The one practical fact is that, if the doses are skilfully regulated, there is no appreciable loss of muscular power. In the first stage, the machinery really works more rapidly under scopolamin-morphine than under normal conditions, since the woman, in her twilight state, does not consciously attempt to hold back the contractions.

This, then, was the Twilight Sleep: a condition which the obstetricians who made such failures a few years ago did not understand. Likewise, they did not understand the sign that marked the attainment of this crepuscular condition. We can read most diligently the scientific papers put out in this country in 1907 and 1908 without finding any reference to what is now the distinguishing feature of the treatment — the memory test. Krönig and Gauss insisted as strongly nine years ago as they do now that their whole method stood or fell by this memory test. The drugs affect different women differently: a small dose induces Dämmerschlaf in one patient, while another requires a dose considerably larger. Any physician who seeks to standardize the treatment comes to grief. How, then, is he to know that his patient has reached the twilight stage? It is purely a question of remembering or forgetting. If the patient remembers, the Dämmerschlaf is not complete and other doses are required. If she forgets, then this mental condition has been attained. The test is as elusive as it is decisive. Other mental symptoms are not safe guides. The patient may seem fairly conscious; she may ask rational questions, quietly follow the attendant's spoken instructions, and still have lost all faculty of memory. It is only when she fails to remember an object shown her a short time before that the drugs have filled their appointed mission.

American Women Demand Twilight Sleep

In the last six months, however, Americans in all parts of the country have been doing this. The pressure came from the women themselves. The wide popular exploitation had precisely the effect which the medical profession had so greatly feared: it prompted women to demand the treatment. Considerably against their will, therefore, medical societies began to debate the new procedure. Physicians, sometimes almost under the compulsion of their patients, began to sail for Germany. At one time the hotel corridors of Freiburg were fairly jammed with medical men from this country. Energetic and unprejudiced obstetricians, here and there, attempted to deliver women in Twilight Sleep. Apparently the Jewish Maternity Hospital, in New York, was the American pioneer. Its early experiments carry their lesson. They illustrate that detailed knowledge is essential to success, and that it is necessary to follow scrupulously the Freiburg instructions. The first fifteen cases proved failures. The drug used was unstable and deteriorated, and the practitioners erred in other ways. When these mistakes were corrected, success proved almost continuous. The first report published was that of one hundred cases at the Jewish Maternity and Lebanon hospitals in New York. In eighty-three cases there was amnesia with analgesia—complete forgetfulness with diminished pain; in eight there was analgesia without amnesia; and in nine the drug did not produce the desired effect. This first experiment, therefore, gave more than ninety per cent of successes. Two babies died — both from causes in no way connected with the drug. The Jewish Hospital has since reported two hundred cases, in which the general percentages of success remain about the same as in the figures already given.

Three Thousand Scopolamin-Born Babies in America

In the last eight months there have probably been three thousand scopolamin-morphine babies born in the United States—one third as many as Freiburg has had in ten years. In all the largest cities—New York, Cleveland, Chicago, Washington, St. Louis, Atlanta, San Francisco, Philadelphia, Cincinnati, Milwaukee, Baltimore, Boston — representative obstetricians are using the method. New York is unquestionably the center of interest. The greatest hospitals there are conducting Twilight Sleep cases almost every day. They include the Lying-in Hospital, the Sloane Maternity, Gouverneur, Long Island College, Manhattan, Sydenham, Harlem, and the Jewish Maternity. Up to this writing, only five hospitals in New York and elsewhere have published their scientific reports.

…

Childbirth Without Shock

After all this respectable testimony, it is absurd to suppose that there is no merit in this new procedure. What, then, are its advantages? What its disadvantages? It is hardly necessary to answer the first question in detail. The mere fact that it greatly diminishes pain, and quite successfully obliterates all memory of it, is sufficient. But it does more than this. The agony of childbirth is a terrible thing in itself; that, however, is temporary, and finds its compensation in the spiritual exaltation of motherhood. What is not temporary is the nervous shock that so frequently follows, especially in women of delicate nervous organization.

This shock is both "psychic" and "traumatic"; that is, it affects both the mind and the body. Such shock accompanies practically every surgical operation under general ether anesthesia; it produces prolonged physical and nervous exhaustion, and not infrequently death. One of the greatest of modern surgical discoveries is Crile's anoci-association—a method of shockless operation. As part of his treatment in overcoming shock, Crile uses these same Freiburg drugs—scopolamin and morphine. In the production of psychic shock, the chief element is fear. In childbirth, the actual physical suffering in itself causes shock; but an equally potent influence is fear. The woman suffers, not only from her pain, but from the recollection of the previous pain. The constant knowledge of what is coming unnerves her and makes her sufferings far greater than they would normally be. A man seriously injured in a railway accident suffers physical shock; constantly waiting for such an accident to happen would exhaust him nervously almost as much.

Scopolamin-morphine, however, obliterates all memory of previous pains, and so obliterates this factor in shock. Every labor pain, as it arrives, is a complete surprise and is itself immediately forgotten. By itself, likewise, it is immensely less painful than under "normal" conditions. It is thus plain why these Freiburg births are practically shockless. The women awake as from a refreshing sleep, and find their babies already born. They leave their beds much earlier than the ordinary routine permits. This fact has been one of the things that has prejudiced the profession in America against the method.

…

The Method Can Not be Be Used in General Practice

All this emphasizes the other point which certain opponents urge as a disadvantage—that, under present conditions, the method can not be used in general practice. From von Steinbüchel's time to the present, obstetricians have agreed upon one fact: that the use of scopolamin-morphine requires great obstetrical skill and constant individual attention. The average general practitioner, who takes baby cases as part of his daily routine, can not use it. We can not lay too great emphasis on this fact. It requires ideal hospital conditions — conditions that are not to be found in the average home, even of the more prosperous classes.

Any expectant mother who looks to her family physician to give her this treatment, therefore, nourishes a false hope. He can not do it without endangering the welfare of both the mother and the child. One of the practical dangers is that many inexperienced physicians, in their desire to be up-to-date, and in response to their patients' urging, will attempt the method, with deplorable results. In such cases, there will be plenty of blue babies and delirious mothers. That it easily lends itself to quackery, to the establishment of "Twilight Sleep" hospitals purely for commercial purposes, is also plain. But this is no fundamental objection to its use. It simply means that the whole practice of obstetrics must be changed.

The medical profession has for a long time recognized that this is about the most backward department of their science. That ignorant midwives still preside extensively over so important a function fairly measures the extent of this backwardness. It recalls the days when barbers were our surgeons, when cutting off a leg was too undignified a procedure to claim the attention of a real gentleman of science. Anesthetics changed all this and created modern surgery. Quite likely, the discovery of a successful analgesic in childbirth will have the same effect upon obstetrics. The twentieth-century woman will no more think of having an ordinary practitioner attend her in childbed at her own home than a modern man would now call in a barber to "cut him for the stone" in his own bedroom. She will go to a Dämmerschlaf hospital as a matter of course. Superstitious grandmothers and half-crazed husbands will no longer hover about the lying-in chamber; here science, surgical dexterity, and painlessness will prevail.

"Safeguarding American Motherhood" by Anna Steese Richardson (1915)

Introduction

After the popularity of articles about twilight sleep in *McClure's*, Anna Steese Richardson used interest in birth to promote what she called "a message to the American family more important than Twilight Sleep." Specifically, Richardson worked with the Better Babies Movement to raise awareness about the preventable maternal and infant mortality. In this, her second piece in the series, she emphasizes the importance of women understanding the risks of childbirth and the solutions for their safety and that of their babies.

"Safeguarding American Motherhood" (*McClure's Magazine*, July 1915)

"No," said the imperturbable insurance agent to the important policy-holder. "Sorry we can't oblige you, but our company doesn't insure women. We don't believe in it …

"Why? Uh, because every woman is a potential mother, and child-bearing is hazardous."

The young husband didn't argue the point. He decided to look up another company.

"Yes, we're willing to take a risk on a young married woman in perfect health; but—" And the "buts," or clauses protecting the company, were so discouragingly comprehensive that the husband didn't even read them through.

The third agent offered a policy less restricted in the matter of exceptions, but with what seemed to the husband in question a prohibitively high premium.

Each agent offered the same excuse for this discrimination against women — the hazard of motherhood.

Finally the husband heard of a company that would insure any member of the family, the rate for women being only a little higher than that for men.

"It's this way," the agent explained. "We can offer this rate because we look after the women we insure. We educate them to take care of themselves — send them pamphlets on sanitation, hygiene, pre-natal care, etc. Before the babies come, our nurses call and teach the mothers how to protect themselves. Educate women for motherhood, and they're not a bad risk.

"They've stopped the carriage of certain diseases by organizing a swat-the-fly campaign. They've checked infant mortality by pure-milk agitation. We're pre-venting deaths in childbirth by the simple process of educating the women we insure to protect themselves from infection and any other dangers of motherhood. But when a woman is not educated, not made to think along these lines, as a potential mother she is a poor risk."

The young husband took out the policy, convinced that the insurance agent was right. And he was — as far as he went.

Yet — all the pre-natal education obtainable will not save the mother in her supreme hour if complications arise that her physician can not cope with because of lack of skill or experience. Her own knowledge cannot protect her from the results of neglect, ignorance, and uncleanliness on the part of nurse, midwife, or neighbor.

Safety for mothers is built in the form of a pyramid, with intelligence and education as the base, skilled attendance next, and, for the capstone or apex, the State as represented by medical practice laws.

And, until this pyramid is reared all over the land, motherhood will remain a hazardous occupation in the eyes of science, as it does in the vision of that most unemotional, unsentimental of factors, the insurance company.

Reducing the Hazard from Ten in a Hundred to Less than One in a Thousand

Less than fifty years ago puerperal fever was regarded as an unavoidable and frequent complication of childbirth. To-day it is listed among the preventable diseases, and its appearance is a reflection on the skill of the mother's attendants. Up to the latter part of the nineteenth century, it raged in epidemic form through American homes, carrying off ten mothers in every hundred. To-day, by the aid of science, its toll has been reduced to less than one mother in a thousand.

In 1843 Dr. Oliver Wendell Holmes, in a paper on "The Contagiousness of Puerperal Fever," said:

> 'The disease is so far contagious as to be frequently carried from patient to patient by physicians and nurses.'

This statement created a sensation, and precipitated a controversy quite as violent and bitter as that produced by the article on Twilight Sleep in *McClure's Magazine* for June, 1914. The medical contemporaries of Dr. Holmes were so incensed by his arraignment of the profession that they were blinded to the high scientific value of his theory.

…

Women at Last Waking to Their Situation

The women themselves are demanding education. The chief of a health board in a Western State recently wrote to the editor of *McClure's* as follows:

> For the first time, I have been asked to address organizations of women on pre-natal care of the mother. Now that the clubwomen, with their enormous influence and great following, have dared to ask for information concerning their own care, I have faith that we may be able to stamp out the midwife and the careless, unskilled practitioner, who exist only because women have not been willing to pay what expert care in child-birth must cost.

Dr. J. Morris Slemons, associate professor of obstetrics at Johns Hopkins University, has written an invaluable book called "The Prospective Mother." In an introduction written by Dr. J. Whitridge Williams, also of Johns Hopkins, appear the following significant statements:

"There are two points which I desire to impress especially upon the readers of this book. Firstly, that the advance of the science of obstetrics, and consequently improvements in its practice, must depend greatly upon the cooperation of intelligent women. They must come to realize that they will secure the best treatment only as they demand the highest standard of excellence from their attendants; and they can aid in securing this for their poorer sisters and their children by interesting themselves in obstetric charities.

Secondly, they must realize that real progress in the science of obstetrics can be expected to proceed only from well equipped clinics connected with strong universities and in charge of thoroughly trained and broad-minded men. As yet, such institutions scarcely exist in this country.

It was in a clinic so endowed and rendered independent and efficient at Freiburg, Germany, that Twilight Sleep was worked out successfully, and to such clinics American women must look for safety in motherhood.

How can American women cooperate to insure to themselves and their daughters this safety? One way would be through the women's clubs.

It is said that there are six million federated club-women in the United States. If these six million organized thinkers and workers would cooperate with obstetricians, family physicians, hospital directors, and health officers in their States, they could speedily raise the national standard in obstetrics. By means of Safety First for Mother mass meetings, the federated clubs could inaugurate great campaigns for the reduction of mortality and disease among mothers and babies. Such campaigns could be carried on also by the National Congress of Mothers and Parent-Teachers Association, which claims a membership of 100,000 mothers, and by the hundred thousand women interested in the mother clubs and cradle rolls of churches.

Health officials in forty States of the Union are united in the belief that mortality and morbidity among mothers and infants can be reduced only through stricter laws governing those who attend women in confinement. In this connection, Dr. G. A. Jordan, Assistant Health Commissioner of St. Louis, says:

> A strict supervision by the body issuing certificates allowing persons to practise medicine and midwifery is needed, in the endeavor to eliminate all persons who are incompetent, and only to allow this practice to those persons who are qualified to perform the work properly. Neglect of surgical cleanliness is perhaps responsible for more deaths among women and blindness in babies than any other one thing, and too much stress can not be laid on this matter.

"Our operating surgeons," writes Dr. Horace G. Norton, Secretary of the State Board of Medical Examiners for New Jersey, "state that they find a large percentage of cases for operation and death following confinement cases to have been attended by ignorant and unclean midwives."

It is a mistake for Americans to think that midwives practise only among foreigners. A physician living in a State that prides itself on its intense Americanism says:

> We have no laws governing midwives, because we do not consider them advisable in the American home, nor as factors in medical progress. Therefore we ignore them.

A health officer in this same State writes:

> While we have not the congested districts of Chicago and New York, with their foreign population, the practice of midwifery is equally dangerous here, though our women are called 'monthly nurses.' Especially in our scattered farming districts, neighbors depend upon each other to an alarming extent. Many of our farm women, realizing the seriousness of the situation and their distance from physicians, have really made a study of home obstetrics and try conscientiously to serve each other well.

Suggestions from Various Health Officials

Health officials the country over are discussing the best method of handling the problem. Some think that midwifery should be abolished by drastic laws. The majority contend that this would rob thousands of women of the only form of attendance they can afford, and that a profession that serves from forty to fifty per cent of the mothers in America can not be abolished by the mere enactment of laws.

The danger from the practice of obstetrics by unskilled general practitioners corresponds with that from the practice of midwifery. An eminent authority on public health and vital statistics, whose name, for obvious reasons, is not given, writes:

> 'I question the justice of any organized campaign against the practice of midwifery when the State is so lax in its supervision of obstetrics as practised by un- skilled and sometimes unscrupulous graduates of medical colleges. As an example, we refuse to issue a license to graduates of three medical schools, yet just across the State line these men are practising in obstetrics. No doubt the same conditions exist in other States. A clean, conscientious, progressive midwife, who recognizes the fact that her services are justified only in normal labor, and who sends for an expert practitioner when complications arise, is less of a menace in the community than the slovenly, unskilled general practitioner whose diploma and license give him the right to interfere with labor when interference is undesirable or worse.

An editorial in the Bulletin of the Lying-in Hospital of New York, for March, 1913, contains this statement:

> The public thus far has failed to realize the need for proper and efficient care during the most important period of a woman's life, and we find this lack not only among the poorer classes but even in the so-called better circles .... Among the better classes the same lack of appreciation is expressed in the size of the fee which most families grudgingly pay for attendance in confinement.

Dr. George W. Kosmak, in addressing the Academy of Medicine of Syracuse, referred to the main cause of invalidism among women, and said:

> Acknowledging that the above is true, can we physicians flatter ourselves with the idea that we have afforded to woman as a mother the attention which she deserves? Have we not been satisfied to treat the results and consequences of pregnancy and labor, rather than to do away with the causes? The attendance on a woman during pregnancy and labor is not considered an agreeable branch of medicine by most practitioners, and the family doctors, so-called, have usually regarded it necessary to take care of confinement cases in order to retain their hold on the family. ... Fortunately, the medical student of to-day is better equipped to do this work, because he has been favored with actual clinical experience in obstetrics during his college course or soon after.

In its passion for specialization, the American public has given the skilled obstetrician the high position and the fee that his standard of work have earned; but to the general practitioner in obstetrics, in whose hands rest the true strength and safety of the nation, it renders neither appreciation nor reasonable remuneration.

A very real problem, then, that confronts America to-day is the education of the average family in the right of the mother to expert care. The moderately prosperous, intelligent American family is gradually awakening to the realization that motherhood must be safeguarded.

...

The New York State Department of Health is developing the most progressive step ever taken along the line of pre-natal education. Dr. Linsly R. Williams writes:

> The Department has under consideration the advisability of sending to every woman, on receipt of her marriage certificate, a circular of instruction, informing her how to care for herself during pregnancy. In order to do this, an appro-

priation of fully $5,000 a year would be needed, and it is our belief that it may in the future be possible to do this.

The health boards are not alone in this work of educating mothers. One of the big insurance companies not only supplies its women policy-holders with expertly prepared literature on care before, during, and after confinement, but it actually furnishes nurses and lecturers who coöperate with municipal and charity workers in educating women in pre-natal care.

University extension courses, particularly in agricultural colleges, include lectures on pre-natal care. The University of Minnesota is reaching the wives and daughters of farmers. Lectures are given in farming centers by Miss Dorothy Motl, her object being not only to teach the mother pre-natal care, but to impress upon those who, in the absence of a physician, officiate at births, the importance of aseptic methods.

Physicians have discussed Safety First for mother in their conferences. Welfare workers have pleaded for it. Health officials have fought for it. The way to insure it is through educating the mothers to demand it.

"Every Woman's Chance to Serve Humanity" by Anne Martin (1920)

Introduction

Just as the Nineteenth Amendment was ratified and guaranteed the right to vote for American women, Anne Martin presented this essay to the readers of women's domestic magazine *Good Housekeeping*. In it, she suggests women should use their new political power to lobby for specific legislation to protect against maternal and infant mortality. She writes on behalf of the Children's Bureau, a federal agency created in 1912 to focus on improving the lives of children and families.

"Every Woman's Chance to Serve Humanity: An Everlasting Benefit You Can Win in a Week" (*Good Housekeeping*, February 1920)

Last year our government spent $47,000,000 to protect farmers against avoidable losses of hogs, corn, and cattle. In the same period it spent, in an effort to prevent the avoidable loss of mothers and babies, just $47,000,000 less.

And we lost 250,000 babies, and nearly 23,000 mothers died in childbirth. Such discrimination in favor of hogs and corn should cease. A bill now before Congress (Senate Bill 3259; House Bill 10,925) will stop it if it is enacted into law. The bill is sponsored by the Children's Bureau; it is a good bill and should pass. But it won't pass unless the women of the country let Congress know that it must pass. Through lack of public interest a similar bill died in the Sixty-fifth Congress; if this one fails it will be the people's fault. They get from Congress what they demand. Read Miss Martin's stirring article, fill out the blanks on page 81, get as many signers as you can, and send them in promptly. The nation depends on mothers; now is the time to protect them. Do your part today. You will serve humanity in a way that will profit it for generations.

Protection of maternity and infancy by the state is recognized as a principle of government in every great country in the world except our own. This is a serious indictment. Women are regarded as the natural conservers of human life. Our enfranchisement has been urged not only because it is just, but because the weapon of the vote will arm us more effectively to protect women and children, to improve the race. Now that American women are practically enfranchised, will they use their political power for this purpose? Are they going to make good the promises made for them? The greatest woman's issue and the most needed conservation measure is immediate governmental action for the protection of maternal and infant life and health. Our great loss of soldier life on European battlefields demands the instant attention of our government to the constant and even greater loss of mother and child life at home. Governments of leading foreign countries are already far ahead of the United States in provisions to care for expectant mothers and to safeguard the health and lives of mothers and babies. Human life with them has gained a new value; the importance of the service to the state that women render in bearing children has received a new emphasis. Since the war began European belligerent nations have increased their efforts to save the lives of mothers and babies. The United States government, however, has accepted comparatively calmly its casualty list of nearly 300,000 men. No steps have yet been taken to compensate future generations for the death and disablement of this large number of carefully selected American youths.

No effective steps have been taken to lower our appallingly high maternal and infant death-rate as revealed in a series of startling investigations conducted by the Children's Bureau. The facts gathered in these investigations have become matters of common knowledge, but neither Congress nor the people have been roused to action.

Infant mortality rates are higher in the United States than in ten other leading countries, among them New Zealand, Norway, Sweden, Australia, France, Switzerland, and even Ireland. Of the 2,500,000 babies born in this country every year, 250,000 die within twelve months of birth. Within the first year after birth the United States loses one out of every ten babies born: New Zealand loses only one out of twenty. At least one-half of these 250,000 deaths occur within the first six weeks of life and are due directly to the poor condition and neglect of the mother before. During, and after childbirth. Many thousands of babies that live suffer all their lives from ailments that could have been prevented by proper care of the mother during this period. Although it is now generally known that prenatal, natal, and after care of the mother greatly increases the child's chance of life and health, no provision for such care has yet been made by our government.

Nearly 16,000 women die every year in the United States from causes arising from childbirth; these deaths are almost entirely preventable. Unnumbered tens of thousands suffer impairment of health from these same causes. More American women between the ages of fifteen and forty-four die every year from conditions caused by childbirth than from typhoid fever or any other disease except tuberculosis. From the latest available figures more new mothers die in this country than in thirteen other principal countries, and there is no decrease in the rate from year to year, while deaths from typhoid fever and other diseases have been greatly reduced. Sweden, Norway, Italy, France, Prussia, England and Wales, Scotland, New Zealand, Ireland, Hungary, Japan, Australia, and Belgium all have a lower maternal death-rate.

The European movement for the protection of maternity and infancy began many years before the war. It sprang in large part from a realization that the health of the industrial population is one of the greatest responsibilities and assets of the state. In 1884 Germany established a national insurance system providing aid to mothers; Austria and Hungary soon followed. Italy and New Zealand took action in 1910, Great Britain in 1911, Russia, Sweden, and Australia in 1912, France in 1913; so that at the beginning of the war practically all the leading countries except the United States had adopted some system of maternity relief.

The methods adopted by these countries are different, but the principle recognized in all of them is that both mother and child are given a better chance of life and health by relieving the mother of financial anxiety and providing the means for rest and care before and after her baby's birth. One method provides the mother before and after childbirth with helpful advice, skilled nurses. and medical attendance, which she pays for if she is able. This system has been most successfully developed in New Zealand, largely subsidized by government funds and greatly assisted in its operation by the unofficial action of the New Zealand Society for the Health of Women and Children. Other countries follow the plan of giving a sum of money to the mother at childbirth. Australia gives every mother $25 and spends annually more than $3,000,000, a sum representing three percent of the consolidated revenues of the government, for these subsidies to mothers. France has a system of daily allowances to the mother before and after childbirth, spending more than $2,000,000 annually on these maternity benefits.

A third method is that of insuring mothers working in certain specified industries and occupations. An insurance fund is created by the payment in advance of small sums at stated intervals by the persons insured and by their employers, with subsidies in most cases from the state itself, so that money, nursing, medical and hospital care are available for the mother when the baby comes. Italy, Germany, Austria, Hungary, Great Britain, Switzerland, Russia and Sweden have long had insurance systems.

It is noteworthy that these systems of maternity benefits vary from those under which every woman, regardless of her financial and social status, receives a fixed sum at the birth of a child, to those under which mothers working in certain industries receive benefits from insurance funds largely subsidized by the state. A significant tendency in recent legislation is to include all industries and all occupations in maternity benefit systems. Peculiarly significant also is the attitude of the International Congress of Working Women, which assembled in Washington in November, with delegates present from seventeen foreign countries. When the point was raised by the Italian, Belgian, Czecho-Slovakian, and Polish delegates as to what women should be included in maternity aid systems, Miss Julia Lathrop, Chief of the Federal Children's Bureau, urged the inclusion not only of working women and of workingmen's wives, but of all women. She pointed out that women in the home have to work longer hours than factory women, often under harder conditions, and should benefit by all systems of aid to maternity. The Congress agreed that the period of rest for all employed women should be extended to six weeks before and six weeks after childbirth, and most of the countries represented favored, in addition to free medical, surgical, and nursing care at childbirth, the payment of a money allowance from the state sufficient to support both mother and child during the twelve weeks' period. The Congress was unanimous in the opinion that maternity aid must not be regarded in any sense as a charity, but that it should be subsidized and administered by the state as one of its most important duties, and that such aid should be open to all women.

The list of countries providing some form of government aid to mothers now includes France, Germany, Austria, Czecho-Slovakia, Great Britain, Italy,

Luxemburg, Holland, Denmark, Australia, New Zealand, Norway. Russia, Poland, Sweden, and Switzerland—in fact. All of the large and most of the small countries of the so-called "civilized" world, except the United States.

In view of the bad conditions in our own country, the operation of these laws has a special interest for us. New Zealand's system is most successful, having achieved for that country the lowest infant mortality rate of any country in the world. It provides instruction and nurses for expectant mothers, even for those living in the remote "back blocks," and skilled care at government maternity hospitals. The mothers use the system as they would use public schools, or good roads, or any other public utility.

Canada, with vast and sparsely-settled regions very like those in our northern and western states, has recognized the necessity for providing nursing and hospital care for prospective mothers living in these areas. The western provinces have already developed successful plans for rural nursing and hospital care, supported by the provincial governments.

France leads other countries in infant welfare work. She had protective laws on her statute books as early as 1811, in the time of Napoleon. Between 1874 and 1913 various laws were enacted to aid maternity and infancy. The law of 1913 provides a daily allowance for the mother four weeks before and four weeks after childbirth, and an additional allowance if the mother nurses her child. The government's concern for the health of expectant and nursing mothers was. Pot relaxed during the war. One of the first acts of the military government of Paris early in the war was to organize a central office of maternity aid "to assure to every woman who is pregnant, or who has a baby less than three years old, the social, legal, and medical protection to which she has a right in a civilized society—to be sure that no mother is ignored and no child forgotten." Asa result of this government policy France has a lower maternal and infant death-rate than many other countries, including the United States.

England and Wales achieved, in 1916, the lowest infant mortality rate in their history, in spite of the war-time conditions, and have a lower rate of maternal mortality than the United States. The national insurance act in operation since 1912 is undoubtedly a factor in securing this result. Nearly all the British writers on the subject emphasize as perhaps the greatest advantage of the maternity benefit to the mother, the elimination of anxiety about increased expenses at the time of childbirth. The need for money to meet these expenses had previously forced her to work up to the last possible moment, which, of course, was bad for both mother and child. In 1918, during the crisis of the war, the government assumed the entire cost of the so-called "sickness benefit for women during pregnancy." A special woman's fund was established by annual appropriations which may amount to $1,216,625.

Thus the governments of other countries are meeting their responsibility to maternity and infancy and increasing their efforts to repair the ravages of war by safeguarding the lives of the next generation, while the United States government is neglecting the whole problem except for the gathering of statistics by the Children's Bureau—and the high death-rate continues. The real tragedy in this country lies in the fact that almost all these lives of mothers and children lost every year could be saved. Can our nation afford such waste of human resources involved not only in the large number of deaths, but in the impaired health and lowered vitality of many mothers and babies that live? Governmental ignorance, apathy, and neglect are directly responsible. The lesson to be learned is the immediate institution of higher standards of care during this period. Our government spent last year more than $47,000,000 through its Department of Agriculture to prevent avoidable losses of crops, cattle, and hogs, and to produce healthy plants and animals; it is its equally imperative duty to make adequate provision to prevent avoidable losses of human life and to produce healthy human beings.

Investigations in Rural Districts

Investigations carried on by the Federal Children's Bureau in rural areas in Wisconsin, Kansas, North Carolina, and Montana have revealed a higher maternal mortality rate than in the United States as a whole; the rural districts are in the greatest need of help. The rate found in Montana was double the average for the United States, and the records of other sparsely settled states, where available, show a high maternal death-rate. The number of babies' deaths arising from the care and condition of the mother 1s as high proportionately in these country districts studied as in cities, where overcrowding and attendant evils com- plicate the problem. A majority of the mothers interviewed in the rural areas of these states received no advice or prenatal care whatever, although many tried to secure information by sending for books and magazines. Owing to the lack of any provision for assistance nearly all worked until the last day at heavy tasks, like carrying water, and with the exception of the Kansas area studied, more than half of these-mothers had no trained attendance of any kind at the birth of the baby, or after care, or help with their housework, washing, and chores, which many had to resume within two weeks or even less. One-fifth of the women in the Montana area were attended only by their husbands when the child was born, and three were entirely alone and delivered themselves.

Those who know our sparsely populated northern and western states know also the cruel circumstances under which most mothers must bear their children—in remote and isolated cabins, on desert or prairie homesteads, or in the primitive surroundings of new mining or lumber camps—but how many of us have realized that these circumstances produce great loss of life of mothers and babies in these regions? The absence of any organized effort to meet the imperative need for instruction of expectant mothers in prenatal and infant hygiene, the difficulty of securing household help and proper food and water, combined with the inaccessibility and often entire lack of hospitals, doctors, and nurses are of course the chief factors in the high death-rate. Pure country air and an out-of-door life do not make up for these deficiencies. The expense of securing adequate care for expectant mothers and babies in distant and newly settled areas is naturally much greater than in cities: by the very fact of their remoteness and the high number of deaths these are the districts where care is most needed; and the families living in these districts are usually the least able to obtain it without financial aid and socialized effort.

Precedents Are Abundant

Here lies women's of opportunity to impress the issue of governmental aid for maternity and infancy upon the minds of political leaders. We have abundant precedent for federal aid to state work in rural areas in existing laws for encouraging scientific farming, teaching home economics, building good roads, and protecting the health of domestic animals. Through the Smith-Lever act, based on the belief that demonstration is the surest way to teach, cooperating federal and state agencies are already bringing the best knowledge of scientific farming and home economics to the farmer and his wife in their homes. Women voters can perform no greater human service than to insist that the same agencies be employed to bring to women on farms and isolated homesteads, in mining camps and other remote settlements, and in crowded industrial districts, knowledge and aid for their own health and for their babies during the period when they most need it.

The first practical measure to accomplish this purpose was introduced into the Sixty-fifth Congress by Miss Jeannette Rankin, on behalf of the Children's Bureau. It provided for instruction in the hygiene of maternity and infancy and for proper care of maternity and infancy in rural districts; provision was made for cooperation with the states in the promotion of such instruction and care. Hearings were held upon this bill before the House Committee on Labor in January, 1919, but it progressed no further than a committee report and died with the Sixty-fifth Congress.

Sponsored by Miss Julia Lathrop, a new bill has been introduced into the Sixty-sixth Congress by Senator Sheppard of Texas. It was referred to the Committee on Public Health and National Quarantine, of which Senator France of Maryland is chairman. Representative Towner of Iowa has recently introduced it also into the House, where it was referred to the Committee on Interstate and Foreign Commerce, of which Representative Esch of Wisconsin is chairman. It is entitled "A Bill for the Public Protection of Maternity and Infancy, and Providing a Method of Cooperation Between the Government of the United States and the Several States." In this bill we have the most far-reaching conservation measure before the American people. Its enactment will undoubtedly save as many lives every year as comprised our total casualty list of nearly 300,000; four times as many lives can be saved annually as we lost in battle. Because of its vital importance to mothers and babies, women voters should study its every detail. Unlike the first bill, not only mothers in rural, but those in industrial districts—all mothers in the United States, in fact—may avail themselves of its benefits, subject to the acceptance of the terms of the act by the state in which they live. The bill provides an annual appropriation of $480,000, $10,000 of which shall be paid annually to each state accepting the terms of the act, for the purpose of printing and distributing information and providing other necessary facilities. For the year 1921, an additional sum of $2,000,000 is appropriated, to be increased by $400,000 every year until 1926, when the sum of $4,000,000 is reached, and thereafter $4,000,000 is to be annually appropriated. This money is to be apportioned on the basis of population to those states which appropriate a sum equal to that received from the government.

...

Administration of the Act

The act is to be administered by cooperation of the Federal Board with the state boards of maternal and infant hygiene, but no state shall receive its benefits until careful plans for carrying it into operation have been submitted to and approved by the Federal Board. These plans must include provision for popular instruction in the hygiene of infancy and maternity and related subjects, particularly in regions where such facilities are not otherwise accessible. This instruction is to be carried out through public health nurses and consultation centers, and through qualified lecturers in extension courses provided by the state universities, land grant colleges, and other public educational institutions. The plans must also include provision of medical and nursing care for mothers and infants at home or at a hospital when necessary, especially in remote areas.

In a recent interview Senator Sheppard said of the measure he introduced: "The unborn can not help themselves. We can not assure 'life, liberty, and the pursuit of happiness' to the people of the next generation, unless we of this generation give them a fair chance of health at birth. The lives of the mothers and children now needlessly lost must be saved, and health and vigor must be assured to those that live by government aid to mothers and children before and after birth. Only the government can perform this duty. And the women voters are the greatest force we have in the nation to make the government perform it."

When Miss Lathrop discussed this measure before the International Congress of Working Women, she emphasized as one of the chief duties of enfranchised women the reduction of the great maternal and infant loss of life in this country.

"There are some things for which we can not blame men, some inequalities which have existed because women have made no demands," said Miss Lathrop.

"In the new partnership between men and women which now supplants the ownership, the headship of men, the first and simplest duty of women is to safeguard the lives of mothers and babies, ... to develop the perfect dignity of motherhood. Motherhood has too long suffered from sheer sentiment and has not been treated with common sense. True sentiment is based on respect and affection and leads to action. We are learning to abandon the old fatalistic cry which science refuses to accept, "The Lord gave, and the Lord hath taken away; blessed be the name of the Lord." As true sentiment and respect for motherhood develops, we shall depend upon scientific knowledge and make it universally available.

"As women now emerge into joint control of the resources of the world, they will find themselves forced to insist that mothers shall no longer make bricks without straw, that the scientific means for safeguarding her children must be at the command of every mother."

In these words the woman who has laid the foundation for governmental protection of maternity and infancy in the United States, appealed to the women of seventeen foreign countries, and to the women of our own country, to do their part. When it is squarely presented to them, American women voters will unite upon this great human issue. They will insist that Congress take instant action. How can this insistence be made effective? From every woman's organization, from every household throughout this broad land, from every woman in the country, letters and telegrams should at once be sent to her two senators and to her congressman, to Senator France, and Representative Esch, chairmen of the committees which have the bill in charge, and to Senator Sheppard and Representative Towner, demanding an immediate and favorable report of the bill for the public protection of maternity and infancy (known as Senate Bill 3259; House Bill 10,925), and its speedy passage by this session of Congress. Without insistent and nation-wide pressure it will not attain momentum enough to pass Congress. It is unfortunate, but true, that the history of political reform in representative governments is the history of unceasing, popular demand upon inert or unwilling majorities in power. They must be shown. However just the demand, Congress has not moved, and it will not move until political advantage is seen through granting that demand.

If, unhappily, the bill for the public protection of maternity and infancy should fail of passage this session of Congress, as it failed in the Sixty-fifth Congress, because of lack of sufficient pressure throughout the country, women will surely make it an issue in the autumn campaign.

A Practical Working Plan

How can we get the measure before the women of the nation, and how shall we force it into the platforms of the political parties?

This is a comparatively simple thing to accomplish. The leaders of the Republican and Democratic parties recognize the fact that the party which secures a large proportion of the more than fifteen million women's votes will carry the election. They are already laying plans to win this vote by offering issues they believe will appeal to women. Let us take immediate steps to offer our own issues to the parties. This can be done by calling a national conference of women, composed of authorized representatives of the leading national women's organizations which have state branches, such as the Federation of Women's Clubs, the National Congress of Mothers, the national suffrage organizations, the Women's Christian Temperance Union, the Consumers' League, the Federation of Business and Professional Women, the Young Women's Christian Association, the National Women's Trades Union League, and many others.

At this conference there is no doubt that women will realize their great opportunity and responsibility and adopt as the chief plank in their platform government protection of maternity and infancy, as provided in the bill of the Children's Bureau introduced by Senator Sheppard. A Woman's National Committee on which every state is represented should be elected to attend the national conventions next summer, there to urge their demand upon all political parties. Backed by the leading woman's organizations of the country, representing from fifteen to twenty million women voters who will help elect more than a majority of the electoral college and who hold the election in their hands, is it conceivable that the platform of the Woman's National Committee will be rejected? The party taking such a course would be certain of defeat, and the party supporting women's demands would come into power. Undoubtedly all national conventions will accept it. That our platform may become a sincere "program," and not suffer the fate of election promises of the past, it will then be for us to pledge personally all candidates for president and for Senate and House to do their utmost to enact into law, if elected, the maternity and infancy bill; it will be for us to see that none but genuine supporters of the measure *are* elected.

Only four million women could vote in 1916; yet by almost precisely such methods we succeeded in making the national woman suffrage amendment a political issue in the last presidential election, and it has now been passed by Congress. With four times as many women voters in 1920, we can surely make an equally good fight for the lives of the mothers and babies of this country, and for the health of the next generation.

"Infant Death Rate Reaches High Mark" (1926)

Introduction

In this article, the *New York Times* presents the shocking statistics about how the United States compared with other nations in terms of infant and maternal mortality. In comparison with many nineteenth-century pieces on this topic, the title begins with infant deaths rather than maternal deaths, though both are important to the larger crisis presented here.

"Infant Death Rate Reaches High Mark: Nation Compares Unfavorably with Many Others, Children's Bureau Survey Shows. Same is True of Mothers" (*New York Times*, 30 August 1926)

About 100,000 infants under one month of age die in the United States every year, according to a report of the Children's Bureau of the Department of Labor, prepared by Dr. Robert Morse Woodbury. He adds that maternal mortality rates in this country are among the highest in the world and that the annual ratios since 1900 have risen.

Through this report, just made public, the Children's Bureau is putting forward a national program to decrease maternal mortality.

The report assembles and analyzes American and foreign data on deaths of mothers in child-birth, and shows the need for organized counteracting efforts.

"A very considerable proportion of all deaths of infants under one year of age occur during the first month of life, from causes which have their origin in the care and condition of mothers during pregnancy and confinement," says the report.

Dr. Woodbury estimates the total annual number of maternal deaths in the United States to be 18,281 on the basis of 1921 birth registration area statistics.

However, a survey of sources of error in certifications of death throughout the area leads him to the conclusion that the true number of maternal deaths is probably as much as 12 per cent. in excess of those reported, making an estimated yearly death toll of more than 20,000 women. The maternal mortality rate in 1921 was 6.8 per 1000 live births. The provisional 1924 rate was 6.6.

Figures showing the trend of maternal mortality over a twenty-two-year period in the United States, if accepted at their face value, would show an increase in the maternal death rate from 13.3 per 100,000 population in 1900 to 16.9 in 1921, according to the report.

Comparison of the United States rates with those of other countries shows that the United States ranks among those having the highest rates, such as New Zealand and Chile. Among the countries having rates less than half that of the United States are Denmark, Finland, Italy, Japan, the Netherlands, Norway, Sweden and Uruguay.

Cities showed a higher maternal mortality rate than rural districts in the United States, according to the 1921 figures, but to some extent this difference was accounted for by the fact that many of the more difficult or complicated cases were brought from rural regions into cities to secure the better medical and hospital facilities there.

Twilight Sleep by Edith Wharton (1927)

Introduction

In this novel, Edith Wharton presents the lives of a Jazz Age family in New York. The novel's title draws on the method of pain management for childbirth that was wildly popular in the previous decade. In the opening chapter, excerpted here, one of the main characters, flapper Lita Wyant, describes her feeling about childbirth, which is reinforced by her mother-in-law, Mrs. Manford. Here, though, twilight sleep is also a metaphor for the characters' larger avoidance of pain and difficult in 1920s America.

Excerpt from Chapter 1

Lita, in spite of her soft curled-up attitudes, was not only a tireless dancer but a brilliant if uncertain tennis-player, and an adventurous rider to hounds. Between her hours of lolling, and smoking amber-scented cigarettes, every moment of her life was crammed with dancing, riding or games. During the two or three months before the baby's birth, when Lita had been reduced to partial inactivity, Nona had rather feared that her perpetual craving for new "thrills" might lead to some insidious form of time-killing—some of the drinking or drugging that went on among the young women of their set; but Lita had sunk into a state of smiling animal patience, as if the mysterious work going on in her tender young body had a sacred significance for her, and it was enough to lie still and let it happen. All she asked was that nothing should "hurt" her: she had the blind dread of physical pain common also to most of the young women of her set. But all that was so easily managed nowadays: Mrs. Manford (who took charge of the business, Lita being an orphan) of course knew the most perfect "Twilight Sleep" establishment in the country, installed Lita in its most luxurious suite, and filled her rooms with spring flowers, hot-house fruits, new novels and all the latest picture-papers--and Lita drifted into motherhood as lightly and unperceivingly as if the wax doll which suddenly appeared in the cradle at her bedside had been brought there in one of the big bunches of hot-house roses that she found every morning on her pillow.

"Of course there ought to be no Pain ... nothing but Beauty. ... It ought to be one of the loveliest, most poetic things in the world to have a baby," Mrs. Manford declared, in that bright efficient voice which made loveliness and poetry sound like the attributes of an advanced industrialism, and babies something to be turned out in series like Fords. And Jim's joy in his son had been unbounded; and Lita really hadn't minded in the least.

References

Caton, Donald. 1999. *What a Blessing She Had Chloroform: The Medical and Social Response to the Pain of Childbirth from 1800 to Present.* New Haven: Yale University Press.

Doyle, Nora. 2018. Maternal Bodies: Redefining Motherhood in Early America. Chapel Hill: University of North Carolina Press.

Ehrenreich, Barbara, and Deirdre English. 2010. *Witches, Midwives, and Nurses: A History of Women Healers.* 2nd ed. The Feminist Press at CUNY.

Epstein, Randi Hutter. 2010. *Get Me Out: A History of Childbirth from the Garden of Eden to the Sperm Bank.* New York: W. W. Norton & Company.

Filippini, Nadia Maria. 2021. *Pregnancy, Delivery, Childbirth: A Gender and Cultural History from Antiquity to the Test Tube in Europe.* Translated by Clelia Boscolo. London: Routledge.

Fox, Sarah. 2022. *Giving Birth in Eighteenth-Century England.* London: University of London Press.

Hanson, Clare. 2004. A Cultural History of Pregnancy: Pregnancy, Medicine and Culture, 1750–2000. Houndmills: Palgrave Macmillan.

Klepp, Susan E. 2009. *Revolutionary Conceptions: Women, Fertility, and Family Limitation in America, 1760–1820.* Chapel Hill: University of North Carolina Press.

Leavitt, Judith Walzer. 2016. *Brought to Bed: Childbearing in America 1750 to 1950.* New York: Oxford University Press.

Loudon, Irvine. 2000. *Death in Childbirth: An International Study of Maternal Care and Maternal Mortality 1800–1950.* Oxford: Clarendon Press.

Marland, Hilary. 2004. *Dangerous Motherhood: Insanity and Childbirth in Victorian England.* Houndmills: Palgrave Macmillan.

Marsh, Margaret, and Wanda Ronner. 2019. *The Pursuit of Parenthood: Reproductive Technology from Test-Tube Babies to Uterus Transplants.* Baltimore: Johns Hopkins University Press.

Rooks, Judith Pence. 1997. *Midwifery and Childbirth in America.* Philadelphia: Temple University Press.

Simonds, Wendy, Barbara Katz Rothman, Bari Meltzer Norman. 2002. *Laboring On: Birth in Transition in the United States.* New York: Routledge.

Wertz, Richard W., and Dorothy C. Wertz. 1989. Lying-in: A History of Childbirth in America. New Haven: Yale University Press.

3

Contraception & Abortion

Introduction

Contraception and abortion are the topic of contemporary debate in the United States, but discussions about their availability and legality can be traced back thousands of years. The efforts to prevent or terminate pregnancy have been the work of both the medical profession and uncredentialed practitioners as well as in the hands of individuals and couples seeking to control fertility or the size of their families. Over time and in different situations, the methods employed have varied widely from behavioral approaches—including abstinence, coitus interruptus, barrier methods, and lactational amenorrhea—to treatments—including herbal potions, chemical or hormonal pills, and surgery. Social, cultural, political, and religious beliefs have evolved to address issues around population growth or control, the rights of women or of embryos and fetuses, and the scientific and medical developments that provide people with fertility control.

History of Methods for Preventing and Terminating Pregnancy

Though modern medicine has provided new methods for preventing and terminating pregnancy, "there was always a concern to influence or shape fertility, to reduce or increase conceptions or births" (McLaren 1990, p. 3). The societal and personal motivations for controlling fertility may vary, but this long history has been a series of advances and responses to those advances until "family planners of the 1950s…popularized the idea of science's recent, sudden triumph over fertility" (2). Historically, the approaches to this were not clearly divided between contraception and abortion; instead, both existed on what McLaren (1990) calls "a continuum of fertility-regulating strategies" that has been replaced with a twentieth-century view that abortion is used primarily after the failure of contraception methods (8). Linda Gordon (2002) uses the phrase "birth control" to refer to this full range, "mean[ing] any kind of action taken to prevent having children, including not only abortion and infanticide but also periodical and even sustained sexual abstinence if it is done with that intent" (p. 370, note 6).

This range of approaches to limiting fertility included a wide variety of techniques. Gordon's list of birth control methods includes the following: "infanticide; abortion; sterilization; withdrawal by the male (*coitus interruptus*); suppositories designed to form an impenetrable coating over the cervix; diaphragms, caps, or other devices, which are inserted into the vagina over the cervix and withdrawn after intercourse; intrauterine devices; internal medicines—potions or pills; douching and other forms of action after intercourse designed to kill or drive out the sperm; condoms; and varieties of the rhythm methods, based on calculating the woman's fertile period and abstaining from intercourse during it" (pp. 13–14). Whether any of these methods were effective in their historical uses is less important for understanding this history and the texts presented in this chapter. Instead, they are valuable as "evidence not only of the desire to control reproduction but also of the conviction that it is proper to do so and of the aspiration to do so" (Gordon 2002, p. 14). The sections that follow trace the history of these methods through three types of approaches: natural potions, tools, and techniques; modern pharmaceuticals; and surgical methods.[1]

Natural Potions, Tools, and Techniques

Since the time of the ancient Greeks, solutions for preventing or terminating pregnancies have included the use of herbal potions and other physical tools or techniques that were shared through word of mouth or through medical providers. Many of the same potions could be used as contraceptives or abortifacients. Options for herbal contraception were accompanied by instructions about whether they should be taken before, during, and/or after

---

[1] Detailed histories of these approaches to and methods for contraception and abortion can be found in McLaren's *A History of Contraception* (1991), Gordon's *The Moral Property of Women* (2002), and chapter 5 of Klepp's *Revolutionary Conceptions* (2009).

coitus. In each era and region, different combinations of the available herbs were believed to prevent pregnancy with some ingested orally, others inserted as a pessary or suppository, and others applied externally as poultices. The pessaries worked to block the cervix through oil sometimes combined with a spermicide or through solid items like grass, seaweed, cloths, or wool. For centuries, the most effective of these was the sponge, which "was first used by people who lived by the sea" and "block[ed] the cervix,…absorb[ed] semen and [could] be saturated with a spermicidal fluid" (McLaren 1990, p. 20). Condoms were also tools used for blocking semen and were developed in the sixteenth century to prevent venereal disease. Finally, rhythm (timing intercourse around ovulation or menstruation) or lactational amenorrhea (prolonged breastfeeding) methods relied on more advanced understanding of physiology. Because of misconceptions about fertility and menstruation, rhythm methods were historically ineffective, but extended breastfeeding could work better and was widely practiced. Over the centuries, though, the most commonly practiced method was *coitus interruptus*, or male withdrawal and ejaculation outside of the vagina, but other physical approaches related to the movements of either partner before, during, or after intercourse were sometimes practiced (McLaren 1990).

Because the prevention of pregnancy could be more difficult to achieve due to misconceptions about physiology, the termination of pregnancy was more common. In many ways, abortions were essentially self-induced miscarriages, which meant they were typically more painful and less safe than contraception, but women were also well aware of the risks of childbirth as detailed in Chap. 2. Herbal concoctions could be used to "irritate or poison the body or the digestive system [to] cause the rejection of the fetus as a side effect" or as "mild emmenagogues stimulating the onset of menstruation" (Gordon 2002, p. 16). Other forms of abortions were through insertion of pessaries or apparatuses that would cause early labor, dilate the cervix, and force expulsion of the fetus. While most of the methods to prevent pregnancy could be practiced by individuals or couples with advice, many procedures for terminating a pregnancy were supported by a specialist with knowledge and experience (Gordon 2002).

Modern Pharmaceuticals

Compared with the long history of measures used to control fertility, pharmaceutical solutions are a relatively recent phenomenon, with hormonal birth control through "the pill" becoming commercially available in the early 1960s, emergency contraception or "the morning-after pill" in the late 1990s despite several decades of using high doses of hormones for the same effect, and medical options for terminating pregnancy through RU-486 or "the abortion pill" about 2000. These options represented the first true innovations in birth control in centuries. As they were developed through scientific research and with support from commercial pharmaceutical companies, they gave a sense of medical legitimacy to birth control efforts.

From the 1930s, researchers in several countries began experimenting with the use of estrogen to alter or prevent ovulation, which led to the development of Enovid, the first oral contraception approved by the American FDA in 1960 and the British NHS in 1961. In particular, the work of Gregory Pincus laid the foundation. He met birth control activist Margaret Sanger in 1950, and they engaged Katharine McCormick for financial support as well as research support from obstetrician and gynecologist John Rock and reproductive biologist Min-Cheuh Chang.[2] Their years of work produced a reliable female-controlled form of contraception, but the development included controversial trials that tested on low-income women, mentally ill women, and women of color. Because of the extreme side effects from the high levels of hormones, many women who could do so withdrew from the trials. Still, the pill went onto the market and was incredibly popular (Eig 2014; Engelman 2011).

With this foundation in research on the use of hormones to regulate ovulation, other researchers sought a contraceptive that could be taken post-coitus but prior to implantation. The Yuzpe method developed by Albert Yuzpe in the early 1970s moved away from more intense high-dose estrogen options to use a combination of estrogen and progestin (Ellertson 1996). Other widely used options rely on either levonorgestrel (Plan B) or ulipristal (Ella). Because the regimens developed for postcoital solutions often rely on similar ingredients to pre-coital ones but in different combinations, the side effects are similar and thus are generally accepted by women needing emergency contraception. In addition to pills, intrauterine devices (IUDs) are commonly used for both ongoing and emergency contraception. Many of these use the same hormones as oral contraceptives, though copper IUDs are also used for prevention of both pregnancy and implantation.

The idea of medical abortion, or the use of specific medication for terminating pregnancy, builds on centuries of herbs and poisons that sought to induce menstruation, deliberately avoiding the term abortion. RU-486, also

---

[2] A detailed history of this research and the development of "the pill" is available in Eig (2014) and Engelman (2011).

known as mifepristone, was developed in France in the 1980s and has been licensed in the UK since the late 1980s and in the United States since 2000. Mifepristone blocks the hormones needed to sustain a pregnancy and is also sometimes used as emergency contraception. For a medical abortion, it is often combined with misoprotol taken orally or vaginally, which causes the cervix to dilate and contract to expel the embryo like a menstrual period. Overall, medical abortions are highly effective in terminating pregnancies and offer patients an option that is less invasive and allows for more agency and discretion.[3]

Surgical Methods

Women's surgical options for contraception can range from a tubal ligation that inserts clips onto the fallopian tubes to a full hysterectomy removing all or part of the uterus. This form of fertility control began in the early twentieth century in both the United States and Britain and was often connected with eugenics. Sterilization was initially performed as a treatment for medical conditions like ovarian cysts but was soon applied to population control efforts. By the 1920s, it was promoted as a solution for preventing the birth of "feeble-minded" or "unfit" individuals and encouraging the reproduction of those deemed "fit." These distinctions were often based on race, class, and other social, not clinical, factors. In the mid-twentieth century, surgical sterilization became more widely available and provided an alternative form of birth control for women who did not want more children or with medical conditions that made pregnancy risky (Reilly 1991). The use of sterilization as a form of birth control is controversial because of its applications in limiting the reproductive freedom of marginalized groups, such as women with disabilities and women of color (Roberts 2016).

Until the early twentieth century, most options for terminating pregnancy remained the herbal or mechanical ones described above. However, in the nineteenth century, more physicians and unlicensed practitioners were using instruments to induce a miscarriage, though they could be dangerous for the patients in the same ways as childbirth. In 1843, the metal curette was introduced as a tool for scraping uterine lining and provided a surgical option for terminating pregnancy or for treating a patient after a miscarriage. This tool became part of the dilatation and curettage (D&C) procedure, which continues into the twenty-first century but has evolved by using hormones for

---

[3] Both Adashi et al. (2022) and Brodie (2002) offer more detailed histories of the place of medical abortion through mifepristone in America.

dilating the cervix instead of instruments. Other mechanical systems for inducing menstrual flow and terminating an early pregnancy included vacuuming suction or syringes as well as electricity (Mohr 1978). By the early twentieth century, devices for manual vacuum aspiration were widely available and became a common practice for surgical abortion.

Legality and Beliefs around Contraception and Abortion

Controlling fertility is one of the most controversial and debated topics in the past century with many factors shaping individual beliefs, cultural norms, and national or regional laws. The primary considerations that shape views are when human life is believed to begin and what conception means. Because of the rates of infant and child mortality, historical approaches to this question often marked the moment that human life begins as later than those of the past century. Many ancient societies "simply assumed that life was not present until parturition" or birth, which was also seen in their acceptance of exposing unwanted children by abandoning infants in nature (McLaren 1990, pp. 32–34). For centuries, pregnancy was suspected by the cessation of menses and other physical symptoms, but inducing a miscarriage was not considered an abortion in a legal or religious sense until the moment the pregnant woman could feel fetal movement, which was called quickening and occurred around the fourth month of pregnancy or in the second trimester.

Another consideration shaping these views lies in the reasons for preventing or terminating pregnancy, whether economic, medical, or personal. Limiting the number of children, through contraception or abortion, reduces the financial burden on parents to provide for them. This need for limitation could be extended more broadly in societies or groups facing over-population, which could strain the resources for the entire community. Sometimes, however, the desires of the family and society were in tension, as communities sought to expand their population while individual households could not afford to do so. Pregnancy, childbirth, and childrearing could strain the mother's physical and mental health, particularly in cases where women bore children in short succession, so contraception was a valuable recourse. In some cases, pregnancy or childbirth could put the mother's life at risk (see Chap. 2 for more discussion of maternal mortality), necessitating a decision between terminating the pregnancy and risking the mother's life. Behind many personal or social reasons was the debate about the purpose of sexual intercourse, whether only procreation or if pleasure could be a factor at all. For men and women, the risks of intercourse outside of or before marriage could be resolved with contraception or abortion.

Language used to describe pregnancy, contraception, and abortion reveals quite a bit about individual or societal beliefs. Letters submitted to Margaret Sanger's *Birth Control News* described pregnancy with such phrases as "'caught' or had 'fallen', 'am that way again', 'my monthly courses are ten days late', 'am a month over my time', 'am four months on the way', 'am two months on the road'," which McLaren (1990) notes "implied a process which might or might not be terminated." Instead of using the term abortion which implied a surgical procedure, the women described efforts to "'restore her menses' or 'make herself regular'" (pp. 230–1). Other terms for the termination of a pregnancy included "'bring me round', 'put me on my way' or to 'put me right'" (Brookes 1988). Language to represent the object of abortion worked similarly, as uses of scientific terms like embryo or fetus are replaced with baby or child by those who oppose abortion.

In the sections that follow, the beliefs around contraception and abortion are discussed as they relate to laws and criminalization, the influence of eugenics, and the connections to voluntary motherhood and feminist movements.

Legal History

Before the nineteenth century, abortion was not explicitly illegal in Britain or America. Many of the early laws about abortion focused on termination of a pregnancy after quickening. In Britain, the 1803 Lord Ellenborough Act and 1828 Lord Lansdowne's Act made an abortion illegal with post-quickening penalties ranging from imprisonment to execution. These were refined by the 1861 Offences Against the Person Act to distinguish between the penalties for pre- and post-quickening abortions, which also allowed doctors to use their discretion when the life of the mother was at risk. The 1929 Infant Life (Preservation) Act further clarified to make abortion legal if performed by a registered medical practitioner with the intention of preserving the life of the mother. Even with these laws in effect, a British interdepartmental committee on abortion found in 1937 that "Many mothers seemed not to understand that self-induced abortion was illegal. They assumed it was legal before the third month, and only outside the law when procured by another person" (qtd. in McLaren 1990, p. 228).

In America, the first law criminalizing abortion was passed in Connecticut in 1821 with a number of other states passing similar rules in the following two decades. The Connecticut law forbade abortion after quickening but specifically addressed attempted murder of a mother by using abortifacients as poison. Notably, it did not include punishment for the mother. An 1830 revision added instrumental abortion, making the termination of any pregnancy illegal after quickening but not before it (Mohr 1978). The laws in other states varied on the allowances before quickening and whether procedures to save a woman's life were exempt, though many of these laws were difficult to prosecute (Brodie 1994). In the 1870s, a federal law named for Anthony Comstock was passed to prohibit "the interstate trade in obscene literature and materials," which specifically included any information or items related to contraception or abortion. Again, state laws varied in their local versions (Brodie 1994, pp. 255–7). In essence, these laws forced many efforts toward contraception or abortion underground—or forced people to be creative in these efforts—for more than a century. As the texts in this chapter demonstrate, however, many individuals and groups continued their work to spread information about fertility control throughout that period.

The reversal of these efforts came a century later. In 1967, the Abortion Act made abortion legal in England, Scotland, and Wales (but not Northern Ireland) before 24 weeks and with agreement from two doctors that continuing the pregnancy would pose a risk to the physical or mental health of the mother or that there was a risk of serious fetal abnormality. Then, in 1973, the landmark United States Supreme Court case Roe v. Wade superceded most state laws criminalizing abortion, holding that a woman had a constitutional right to choose to have an abortion but that states could regulate abortion after the first trimester of pregnancy. The 2022 Supreme Court decision in Dobbs vs. Jackson Women's Health Organization returned power to the states, reactivating dormant state laws criminalizing abortion and initiating a wave of legal and political efforts to protect or restrict women's rights.

Eugenics

Eugenics is a concept that formally began in the nineteenth century with the application of ideas from Charles Darwin's *Origin of Species* by Sir Francis Galton, who believed in improving the human race by selective breeding. The idea gained momentum in the early twentieth century, particularly in the United States, where it was embraced by many scientists and policymakers and aimed to promote the reproductive success of certain groups while limiting the reproduction of others deemed "unfit" or "undesirable," such as people with disabilities, those deemed "feeble-minded," or members of minority groups. Some advocates saw contraception and abortion as tools of eugenics to control population growth and prevent the propagation of undesirable traits. In particular, Margaret Sanger and Marie Stopes, prominent birth control activists, were both associated with the eugenics movement.

Women's Rights and Feminism

From their beginnings in the mid-nineteenth century, the women's rights movements in Britain and America have recognized the importance of reproductive control with language about choice that derives from the concept of voluntary motherhood. However many of the nineteenth-century women's rights and voluntary motherhood advocates promoted periodical abstinence, rather than contraception and abortion, in controlling family size as a way to both encourage sexual purity and provide women with power over their family role (Gordon 2002). After the turn of the twentieth century, social limitations changed to allow women more sexual freedom, particularly in large cities. In describing this period as a sexual revolution, Gordon (2002) cites two studies that indicated "women born between 1890 and 1899 (women, therefore, coming to sexual maturity between 1910 and 1920) had twice as high a percentage of premarital intercourse as those born before 1890" (pp. 130–1). In the same period, many of those advocating for birth control—a term coined by Sanger in 1915—were also associated with the women's rights movement. Sanger argued that women's access to birth control was essential to their ability to control their own lives and destinies. The second wave of feminism became closely tied with a larger interest in reproductive rights, which included both contraception and abortion as central parts of women's liberation. This included fights for access to oral contraception through "the pill" and for legalizing abortion.

Themes and Topics in Selections

Across the texts presented in this chapter, several key ideas recur and offer the opportunity for comparison.

Moral, Social, and Legal Perspectives

Nearly all of the texts included in this chapter deal with the moral, social, and/or legal perspectives on fertility control. In particular, the periodical press covered (and often sensationalized) the legal ramifications for doctors and unlicensed practitioners who performed abortions, and the impact of the Comstock Act (and Anthony Comstock himself) is evident through the prosecution against writers and abortionists as well as in a fictional character's name. Many of the health guides for women turned from medical suggestions in other sections to moral views in coverage of fertility, with only a few directly suggesting strategies for preventing pregnancy and being prosecuted for it. Several doctors quoted in these selections boast about their practice of giving placebos to women who request abortifacients, manipulating patients and delaying their treatment until too late to terminate the pregnancy. Writers promoting access to birth control strategies often framed their efforts as a solution for preventing women from abortion. Over time, discussion of fertility control became more direct, in spite of the fact that the Comstock Act technically continues into the twenty-first century.

Fertility Control and Marriage

A woman's relationship status often shaped her experience of contraception and abortion but in complicated ways. Though some believed it was the responsibility of married women to bear children, most guides to contraception directed their advice to married women, suggesting that unmarried women were not sexually active. The unmarried women who seek abortions are tragic figures even if they do not die from the abortion, including characters in *Maria*, *Waste*, "A Sunday Morning Tragedy," and *Summer*, as well as Elizabeth Peer in the news coverage.

The Perception of Danger

Written portrayals of fertility control, particularly those of abortion, present the dangers of the procedure; however, as Chap. 2 illustrates, childbirth was not an entirely safe alternative. Prior to the widespread acceptance of antiseptic practices, instrumental or surgical abortion included the same risks of infection as childbirth, and opponents used that danger to create fear among women. In some ways, abortion could be a safer alternative for women who might have medical difficulties in enduring childbirth, but while abortion was illegal, the practitioners, licensed or not, were secretive in their treatments and not always aware of or following best practices for the safety of their patients. In spite of those dangers, many of the fictional portrayals in the early twentieth century included characters, particularly men who will benefit from terminating the pregnancy, downplaying the dangers to the women who will undergo the procedure.

Maria: Or, The Wrongs of Woman by Mary Wollstonecraft (1798)

Introduction

In this novel, Mary Wollstonecraft adapts the views from *A Vindication of the Rights of Woman* into fictional form through the story of a woman whose abusive husband has her imprisoned in a mental health institution. There she encounters a few characters who share their stories. In this excerpt, a servant in the institution named Jemima shares her story of her sexual assault and decision to terminate the resulting pregnancy. The entire excerpt included here is quoted from Jemima's first-person point of view.

Excerpt from Chapter 5

"At sixteen, I suddenly grew tall, and something like comeliness appeared on a Sunday, when I had time to wash my face, and put on clean clothes. My master had once or twice caught hold of me in the passage; but I instinctively avoided his disgusting caresses. One day however, when the family were at a methodist meeting, he contrived to be alone in the house with me, and by blows—yes; blows and menaces, compelled me to submit to his ferocious desire; and, to avoid my mistress's fury, I was obliged in future to comply, and skulk to my loft at his command, in spite of increasing loathing.

"The anguish which was now pent up in my bosom, seemed to open a new world to me: I began to extend my thoughts beyond myself, and grieve for human misery, till I discovered, with horror—ah! what horror!—that I was with child. I know not why I felt a mixed sensation of despair and tenderness, excepting that, ever called a bastard, a bastard appeared to me an object of the greatest compassion in creation.

"I communicated this dreadful circumstance to my master, who was almost equally alarmed at the intelligence; for he feared his wife, and public censure at the meeting. After some weeks of deliberation had elapsed, I in continual fear that my altered shape would be noticed, my master gave me a medicine in a phial, which he desired me to take, telling me, without any circumlocution, for what purpose it was designed. I burst into tears, I thought it was killing myself—yet was such a self as I worth preserving? He cursed me for a fool, and left me to my own reflections. I could not resolve to take this infernal potion; but I wrapped it up in an old gown, and hid it in a corner of my box.

"Nobody yet suspected me, because they had been accustomed to view me as a creature of another species. But the threatening storm at last broke over my devoted head—never shall I forget it! One Sunday evening when I was left, as usual, to take care of the house, my master came home intoxicated, and I became the prey of his brutal appetite. His extreme intoxication made him forget his customary caution, and my mistress entered and found us in a situation that could not have been more hateful to her than me. Her husband was 'pot-valiant,' he feared her not at the moment, nor had he then much reason, for she instantly turned the whole force of her anger another way. She tore off my cap, scratched, kicked, and buffeted me, till she had exhausted her strength, declaring, as she rested her arm, 'that I had wheedled her husband from her.—But, could any thing better be expected from a wretch, whom she had taken into her house out of pure charity?' What a torrent of abuse rushed out? till, almost breathless, she concluded with saying, 'that I was born a strumpet; it ran in my blood, and nothing good could come to those who harboured me.'

"My situation was, of course, discovered, and she declared that I should not stay another night under the same roof with an honest family. I was therefore pushed out of doors, and my trumpery thrown after me, when it had been contemptuously examined in the passage, lest I should have stolen any thing.

"Behold me then in the street, utterly destitute! Whither could I creep for shelter? To my father's roof I had no claim, when not pursued by shame—now I shrunk back as from death, from my mother's cruel reproaches, my father's execrations. I could not endure to hear him curse the day I was born, though life had been a curse to me. Of death I thought, but with a confused emotion of terror, as I stood leaning my head on a post, and starting at every footstep, lest it should be my mistress coming to tear my heart out. One of the boys of the shop passing by, heard my tale, and immediately repaired to his master, to give him a description of my situation; and he touched the right key—the scandal it would give rise to, if I were left to repeat my tale to every enquirer. This plea came home to his reason, who had been sobered by his wife's rage, the fury of which fell on him when I was out of her reach, and he sent the boy to me with half-a-guinea, desiring him to conduct me to a house, where beggars, and other wretches, the refuse of society, nightly lodged.

"This night was spent in a state of stupefaction, or desperation. I detested mankind, and abhorred myself.

"In the morning I ventured out, to throw myself in my master's way, at his usual hour of going abroad. I approached him, he 'damned me for a b———, declared I had disturbed the peace of the family, and that he had sworn to his wife, never to take any more notice of me.' He left me; but, instantly returning, he told me that he should speak to his friend, a parish-officer, to get a nurse for the brat I laid to him; and advised me, if I wished to keep out of the house of correction, not to make free with his name.

"I hurried back to my hole, and, rage giving place to despair, sought for the potion that was to procure abortion, and swallowed it, with a wish that it might destroy me, at the same time that it stopped the sensations of new-born life, which I felt with indescribable emotion. My head turned round, my heart grew sick, and in the horrors of approaching dissolution, mental anguish was swallowed up. The effect of the medicine was violent, and I was confined to my bed several days; but, youth and a strong constitution prevailing, I once more crawled out, to ask myself the cruel question, 'Whither I should go?' I had but two shillings left in my pocket, the rest had been expended, by a poor woman who slept in the same room, to pay for my lodging, and purchase the necessaries of which she partook.

"With this wretch I went into the neighbouring streets to beg, and my disconsolate appearance drew a few pence from the idle, enabling me still to command a bed; till, recovering from my illness, and taught to put on my rags to the best advantage, I was accosted from different motives, and yielded to the desire of the brutes I met, with the same detestation that I had felt for my still more brutal master. I have since read in novels of the blandishments of seduction, but I had not even the pleasure of being enticed into vice.

"I shall not," interrupted Jemima, "lead your imagination into all the scenes of wretchedness and depravity, which I was condemned to view; or mark the different stages of my debasing misery. Fate dragged me through the very kennels of society: I was still a slave, a bastard, a common property. Become familiar with vice, for I wish to conceal nothing from you, I picked the pockets of the drunkards who abused me; and proved by my conduct, that I deserved the epithets, with which they loaded me at moments when distrust ought to cease.

"Detesting my nightly occupation, though valuing, if I may so use the word, my independence, which only consisted in choosing the street in which I should wander, or the roof, when I had money, in which I should hide my head, I was some time before I could prevail on myself to accept of a place in a house of ill fame, to which a girl, with whom I had accidentally conversed in the street, had recommended me. I had been hunted almost into a fever, by the watchmen of the quarter of the town I frequented; one, whom I had unwittingly offended, giving the word to the whole pack. You can scarcely conceive the tyranny exercised by these wretches: considering themselves as the instruments of the very laws they violate, the pretext which steels their conscience, hardens their heart. Not content with receiving from us, outlaws of society (let other women talk of favours) a brutal gratification gratuitously as a privilege of office, they extort a tithe of prostitution, and harass with threats the poor creatures whose occupation affords not the means to silence the growl of avarice. To escape from this persecution, I once more entered into servitude."

"Fruits of Philosophy" by Charles Knowlton (1832)

Introduction

In this pamphlet, Dr. Charles Knowlton provides information for married couples to control reproduction. Though originally published anonymously, a second publication with Knowlton's name led to his arrest and imprisonment for violation of American obscenity laws. His various legal battles increased the popularity of the volume. In the first chapter, Knowlton describes the political goal of avoiding overpopulation and the social one for families being able to control when they have children and how many. The second chapter provides vivid detail on the female reproductive system using scientific terms, emphasizing the importance of dispelling misunderstandings about the anatomical structure and how conception occurs. The excerpt here is from the second half of the third chapter, which begins with promoting conception for those with sterility or infertility before sharing this discussion of preventing conception.

Excerpt from Chapter III. Of Promoting and Checking Conception.

…

Occasional nocturnal emissions, accompanied with erection and pleasure, are by no means to be considered a disease, though they have given many a one such uneasiness. Even if they be frequent, and the system considerably debilitated, if not caused by debauch, and the person be young, marriage is the proper measure.

There have been several means proposed and practiced for checking conception. I shall briefly notice them, though a knowledge of the best is what most concerns us. That of withdrawal immediately before emission is certainly effectual, if practiced with sufficient care. But if (as I believe) Dr. Dewees' theory of conception be correct, and as Spallanzani's experiments show that only a trifle of semen, even largely diluted with water, may impregnate by being injected into the vagina, it is clear that nothing short of entire withdrawal is to be depended upon. But the old notion that the semen must enter the uterus to cause conception, has led many to believe that a partial withdrawal is sufficient, and it is on this account that this error has proved mischievous, as all important errors generally do. It is said by those who speak from experience that the practice of withdrawal has an effect upon the health similar to intemperance in eating. As the subsequent exhaustion is probably mainly owing to the shock the nervous system sustains in the act of coition, this opinion may be correct. It is further said that this practice serves to keep alive those fine feelings with which married people first come together. Still, I leave it for every one to decide for himself whether this check be so far from satisfactory as not to render some other very desirable.

As to the baudruche, which consists in a covering used by the male, made of very delicate skin, it is by no means calculated to come into general use. It has been used to secure immunity from syphilitic affections.

Another check which the old idea of conception has led some to recommend with considerable confidence, consists in introducing into the vagina, previous to connection, a very delicate piece of sponge, moistened with water, to be immediately afterward withdrawn by means of a very narrow ribbon attached to it. But, as our views would lead us to expect, this check has not proved a sure preventive. As there are many little ridges or folds in the vagina, we cannot suppose the withdrawal of the sponge would dislodge all the semen in every instance. If, however, it were well moistened with some liquid which acted chemically upon the semen, it would be pretty likely to destroy the fecundating property of what might remain. But if this check were ever so sure, it would, in my opinion, fall short of being equal, all things considered, to the one I am about to mention—one which not only dislodges the semen pretty effectually, but at the same time destroys the fecundating property of the whole of it.

It consists in syringing the vagina immediately after connection with a solution of sulphate of zinc, of alum, pearl-ash, or any salt that acts chemically on the semen, and at the same time produces no unfavorable effect on the female.

In all probability a vegetable astringent would answer—as an infusion of white oak bark, of red rose leaves, of nut-galls, and the like. A lump of either of the above-mentioned salts, of the size of a chestnut, may be dissolved in a pint of water, making the solution weaker or stronger, as it may be borne without any irritation of the parts to which it is applied. These solutions will not lose their virtues by age. A female syringe, which will be required in the use of the check, may be had at the shop of an apothecary for a shilling or less. If preferred, the semen may be dislodged as far as it can be, by syringing with simple water, after which some of the solution is to be injected, to destroy the fecundating property of what may remain lodged between the ridges of the vagina, etc.

I know the use of this check requires the woman to leave her bed for a few moments, but this is its only objection; and it would be unreasonable to suppose that any check can ever be devised entirely free of objections. In its favor it may be said, it costs nearly nothing; it is sure; it requires no sacrifice of pleasure; it is in the hand of the female; it is to be used after, instead of before the connection, a weighty consideration in its favor, as a moment's reflection will convince any one; and last, but not least, it is conducive to cleanliness, and preserves the parts from relaxation and disease. The vagina may be very much contracted by a persevering use of astringent injections, and they are constantly used for this purpose in cases of *procidentia uteri*, or a sinking down of the womb; subject as women are to *fluor albus*, and other diseases of the genital organs, it is rather a matter of wonder that they are not more so, considering the prevailing practices. Those who have used this check (and some have used it, to my certain knowledge with entire success for nine or ten years, and under such circumstances as leave no room to doubt its efficacy) affirm that they would be at the trouble of using injections merely for the purposes of health and cleanliness.

By actual experiment it has been rendered highly probable that pregnancy may, in many instances, be prevented by injections of simple water, applied with a tolerable degree of care. But simple water has failed, and its occasional failure is what we should expect, considering the anatomy of the parts, and the results of Spallanzani's experiments heretofore alluded to.

This much did I say respecting this check in the first edition of this work. That is what I call the chemical check. The idea of destroying the fecundating property of the semen was original, if it did not originate with me. My attention was drawn to the subject by the perusal of "Moral Physiology." Such was my confidence in the chemical idea that I sat down and wrote this work in

July, 1831. But the reflection that I did not know that this check would never fail, and that if it should, I might do someone an injury in recommending it, caused the manuscript to lie on hand until the following December. Some time in November I fell in with an old acquaintance, who agreeably surprised me by stating that to his personal knowledge this last check had been used as above stated. I have since conversed with a gentleman with whom I was acquainted, who stated that, being in Baltimore some few years ago, he was there informed of this check by those who have no doubt of its efficacy. From what has as yet fell under my observation, I am not warranted in drawing any conclusion. I can only say that I have never known it to fail. Such are my views on the whole subject, that it would require many instances of its reputed failure to satisfy me that such failures were not owing to an insufficient use of it. I even believe that quite cold water alone, if thoroughly used, would be sufficient. In Spallanzani's experiments warm water was unquestionably used. As the seminal animalcule are essential to impregnation, all we have to do is to change the condition of, or, if you will, to kill them; and as they are so exceedingly small and delicate, this is doubtless easily done, and hence cold water may be sufficient.

What has now been advanced in this work will enable the reader to judge for himself or herself of the efficacy of the chemical or syringe check, and time will probably determine whether I am correct in this matter. I do know that those married females who have much desire to escape will not stand for the little trouble of using this check, especially when they consider that on the score of cleanliness and health alone it is worth the trouble.

A great part of the time no check is necessary, and women of experience and observation, with the information conveyed by this work, will be able to judge pretty correctly when it is and when it is not. They may rest assured that none of the salts mentioned will have any deleterious effect. The sulphate of zinc is commonly known by the name of white vitriol. This, as well as alum, have been extensively used for leucorrhæ. Acetate of lead would doubtless be effectual—indeed, it has proven to be so; but I do not recommend it, because I conceive it possible that a long continued use of it might impair the instinct.

I hope that no failures will be charged of efficacy of this check which ought to be attributed to negligence or insufficient use of it. I will therefore recommend at least two applications of the syringe, the sooner the surer, yet it is my opinion that five minutes' delay would not prove mischievous—perhaps not ten.

"Periodical Coverage of Madame Restell" (1841–1878)

Introduction

In the nineteenth century, Madame Restell provided birth control, abortions, and medical support to thousands of women from a boarding house on Fifth Avenue in New York City. Her business was incredibly successful, and she was highly visible in her location and her general display of wealth. Over the course of her forty years in business, she was arrested multiple times and continued updating her business model around the evolving social views and legal restrictions around preventing and terminating pregnancy. These articles represent several of those moments including her 1841 trial, an interview after her 1878 arrest, and a story after her 1878 suicide the day her trial was set to begin.

Untitled Article (*The New World*, 27 March 1841)

The notorious wretch, calling herself Madame Restell, and having a reputed husband named Charles Lohman, has been arrested for the probable murder of a Mrs. Purdy. The circumstances are too horrible and too disgusting for repetition in this journal; but it seems that Mrs. Purdy was a respectable married lady. She did not wish to become a second time a mother, and so, by the advice of some female devil, consulted this Madame Restell. She was, however, first induced to do so by reading an advertisement in the *Sun* newspaper. The first cause, therefore, of her probable death, is the advertisement. We believe that the *Herald* and the *Sun* are the only newspapers in New York that have dared to issue the damnable announcement of this Madame Restell, and of others, who, like herself, publish themselves as the workers of an infamy too horrible for belief. Thus have these two papers lent themselves to be accomplices before the fact to a crime, than which there is no deeper in the catalogue of human guilt.

    The tardy movement and wretched inefficiency of the city magistrates and police have suffered these evils to accumulate till they have at last gathered into a head and broken of themselves. Great sins against society will, by the inevitable destruction they bring upon its members, be overtaken sooner or later by a just retribution.

    There seems not to be the slightest doubt of the guilt of the accused. Mrs. Purdy in the last hours of her life (for it is said by the physicians that her demise is certain,) has sworn to facts that are sufficient, if justice were evenly meted out, to hang all the parties concerned. She has given her deposition to the attending magistrate under circumstances the most solemn and with the deep conviction that but a few short moments must elapse before she goes to give her account at the bar of God. Her repentance is bitter and sincere; and the only consolation of her friends is derived from that high promise, which declares "though thy sins be as scarlet they shall be white as snow."

The accused was arrested and brought to the bedside of her dying victim, and there solemnly recognised. Madame Restell is now in custody and will be tried for this murder. Other crimes of as black a dye will unquestionably be brought to light. In conclusion, we have but one question to ask—How can those, whose duty and whose obligation it is to guard public morality, hold themselves guiltless of the results of their negligence?

"Madam Restell Still in Prison: Ransacking the City to Find a Man Who Will Put His Name on Her Bail Bond" (*The Sun*, 13 February 1878)

Madame Restell's lawyer made a total change of front yesterday, necessitating an appeal to the discretion of the court before which she was originally taken, and leading up to a further move before the Supreme Court to-day. The prisoner waived examination before Justice Kilbreth on Monday, and he held her in default of $10,000 bail. Her lawyer, Judge Mackinley, spent all Monday evening in an unsuccessful search for bail, and yesterday his efforts in that direction were renewed.

Mrs. Foster, the Matron of the City Prison, made Madam Restell as comfortable as she could. and as the prisoner was held in default of bail only, she was entitled to all the consideration her money could buy. The prison doors were closed at the usual hour, and Warden Quinn saw to it that the regulations were enforced in Restell's case precisely as in all others. She slept like a top, and enjoyed her breakfast in the pleasurable anticipation of a speedy release.

Meantime Mr. Mackinley concluded that it would be better to have an immediate examination, and so told his client. At first she was inclined to adhere to her original determination, but at length she yielded. Mr. Mackinley then appeared before Justice Kilbreth and informed the Court that his client desired an examination before it, and offered bail pending the same. The Justice, who looks enough like Peter B. Sweeny to be his twin, granted the request for an examination, but declined to take bail pending it.

In this way matters stood at the close of the court yesterday afternoon, at which time the counsellor called at the City Prison, and gave Madame Restell the decision.

The examination is set down for Friday next, at 10 o'clock A. M., and, according to Justice Kilbreth, until that time Madam Restell must remain in the City Prison. In order to obviate that, Mr. Mackinley will move in Supreme Court, Chambers, to-day, for an order compelling Justice Kilbreth to reduce the amount of bail demanded, and directing him to accept bail pending the examination.

In view of the notoriety attaching to the prisoner, and the insinuations made against Anthony Comstock, the writer sought interviews with both the detective and the prisoner.

Mr. Comstock is a special agent of the Post Office Department, and acts as a detective and moral censor in the interest of the Society for the Suppression of Crime. He is of medium height, English in look, stout built, and dresses with care. In answer to a question as to his motive he said:

"There were several motives leading up to this very important arrest. In the first place, she flaunts her nefarious avocation in the face of the world, advertises openly, and makes no secret of her operations. In the second place, many reputable physicians have told me that she is doing grievous injury to the community. In the third place, it has been thrown in my teeth repeatedly that while I break up weak and inconspicuous abortionists, and send the poor devils to prison, I either dare not arrest the most notorious of them all, or else I have been bribed. This, of course, injures the service, and it could not be tolerated."

"In there any individual back of you in this arrest?"

"Literally no one, I know Restell says there is, but that's bosh. I have done it on my own any responsibility."

"Can you show her agency in the business for which she is arrested?"

"Certainly. I went three times to her office. Each time I saw her I told her I wanted to procure preparations for an unlawful purpose, and she sold them to me with her own hands."

"Did she offer to pay you for release?"

"No; she knows better than that. We have simply made a long contemplated arrest in the firm determination to bring her to a dead stop. I found all the evidence I wanted on her premises, and the analyses will show the character of her medicines."

Madame Restell found yesterday afternoon in the Matron's room of the City Prison, Warden John Quinn was escorting some lady visitor through the prison, and when he entered the room Madam Restell threw several folds of a brown veil over her face. She wore a fashionable hat, diamond earrings, an embroidered velvet sack, and a black silk dress, Although she is 65 years of age, time has dealt very gently with her, her hair being black and thick, her eye full and sharp, and her general look that of a contented and well-to-do keeper of a fashionable boarding house. She was as calm and mild as a morning in June, betraying no emotion whatever, save now and then a gleam of indignation at "Comstock's trick," and regret that her granddaughter should be left alone so long. She said, "This man has made a mistake, He came to see me, told me a long yarn about his wife, and asked for a preparation and pills. Of course I gave, or rather sold them, to him. Then he ran off and had them analyzed, which was an entirely unnecessary and foolish expense, as I would have given him the prescription cheerfully, They are put up by the druggist, and there is no secret about it."

"Has Comstock any personal feeling against you?"

"I think not; but he is in this nasty detective business, you know. There are a number of little doctors who are in the same business behind him. They think if they can get me in trouble and out of the way they can make a fortune, If the public are determined to push this matter they will have a good laugh when they learn the nature of the terrible items of the preventive prescriptions. Of course, if there's a trial it will all come out."

"But Mr. Comstock found other articles in your house?"

"Of course he did. He ransacked my house, my pantry, my wine cellar, and even my kitchen. But what did he find? Nothing but sundry toilet articles sold by every druggists in the city. I can bring five hundred druggists to testify that they sell precisely what Comstock found in my house. For that matter, he bought none of them, I presume I have a right to keep such things if choose. No; they are envious because I have a fine house in such a splendid location."

"Is it so large that you possibly have room for boarders?"

"Not one. I haven't had a patient in the house since we moved to the up-town house."

"Why is it you can't get bail?"

"Oh, I suppose people are afraid. Here I have all, and more than is needed or asked, exorbitant as it is. I have sent here, there, everywhere; but one man is out of town, another has a partner, a third owns property in Kings county only, and they are all unable to do me the service, The object of bail is to secure attendance at a certain time. They know very well I am here, and mean to stay—if they doubt it, why not take the money? What a lot of little lawyers there were in the court. They bugged about me like flies, but of course I took no notice of them. The papers have treated me very fairly, though I really can't see the use in reviving that affair of thirty years age."

Three lawyers well known in and about the City Prison said that they could get bail for the prisoner in fifteen minutes, all that was necessary being a deposit in their hands of the Madam's bonds. She seemed to view them as safer in her own hands.

At 5½ o'clock Warden Quinn directed the doors to be closed, the bolts shut, and all communication with the outer world to cease. The matronly prisoner was marched back to the women's prison and thence to her apartment, where she removed her outer clothing and proceeded to make herself at home with the news-papers and a cup of tea,

To-day the authority of the Supreme Court is to be appealed to, and on Friday next Judge Kilbreth will listen to the formal examination.

"The Restell Tragedy" (*The American Socialist*, 11 April 1878)

The death of Madame Restell, who has been prominently before the public in odious ways for a long generation, has been a subject of much attention and comment during the past week. There seems to be some reäction of public sentiment in her favor, or at least a persuasion toward charity for her, in consequence of the dreadful tragedy of her "taking off." The allowance of extenuation given to her is mostly summed up in the plea that she had many and respectable accomplices in her crimes. Thus the *Graphic* says in its "History of the Day:"

"Ann Lohman, *alias* Mme. Restell, cuts her throat in a bath tub. Frightened to her death by fear of trial. Occupation 'infamous and murderous.' She murdered to order at solicitation of people who wanted murder done. Had several hundred, possibly thousands, of accomplices in crime, many of whom belonged to 'good society.' Popular sentiment places all the infamy on Restell's head and regards accomplices with indifference. Conundrum: Which is the most & murderess, the woman who hires an assassin to murder her child, or the assassin who strangles it?"

A valued correspondent of ours asks us to ventilate some merciful reflections on Madame Restell, which we do for the sake of the historical reminiscences which accompany them. She says:

"Nobody dares to compassionate this old lady, though she has fallen among thieves and been literally murdered. She may have been a bad woman, very bad, but the good Samaritan made no deep scrutiny into the character of the man to whom he showed mercy, and I am not ashamed to say that my feelings are touched in view of this woman's fate, and I am led to consider what extenuation there may be of her crimes. Her calling was certainly created by a great demand, and that not from the lower classes—the poor and degraded—but from the highest ranks of society and from professors of religion. We all remember the excitement there was in Massachusetts several years ago about the mania for abortion which prevailed there, and what exposures Dr. Todd made in his 'Serpents in the Dove's Nest,' of the extent of this mania. From another publication under my eye, I give the testimony of two physicians on this subject, one a Boston man of long practice, the other a practitioner of high reputation in a large village of this State. The first says:

"The extent of this practice of abortion has not been exaggerated. It is almost universal among the upper classes. The poor are comparatively free from it; but it increases as you rise among the rich and select circles. It not only lessens the number of children among the wealthy, but the children they do have are often constitutional sufferers from the effects of the medicines and means which have been used to prevent their birth. I often see children bearing marks which I am well satisfied are caused by this unnatural attempt."

The other physician says:

"I am beset day after day by young married women, and old married women, to give them something that will produce an abortion. One young woman, who has been married only a few weeks, and who must be about three months pregnant, insists upon having an abortion and will not take no for an answer. I generally give them some simple medicine that is sure to do no harm, and tell them that if that don't work they will have to endure till the end. There seems to be a perfect monomania in the village and vicinity on this subject. I don't know what to do. If I refuse to do what they ask, they will be sure to go to some one who loves money more than a clear conscience, and so accomplish their purpose."

"The fact that Madame Restell made a fortune by her calling is evidence of a great demand to which she ministered supply.

"Now the demand for any method for abortion is not legitimate—it is horrible; but the demand for some method of controlling propagation *is* legitimate, and will be more and more so to the world's end; and it is certain so long as thins legitimate demand is ruled down, the illegitimate will force supply, and the Restells will have as good a conscience in their calling at least as the rum-sellers and soldiers, If their remedy is successful, the public may reprobate them, but there must be thousands of women and men too who will regard them with secret approbation and gratitude."

So much from our correspondent. Her reference to the excitement about abortions which shook Massachusetts and the churches of the whole country ten years ago, recalls to mind the following paragraph from the *American*

Agriculturist, published in the midst of that excitement. It gives valuable information of the literature of the subject:

"The *murder* of the unborn is beginning to attract, in some degree, the attention which its great importance imperatively demands. The prevalence and recent great increase of this crime, the general ignorance as to its criminality and of its terrible consequences upon the guilty actors themselves, forbid longer silence on the part of medical men, ministers and editors, who have until now feared lest public effort should make known and increase an evil which it aimed to diminish, Dr. Storer's Essay, 'Why Not,' published by Messrs. Lee & Shepard, of Boston, should be in the hands of every Physician, Clergyman, Editor, and of all other intelligent persons of either sex, in the country.—(Price 50 cts.) Dr. Todd recently furnished an article on the subject to the *Congregationalist*, at Boston, and we hear he is preparing a longer essay for publication. [This refers to a book afterward published by Dr. Todd entitled '*Serpents in the Dove's Nest.*'] The *Christian Advocate*, of New York, also published an article from an intelligent lady, entitled: 'Fashionable Murder.' The *Northwestern Christian Advocate*, of Chicago, Ill., of March 13, devoted seven and a half columns to a bold and outspoken discussion of the subject, which is being copied at the West and is worthily awakening much attention. We learn that one of the editors, Rev. Arthur Edwards, Chicago, is preparing a cheap pamphlet or tract designed for extensive circulation."

All this shows how large and respectable Madame Restell's constituency must have been ten years ago; and we have no reason to think that it has declined since, though the excitement soon passed away and the exposures ceased. How much the churches who are implicated in her death may have been also implicated in her crimes will be known only in the day of judgment.

Finally, to deal fairly all around, we give place to a communication from another valued correspondent, enthusiastically defending Anthony Comstock, who is the antithesis of Madame Restell, and has been much blamed for his agency in her death, It is best to hear all sides in such affairs. We agree with the moral views of the following letter for the most part—especially with the call for open dealing with the young on the part of parents as the only means to save them from the obscenists:

"EDITOR OF THE AMERICAN SOCIALIST:— I have just read your article on the 'Comstock Laws,' and think you do (unintentional) injustice to Mr. Comstock. You can hardly realize what that heroic man bas done to stem the tide of filth which has been threatening to engulf, and to ruin in body and soul, both the boys and the girls of our land. He has told me personally of facts he has encountered, which, when you had brought yourself to believe them, would first curdle your blood with horror and then make it boil with indignation against the *devils*—that is not too hard a word—in human form who are building up fortunes by corrupting the young, and whom Anthony Comstock has been fighting almost single handed. If I mistake not, he bears on his face to-day a scar received in bringing to justice one of these wretches who, having failed to bribe him, resorted to the knife to effect an escape. You should hear him tell of obscene pictures, books, and articles, sent by means of school-catalogues into the midst of boys' and even girls' schools, and these pictures designed to awaken and pander to an immature and lustful passion. You should read as I have in the various vile 'boys' story papers' advertisements, scarcely veiled even, of the same filthy things.

"Honor then, all honor, to the one man who has had the courage to disregard false shame and grapple with the insidious but monstrous iniquity; and this in spite of the blindness and indifference of parents, and the aggravating delays of the courts, and the often absurdly inadequate penalties awarded to the convicted.

"I say 'false shame;' for let me add a word further upon the root of all the trouble. I sometimes think that nine-tenths of all the crime and misery in the world is more or less directly connected with the sexual function—ignorance, or at any rate violation, of its laws. Eliminate all the jealousies, bickerings, assaults, murders (from the fœtus up to adult life), all the diseases and infirmities of body or mind, all the extravagances, al the thefts, traceable finally to some abnormal exercise of the sexual instinct, and what a marked decrease in the crime-list there would be!

"Now the child is *sure* sooner or later to find out about this part of its organization, and *if it does not learn purely and correctly, it will learn impurely and incorrectly*. Probably not a boy, perhaps not a girl, reaches the age of ten or twelve, without picking up a good deal of information true or false about these matters; information dangerous if false, and even if true made dangerous by the appearance of covering stolen secrets. Why then should not parents, why should not decent people, forestall the ignorant and vulgar informants of the little ones, by explaining to them as early as they can understand it, the nature and purpose of this wonderful portion of our mechanism—fore-arming them against the corruption which threatens at every turn, and freeing the whole subject from its present dangerous fascination by divesting it of its false mystery, which naturally so piques the child's curiosity, and by taking away the temptation to *stolen* knowledge and al necessity of *secrecy* on the child's part, which is itself a fascination? Surely, a new era will begin, if wise and loving fathers and mothers teach their children about these things, and do not wait to let them learn as they may and will from the corrupt world without.

"But while we advocate most earnestly this wise instruction, and deplore the false shame which obstructs it, let us not make the unhappy mistake of hindering, and not rather aiding by every means in our power, the heroic efforts of a man who is patient and persevering enough to ferret out the destroyers of our precious little ones, and daring enough to grapple with them in their very dens of infamy and drag them to the light. But for this man, the notorious woman who has just sought in suicide escape from human punishment might to-day be plying still her nefarious trade.

"Wise and pure instruction let us aim at as the ultimate and complete cure for these evils; but meanwhile let us, even if to do it we have to come dangerously near au infringement of some cherished rights, as of the inviolability of the mails —let us arrest and punish by the strong arm of the law the corrupters of our youth.

"Honor to Anthony Comstock!
"h. d. c.
"*N.Y. City, April 5th,*1878."

If Mr. Comstock could make it clear that his aim is simply to put down obscenity and that he favors the "wise instruction" on the sexual question which our correspondent so earnestly commends, he would unquestionably do much to allay the storm of indignation rising against him; but it has been difficult to discern in his acts and utterances any such wise discrimination.

The Ladies' Medical Friend by W. Hamilton Kittoe (1845)

Introduction

Dr. William Hamilton Kittoe's *The Ladies' Medical Friend* includes information on treating diseases specific to women, information on infant care for mothers, and an appendix of prescriptions. The opening of the book lists his qualifications with M.D. after his name, his role as surgeon and accoucheur, and the location of his home in London as well as the hours he is available to consult patients. The section on pregnancy includes a discussion of the symptoms and treatment for accidental miscarriage (included in Chap. 2 of this volume), which is followed by this brief excerpt about abortion and British legal restrictions.

Excerpt from "Abortion or Miscarriage"

The practice of producing miscarriage, for criminal purposes, has prevailed in all ages. In the early months it is always very difficult to decide whether such an event has or has not taken place. Every woman who attempts to induce abortion, does it at the hazard of her life. "There is no drug," says Male, "which will produce miscarriage in women who are not predisposed to it, without acting violently on their system, and probably endangering their lives." Burns says, "It cannot be too generally known, that when medicines produce a miscarriage, the mother seldom survives their effects." By an act passed in 1803, it was enacted, that any person who should wilfully administer any drug, medicine, or substance, or use any instrument, with the intent to abortion, the person so offending is liable to be fined, imprisoned, stand in the pillory, be publicly whipped, or transported beyond the seas for any period not exceeding fourteen years. The same act directed that a person administering any drug with an intent to procure miscarriage, after quickening, should be punished with death. Setting, however, the illegality of the proceeding out of the question, it is a crime of the most diabolical, revolting, and in-human nature, and what no practitioner possessing the slightest pretensions to honour or respectability would become party to.

"Horrible. Death From Abortion." (1846)

Introduction

This news article presents specific details about the suspected abortion and death of a young woman in New Jersey. The story includes a visit to famous New York City abortionist Madame Costello who advertised her "monthly pills" in New York newspapers for married women who wished to remove the cause of suppression or obstruction of their menstrual cycle. This periodical was part of the nineteenth-century style of journalism that focused on sensational reporting.

Horrible. Death from Abortion. (*National Police Gazette*, 5 December 1846)

Denville, Morris Co., N.J.
Nov 28, 1846

Messrs. Camp & Wilkes.

Gentlemen—I rec'd your letter of the 24th inst. on Thursday evening, too late to reply to it by the next mail which left here on Friday morning, consequently I had to defer sending what you request until next Monday morning's mail (as the mail leaves here but three times a week). You request me to send you a copy of the testimony taken before me in the recent case of the death of a young woman (Elizabeth Peer) &c., which I will do with pleasure. When she first called on Dr. Fairchild last summer, she was afflicted with a complaint in which her internal organs were out of order, and he had great difficulty in restoring them in their proper place, but he finally got them right and got her cured; when she came to him for the purpose of producing an abortion, he first thought she came with the old complaint and wanted to be cured of that; but when she told him what she really did want, he told her he would not do it. And advised her still more, to go on and have her child. And when she spoke of the disgrace and of her character, he told her that it would not be injured any more than it already was, for she had had one before which was the case), but she persisted, and threatened to lay it to him (as he is a young man) but that would not deter him, and he would not do it.

Susan Peer, the mother, was first sworn; says about one week after her sickness she sent for Doctor Van Wyck (Fairchild), which was about four weeks since; she was taken with chills and fever, and in about one week after was taken with vomiting; she got some better in a couple of weeks and then was taken worse, and continued so until her death. She has not lived in the house with her daughter for some time; has lived with Mr. Lindsly; she went to New-York with Elizabeth, but did not know her (E.'s) business in New-York; she (E.) did not tell witness what she went for; she told witness she did not know but she would stay there and work; she left witness a while and then went away, while they were in the city; and she (witness) waited for her about the dock until she came back; and when she came back, she said mother I believe I will go home with you, and they came home together; stopped and got dinner at Newark; came to Morristown with the cars; got a carriage at Morristown, and got home by 8 o'clock in the evening of the same day they left home, they went from here with the stage in the morning to Newark.

[The testimony of Susan Peer, the mother of Elizabeth, as stated above, is certainly, to say the least of it, very strange. I was in hopes that she would relate the circumstance of her going with her daughter to New-York for the express purpose of having the operation performed which produced the abortion, but on that subject she swore through everything, and would not say she knew any thing about it. She bears the name of being a very bad character, and of keeping a house of prostitution for a number of years. I have since been informed that Elizabeth's dying words were to the effect, that she and her mother, went to Madame Cosello's to have it done; and that she (E.) and Costello went into an adjoining room, where she performed the operation, while her mother waited in the next room. When done, Costello came to her mother and told her the job was done, and well done; and that her mother paid Costello thirty dollars for the performing of the operation.]

Dorcas Whitehead, sworn, says she was there engaged to take care of Elizabeth while she was sick; was there three weeks; was there until she died; of the persons who were there while she was there, was Nancy Harriman, Mrs. Lyon, Mrs. Trelease, Widow Cook, Mrs, Southron, and Mrs. Tunis; did not hear Elizabeth say any thing about her situation; did not know she was or had been pregnant; suspected she was.

John S. Pollard, sworn, says he has heard the Doctor speak of his coming up here to see Elizabeth; does not know that he ever heard it said she was advised to go to New-York to get rid of it; saw some person in the stage that looked like Elizabeth and her mother.

Abel Gray, sworn, says he knows nothing about it only by report; heard what was reported that she died by miscarriage; heard she went to New-York for that purpose; heard Mr. Pollard say he heard such report; don't know that he ever heard that any one advised her to go to New-York.

John Blanchard, sworn, he has heard of her miscarriage; knows nothing about it himself; heard about it within two weeks; heard that somebody supposed that somebody said that she had been to New-York.

[This witness is supposed to know a great deal more thon he was willing to tell on the stand; he has often been seen visiting the house, &c.; although he is a man of family, with children grown up.]

John Gray, sworn, says he has heard about, the miscarriage; knows nothing, only what the Doctor told him.

Charles A. Righter, sworn, says he knew nothing of her death before to day; has heard of her being pregnant before she went to New-York; never heard she was to go to New-York; saw her some four weeks ago; saw her at her home; Doctor Fairchild requested him to bring him up, as he had no horse to come with at that time; and he brought the Doctor up from Parsippany to see her; know nothing of any one giving her money to go to New-York.

[This witness it is suspected has given her money to go to New-York.

Nancy Harriman, sworn, says she understood the Doctor said it was an inflammation; Elizabeth told witness that she did not know but something of the kind (pregnancy) was the matter with her; she said nothing about being advised to go to New-York to get rid of it.

[This witness was a very unwilling one, and not until I threatened to commit her would she answer the questions she did; it is supposed she knew a great deal more than she said she did.]

Eunice Trelease, sworn, says she has been there but little; does not know any thing about her situation; only the Doctor said it was inflammation; thought while she was well (in her own mind) that she was pregnant, though her eyes might deceive her.

Nancy Lyon, sworn, says she knows nothing about it, only she told her at one time of a distress about her heart.

Next follows Dr. Fairchild's testimony.

Francis Lindsly, sworn, says he mistrusted she was pregnant, but knew nothing only what he has heard; has heard the Doctor say she had the childbed fever; knows of no one advising her to do any thing to produce the miscarriage.

Another Death from Abortion

We take the following from the "Jerseyman," published at Morristown, N.J. It will be seen that the victim confessed the joint offence to have been committed by herself and Madame Costello, one of the female abortionists of this city, Coroner's Inquest—An inquest was held at Denville, in Rockaway township, on Saturday the 14th inst., before Moses Beam, Esq., on the body of Elizabeth Peer, who died the day preceding. The cause of her death was fully understood, but the object of calling the inquest, we learn, was to endeavor to ferret out the inhuman female in the city of New York who committed this double murder. In this they were foiled, but it was understood pretty evidently that the notorious *Madame Costello* was the operator. Whether it was for the purpose of boasting of the immense business she is now doing at her infamous profession, or to inspire courage in her unfortunate patient, is not known, but this fiend in human shape informed the girl that she had already on that day operated on *four* from Morris county, and *three* from Elizabethtown! Should this be the fact, the police of New York cannot be too watchful over these wholesale murderers and panderers of vice.

We omit the testimony given before the jury, with the exception of the attending physician. The jury rendered a verdict that the deceased came to her death by an abortion, produced by some person to them unknown, in the city of N. York. A publication has gone forth which was evidently intended to create unpleasant feelings in the vicinity, but it only proved another abortion;

neither did the examination cost the county one half the sum there represented "for effect." The following is the testimony of the physician:

Dr. R. V. W. Fairchild sworn—In the month of July, deceased first visited witness and requested him to produce an abortion. Witness refused. She came again about a month afterwards on the same errand. Witness fully stated to her the dangers and impropriety of such an operation. She told him that she had been advised to such a course, and she was determined on it—that she would rather die than suffer the disgrace.

On the 6th or 7th of October, witness was called to her, and found a fœtus of five months in the bed, which he took home. Three days utter, he was again called to see her. Found her bowels uncommonly swollen—pulse small, and 160 to the minute—bilious vomiting, with cold sweat and diarrhea—told her her case was child-bed fever, and that he had no hope. She then stated she had gone to New York to one of those famous female physician houses, and that the membranes were ruptured by an instrument.—After being satisfied that her case was hopeless, she prayed for forgiveness and died at the house of her mother.

The Unwelcome Child; or, The Crime of an Undesigned and Undesired Maternity by Henry Clarke Wright (1858)

Introduction

In this volume, activist Henry Clarke Wright presents the prevention of pregnancy as essential for preventing abortion. Though his text primarily addresses husbands, he advocates for women to have a voice in family planning. He repeatedly emphasizes the morality of those who limit their conception and includes chapters on the damage "undesired maternity" does to mothers and children. In the fifth chapter, excerpted here, Wright includes a narrative from a reader and the story of a couple that followed his advice. He also includes direct addresses to married women and unmarried women with instruction for each group.

Excerpts from Letter V: The Wife's Appeal—The Husband's Response

Dear Friend

In the three preceding letters, I have endeavored to present to you the crime of an undesigned and undesired Maternity, especially in its bearing on the mother and the child. I have shown how it wrongs the mother by crushing out of her heart her love and respect for her husband, and converting them into a settled feeling of bitterness and contempt: and also by filling her with feelings of murderous hostility towards her child, and driving her to deeds which her soul abhors,—thus destroying her self-respect, and making her to seem like a loathsome and degraded object in her own estimation. I have shown, also, how it wrongs the child, by depriving it of a mother's loving sympathy, by forcing it into an existence that is detested by father and mother, by stamping on it, before birth, disease and crime, and tendencies to all that is evil, and thus subjecting it to the detestation of its fellow-beings, in its future manhood or womanhood. The father perpetrates the deepest crime against the child, by committing its ante-natal education to the hands of one to whom its very existence is her abhorrence and loathing. What greater crime could a husband and father commit against his wife and child? None; no, *none*!

THE WIFE'S APPEAL.

In this letter, I will give you the experience of a husband and wife, as given by themselves, and by a mutual friend, who is also a wife and a mother. I extract from their letters with few omissions. See, in the experience of this wife and mother, the deep, unutterable anguish, and the deeper woe of conscious degradation, to which woman, in her mistaken notions of conjugal duty, her fear of losing a husband's love and confidence, and her horror of an undesired maternity, will subject herself Read over her experience, as detailed by her friend and herself, and then say if any crime man can commit, can surpass that which husbands and fathers often do to their wives and children, merely for the momentary gratification of their sensual passions:

"Some fifteen years ago, a man of culture, and engaged in public life, was united in marriage with an intimate friend of mine. With pride and confidence, he selected her from a large and admiring circle of friends, as one embodying his ideal of womanly excellence. My friend was thought a fortunate girl (only seventeen), and many thought him quite as fortunate. They were much in society, and she began to enjoy life intensely.

"She was too much a woman not to desire offspring some time, but she felt unprepared to have maternity forced upon her youth and inexperience. It came at a time when her husband's calling led him much from home, to mix in the society she so much enjoyed, and which she felt was contributing to make her what she so much desired to be,—her husband's fitting and equal companion. It was not without a severe struggle she resigned these advantages and checked her aspirations. However, she submitted, though she keenly felt the sacrifice.

"Though overwhelmed with the greatness of her responsibilities, and an undefined dread of physical suffering, she was determined not to appear weak, but bravely to meet and bear the burden imposed upon her. Her husband was absent when the trial hour came; but when he returned, he took his babe and wife to his bosom with pride and joy, though its gestational development had, apparently, scarcely given him an anxious thought.

"My friend's future looked bright. She did not see or understand the fact, that she was to continue to develop the germs of human beings into life, with little sustaining help from the father, whose caresses generally ended in exhausting her vital powers by passional indulgence. She did not complain, but rather rejoiced, as she saw her other powers of attraction to her husband depart one by one, that she was so organized as to be able to meet what she knew he considered an essential want of his nature.

"Eleven years passed, at which time she gave birth to her sixth child. She was a devoted mother, of a joyous spirit, and possessed of wonderful elasticity. But woman cannot be entirely happy in maternity alone, without the presence and sustaining power of her husband. If she is a true wife, she desires to be more to her husband than merely the mother of his children.

"Her husband made for her a beautiful material home, and seemed happy when with her; but he was much away; he sought other pleasures, social and intellectual, in which she could not participate;— she must stay at home, alone, with her children. Little did he know the trials of patience and strength in his wife, in being compelled to bear the responsibility of the health and training of her little ones alone. The world called her a happy wife, and she felt that she ought to be so; but a dark cloud was coming over her once joyous spirit. She began to realize the fact, so fatal to a wife's happiness, that her husband did not feel her to be his equal, and a fitting companion to meet his social and intellectual necessities. When he brought home a friend, she listened to conversations and discussions in which she could not participate. She felt keenly the growing distance between them, and she knew too well how it had come about.

"She quietly made up her mind to have no more children. How did she propose to bring it about? Not by asking her husband to deny himself his accustomed indulgence; no, that, she thought, would be to cut herself off from her strongest hold on his affection and confidence, and to sever the last link of the chain that bound them together. She did not expect that any precaution would enable her to escape conception. She brought herself to do what was most repugnant to her nature, and which, as she felt, would destroy her self-respect, and make her, in her own estimation, a degraded woman, namely, TO PROCURE ABORTION.

"The first shock given to her constitution by this abuse of her nature was comparatively light. But once did not suffice. As a longer interval passed without a new-born babe than ever before, she had begun to take her place by her husband's side in society, earnestly praying that she might be spared maternity evermore. Her husband delighted to have her with him. He felt that he had a right, by law and the customs of society, to his gratification; he persevered in demanding it, and she continued to yield. Several times in four years did she nip the young flower of foetal life in the bud, and each time told more and more terribly on her constitution, until the power of conception was nearly destroyed, at little more than thirty-five years of age. She was shorn of her Womanhood, and became a sickly, broken-down wife and mother, in the very spring-time, as it were, of her life, being driven frequently to perpetrate a degrading outrage upon herself, or endure a maternity abhorrent to her soul;—and all to gratify the sensual passion of her husband, thinking thereby to secure his affection and respect. How fatally mistaken! By yielding, she strengthened his passion, but not his love.

"Reflecting on her sad experience, in the light of your book on 'Marriage and Parentage,' which I had placed in her hands, she saw clearly where the wrong had been, but for a long time felt powerless to destroy what she regarded as her last hold on her husband. He was absent, and I prevailed on her to write and lay the matter frankly and plainly before him, and send him your book. She was then prostrated in body and soul by the last outrage upon her womanly and maternal nature.

…

"It will do your heart good to know that that husband has, thus far, been true to his pledge; that that wife is now blooming again in comparative health. Hope and triumph are shining in her face, love quickens the intellect, and vitalizes the whole woman. And woman is intuitional, to understand and appreciate a true and noble manhood. You will not wonder, then, that she feels nearer to him, in mind and spirit, than ever before, for now she understands him, and he her. Could they have talked over the subject of passional relations, and understood each other before they entered upon their: marriage life, it had saved her years of anguish. May their history be a beacon light to warn others to shun the rocks and shoals that lie, unseen, in the inner depths of wedded life!

"It may encourage you to know that they owe their salvation to you, though they allow that I have had a hand in it. True, it was through me that the experience of Ernest and Nina came to their knowledge, but I am quite willing that the author of 'Marriage and Parentage should bear the responsibility and have the glory of their redemption. Their names are sacredly private. They would meet you without feeling that you know them. I shall not reveal them further than I have done.

"God speed you in your efforts to vindicate the most sacred and important of all human rights, — the right of woman to say when and under what circumstances she shall assume the office of Maternity, and the right of her child to a joyous welcome into life.

"The crime of an enforced and abhorred maternity! Well and truly do you call it, 'the crime of earth.' In whatever light it is viewed, whether in its bearing on the mother, on the child, on the husband, on home, on society, or on humanity, it is, indeed, the crime of crimes.

"With fervent prayers for the triumph of truth on this subject, I am
Your friend,
------."

My friend, how many wives would appeal to their husbands, if they dared? "Sever the last link of the bond that binds her to her husband!" Mere sensualism "the last link" in such a union! I do not like to talk of chains, links, and bonds, in connection with such a relation. Talk of these in connection with slaveholders and slaves, but let them not sully a relation like this. "The last link," indeed! Yet it is true; it is, often, the first, and last, and only link in the chain that binds the husband to the wife, in what is called marriage. Man seeks woman as a legal wife, that he may legally and respectably give indulgence, without restraint, to his passion. If the wife seeks to preserve her soul and body from desecration, he threatens to leave her, and seek his gratification where he can find it. She submits, to keep him with her; both of them, unmindful and regardless of the results to the mother and the child. "Perish all outward bonds" of marriage at once, rather than that the relation should continue in this way!

Wives! be frank and true to your husbands, on the subject of maternity, and the relation that leads to it. Interchange thoughts and feelings with them, as to what nature allows or demands, in regard to these. Can maternity be natural, when it is undesigned by the father, or undesired by the mother? Can a maternity be natural, healthful, ennobling to the mother, to the child, to the father, and to home, when no loving, tender, anxious forethought presides over the relation in which it originated?— when the mother's nature loathed and repelled it, and the father's only thought was his own selfish gratification; the feelings and conditions of the mother, and the health, character and destiny of the child that may result being ignored by him? Wives! let there be a perfect and loving understanding between you and your husbands, on these matters, and great will be your reward.

Maidens! a word to you. Never enter into the physical relations of marriage with a man, until you have conversed with him freely and fully on maternity, and the relation that leads to it. Learn distinctly his views and feelings, and his expectations, in regard to that purest and most ennobling of all the functions of your nature, and the most sacred of all the intimacies of conjugal life. Your self-respect, your beauty, your glory, your heaven, as a wife, will be more directly involved in his feelings and views and practices, in regard to that relation, than in all other things. As you would not become a weak, a miserable, imbecile, unlovable and degraded wife and mother, in the very prime of your life, come to a perfect understanding with your chosen one, ere you commit your person to his keeping in the sacred intimacies of home. Beware of that man, who, under pretence of delicacy, modesty, and propriety, shuns conversation with you on this relation, and on the hallowed function of maternity. Concealment and mystery, in him, towards you, on all other subjects pertaining to conjugal union, might be overlooked; but if he conceals his views here, rest assured it bodes no good to your purity and happiness as a wife and a mother. You can have no more certain assurance that you are to be victimized, your soul and body offered up, slain, on the altar of his sensualism, than his unwillingness to converse with you on subjects so vital to your happiness. In the relation he seeks with you will he, practically, hold his manhood in abeyance to the calls of your nature and to your conditions, and consecrate its passions and its powers to the elevation and happiness of his wife and children? If not, your maiden soul had better return to God unadorned with the diadem of conjugal and maternal love, than that you should become the wife of such a man, and the mother of his children.

How much of woman's suffering and degradation, under the horrors of an unnatural maternity, are owing to herself, I will not say. My appeal is to husbands, and I would show them the extent of their responsibility in this crime. Doubtless, woman might save herself much anguish and suffering, if she would approach man frankly, in womanly love, tenderness, and dignity, and open to him the depths of her soul in regard to Maternity, and the relation in which it originates. Men are not all below the brutes, in their nature. If woman were true to purity, to justice, to her own nature, and would be just and true to her husband and her children, and freely and lovingly converse with man on these relations and functions, he would, often, with manly pride and affection, respond to her. On no subject would a true and noble man respond to the words of a pure and trusting woman with more manly pride and dignity, and a more conscious self-respect, than on Maternity, and the relation that leads to it. Let wives, then, be true to themselves, if they would have their husbands true to them!

"The Evil of the Age" (1871)

Introduction

This article from the *New York Times* presents the prevalence of unlicensed abortionists practicing in New York City, criticizing the abortionists themselves as well as other periodicals that printed advertisements from them. The article describes the experience of undercover visits to the facilities and quotes from advertisements for some of the most widely known abortionists in the period. Other references to the same people in this chapter include Madame Costello in an 1846 article and Madame Restell in several articles between 1841 and 1878.

The Evil of the Age (*New York Times*, 23 August 1871)

The enormous amount of medical malpractice that exists and flourishes, almost unchecked in the city of New York, is a theme for more serious consideration. Thousands of human beings are thus murdered before they have seen the light of this world, and thousands upon thousands more of adults are irredeemably ruined in constitution, health and happiness. So secretly are these crimes committed, and so craftily do the perpetrators invade their victims, that it is next to impossible to obtain evidence and witnesses. Facts are so artfully, concealed from the public mind, and appearances, so carefully guarded, that very meagre outlines of the horrible truth have thus far been disclosed. But could even a portion of the facts. It has been detected in frightful perfusion, by the agents of the times, be revealed and print, and their hideous truth, the reader with shrink from the appalling picture.

More than once, some of the fearless and eminent of the clergy, have spoken upon this theme from their pulpits. They have declared the existence of these great evils in social life—alike denounced and forbidden by the law of God and man. The records of our criminal courts also occasionally afford indications of the horrible degree in amount of depravity already referred to. Indeed, language can scarcely exaggerate the actual facts. There is a systematic, business in wholesale murder, conducted by men and women in this city, that is seldom detected, rarely interfered with, and scarcely ever punished by law.

The men and women who are engaged in this outrageous business are, with few exceptions, the worst class of imposters. Very few have genuine medical diplomas. Some are, or have been, nurses, and thus picked up fragments of knowledge, but our lamentably devoid of scientific education; in some cases they are ridiculously ignorant of the commonest rudiments of ordinary branches of learning. Some are said to have purchased diplomas, which it is reported can be obtained at certain Pennsylvania and Vermont institutions for $40 each. One man procured the diploma of a deceased physician, erased the name by some chemical process, and inserted his own. These documents are framed, and conspicuously displayed in the "office," to attract the first glance of the dupes, who may enter.

Very rarely, did these persons use their true names. Nearly all have one or more aliases. One fellow who amends "M.D." to his circulars, was recently a cobbling shoemaker—and a very poor one at that. Suddenly he closed his shop, moved to another part of town, and was metamorphosed into a "doctor." Another was formerly a barber. Another was a horse-shoer. Another was a glazier. The female practitioners generally have been nurses or midwives. Often invariably they are in partnership with a man "doctor," and are titled "madame," or in some cases "doctor." Lady patients, of course, prefer to call upon a "madame" in delicate cases, and are willing to converse freely with her. The ice, being broken, the forbidden subject, fully broached, and the purposes of the visit all developed, the "madame" calls in her "husband," (?) the "doctor," (?) who really then assumes the charge of all that is afterwards done. But the "medical treatment" subsequently may be cannot with propriety be here described. Any respectable physician knows the nature of the various methods in vogue. He also knows that they are all illegal, unprofessional, and extremely perilous.

A prominent Christian lady, a doctor, or "doctress," greatly esteemed, for her social virtues, has very often been approached with the most tempting offers of fees for such service, and always argues and dissuade the applicant from thus sinning. And one case where a wealthy man, accompanied by a young girl insisted, she caused his arrest, and although he held a position of wealth and position he was prosecuted. There are a great number of educated, male and female physicians in or near this city, who live and thrive these criminal practices. There are others who are the vilest of quacks. Of the latter there are about two hundred. Most of those have offices where they receive, consult with, and examine patients, but have no nursing rooms attached. The place is cunningly arranged. The outer hall door is open; the inner one is closed. Over the glass is a thick lace curtain, through which a keen-eyed attendant peers. When the enters interest he sums up in his mind what his or her circumstances may be. He then steps into the hall, opens the front room door, and politely ushers them in. Two eye-holes in the folding doors offered the "doctor" a full view from the back room. Similar arrangements are provided at other places, so that a dissatisfied, or incurable dupe may be seen, and the "doctor" can slip out of the back door and be "not it." Sometimes, an ostentatious display of instruments, bottles, and drugs is made for effect. The preliminary conversation is cheerful and polite, but brief. Then to business. As a matter of medical talk follows, then an explanation of symptoms, and examination, and the payment of the fee. A box of pills, a phial of liquid drops, or sometimes powders, are given, and the patient is bowed out.

A retired practitioner told the writer: "I never did any harm to those patients. I knew they were determined to get some one to do what they wished. If it was done, one, or perhaps, two, lives would be sacrificed. So I pretended, and thus saved life. I gave them pills of paste, rhubarb and sugar; and colored water slightly flavored; and when they would return angry, because the desired effect had not been produced, I said, that I must adopt, more severe measures. As you may imagine, I made just as much show in that. I had an arrangement with a clergyman to leave the dates on the certificate, blank! Or, if a wedding was impossible, I advised them to go to nursing rooms, let nature take its course and adopt the 'result.'"

Undoubtedly, a large number of quacks in the country, as well as in the city, practice the same method, and thus the fools and their money are parted. There are others, however, who pursue a widely different course. They compound and prescribe the most dangerous drugs, with reckless disregard of human suffering and life, and venture upon operations that are always hazardous, and not unfrequently fatal. The case of most recent notoriety was that of Dr. "Lookup" Evans, who was recently convicted and sentenced in the court of general sessions to five years' imprisonment in the State Prison. A description of his horrible den in Chatham-street, when pounced upon by the police, has already been given, as nearly as its filthy nature would permit, in these columns. The evidences of guilt found there were of the most conclusive nature. Human flesh, supposed to have been the remains of infants, was found in barrels of lime and acids, undergoing decomposition. He came here from Scotland about 20 years ago, with no medical education whatever. Stubborn energy, active perseverance, and undaunted boldness appear to have forced his guilty success. His first alias was "Old Dr. Ward." Subsequently he assumed a number of others, among which were "Dr. Powers," "Dr. Evans," "Dr. Thompson," "Dr. Elliot," &c. The reckless bravado of this rich may be inferred from the circumstance, that when he was released on bail upon the charge that looked so black against him, he opened an office in Ann-street and Gold-street, and continued to transact a brisk business. He said that he advertised to the extent of $1,000 per week, and received a daily average of 400 letters, most of which enclosed money for "pills." In this nefarious business he had a massive fortune of $100,000, a portion of which is invested in a splendid farm near Jamaica, Long Island. It is believed that his infamous business is even now conducted by hired deputies in Gold-street.

At no. 199 Liberty St. is a sign: "Dr. Mauriceau"–"Office." A gentleman recently called there. He was ushered from one to the next room, and the door between was closed and locked. The person who represented himself as the doctor was a comely exterior, about fifty years of age, and of the bland and courteous manner. He reposed comfortably in an easy revolving chair, and seemed more like a benevolent Samaritan then a designing adventurer. "Are you Dr. Mauriceau?" was asked. "Yes; what can I do for you?" was the smiling reply, accompanied by a keen, penetrating gaze. "I called to ascertain if you could relieve a lady of a physical difficulty," (describing the symptoms of the supposed patient.) "I can, Sir." "Without danger?" "Yes, sir—have had thousands of cases—have them all the time, and never had any trouble at all." "How long will it take, where will she be treated, and what are the terms?" "A week or less, and I can find accommodations, up-town, very elegant, and the terms will be reasonable. But I must see the lady first before I can say anything further."

The history of this man's career is very interesting. His true name is said to be "Loman." "Mme. Restell" is his reputed wife. He was formerly a printer, but his "Madame" induced him to abandon that honorable occupation. Years ago, he published a book, entitled to *Dr. Mauriceau's Medical Companion*. The entire work is said to have been plagiarized from a French author. What medical education he may claim to possess, was picked up in his own haphazard way. The following is a specimen of his advertisement in the New York *Herald*—a paper, which contains strings of disgraceful advertisements:

A GREAT ENSURE REMEDY FOR MARRIED LADIES—the Portuguese female pills always give immediate relief being specially prepared for married ladies. A lady writes: "these pills relieve me in one day, without inconvenience, like magic." Price $5. Dr. A. M. Mauriceau, Office 129 Liberty-street, or sent by mail.

These shameful notices appear in the *Herald* every day. It is said that nearly $60,000 per annum is invested by this couple in advertising.

A lady and gentleman who entered Mme. Restell's house in Fifth-avenue last week, relate the following: "There is a broad, heavily plated sign on the iron gate on one side, labeled 'office.' We descended three steps, and stood in a plain but handsome hallway. A silken cord descended from the ceiling. This we pulled, and almost as soon as the bell tinkled within, the door was opened by a handsome young lady, who we afterward were told was one of 'Madame's' daughters. "Is Mme. Restell in?" we asked. "Yes; walk in." She replied, carefully locking the door. We were ushered into a small darkened room, in the furthest, front corner of the basement, apparently under the great flight of steps at the entrance. We groped our way to the sofa, and had just sat down when the Madame entered herself. 'Well, what can I do for you?' she asked. 'Can you relieve a lady of a physical difficulty?' 'That depends on the circumstances.' A suppositious case was stated, and she probably replied, 'There will be no difficulty about that. Of course, such affairs are expensive, you know. The charge will be —.' Just then a sharp, quick rap, was heard upon the door, and a voice from without exclaimed, 'Ma, I want to speak with you in a moment.' The Madame retired a moment, and we could hear a brief but rapid colloquy. The next instance she returned, and in evident trepidation, said, 'I can sell you some pills, but really, we do no other business. We have had so much trouble about these matters we don't take any more risks. And all the six years that we have lived in this house, there is never a stranger slept under the roof—none in fact, but our own family." Other parties, who have been there had a different experience. Madame was not unsusceptible to the allurements of large fees.

Only the police authorities have anything like an adequate idea of the gigantic dimensions of this evil. Every day adds new indications. That the number of murders from this cause is not generally known is easily accounted for. All the parties interested have the strongest motives to unite in hushing the scandal.

A.—LADIES' PHYSICIAN.—Dr. H. D. Grindle, professor of midwifery, twenty-five years' successful practice in the City, guarantees certain relief to ladies in trouble, with or without medicine; sure relief to the most anxious patient at one interview; elegant rooms for ladies requiring nursing. Office———.

A.—MADAME GRINDLE, Female Physician, guarantees relief to all female complaints; pleasant rooms for nursing.

he foregoing advertisement has for a long time appeared in the columns of the *Herald* and other papers. The history of these two worthies is peculiar. The male member of the firm, if report is correct, knows much more of shoe-making than of medicine. His verbose circular ostentatiously announces him as a "member of the New-York University," &c., with twenty-five years' experience. &c. His diploma is said to have been obtained but four years ago from a New-York Medical College at considerable expense. The nature of his occupation is sufficiently well indicated in the advertisement without the necessity of further description. He and his "Madame" transact an immense amount of business, in which they are reputed to have amassed a handsome fortune. Formerly their premises were in Amity-place, but the house becoming notorious they removed to their present locality in Twenty-sixth street, midway between Sixth and Seventh avenues. The house is of the three-story and basement style, with rear extension. and has a capacity for about twenty patients. It is appropriately surrounded by fashionable markets of infamy. A huge silver plate upon the outer door bears "Dr. Grindle's" name; a sign of similar pattern, bearing the "Madame's" name, glares upon the inner door. The interior is furnished with taste and elegance. The parlors are spacious, and contain all the decorations, upholstery, cabinet-ware, piano, book-case, &c., that is found in a respectable home. A lady and gentleman who recently called there relate the following:

A neat-looking lad ushered us into the parlor. and went after the "Madame." A profusion of circulars were scattered over the centre-tables. some of them being folded as if intended to be mailed. Suddenly the door opened, and the Madame entered. She is fair, fat, forty, and evidently vigorous, and keen in all her actions. She addressed us with primping care, and in a voice as smooth as the flutter of a humming-bird. "My dear friend," she said. " we can do what you hint at. I understand the case. We have had hundreds of them. Poor unfortunate women! How little the world knows bow to appreciate their trials. We think it our mission to take them and save them—a noble work it is, too. But for some friendly hand like ours, how many, many blasted homes, scandalized churches and disorganized social circles there would be. Why, my dear friends, you have no idea of the class of people that come to us. We have had Senators, Congressmen and all sorts of politicians bring some of the first women in the land here. Many— very many aristocratic married women come here—or we attend them in private houses." "What are your charges, Madame?" "Three hundred dollars cover all expenses, and we sec the patient through—unless it occupies more than a week. Then we charge an extra medical fee, and board money." "What about the child ?" "Well, we adopt it out in good bands. One hundred dollars extra, is our fee for that." "But— if— not—a—child—what then?" A quick rolling and flash of her glittering black eyes, a sprightly nod of the head, a finger placed on the lips, a knowing look and "Sh—h!" was the pantomimic reply. "We understand every branch of our business!" she exclaimed, with peculiar emphasis.

She stated that a more aristocratic but expensive nursing place could be furnished in West Twenty-third-street. This place is sumptuously furnished and well kept. "The best of nurses are employed. Chapters of thrilling interest could be written upon the scenes within those elegant rooms. The pale— ghastly pale and remorseful-looking countenances of the suffering are indexes to romances in real life more startling in their stern reality than any web of fiction. How many bitter pangs, scalding tears and moans of agony were there.

The most pitiful sight was that of the babes, sleeping sweetly—evidently under the influence of mild opiates. Fresh and fragrant flowers, and choice fruit were occasionally observed. How many broken hearts and shattered lives these stray points eloquently speak of. But more than that are the parting scenes between mother and child, when the latter is taken away tor adoption. Twenty five dollars per week is charged for board at this place.

A.—Ladies in trouble guaranteed immediate relief, sure and safe; no fees required until perfectly satisfied; elegant rooms and nursing provided. Dr. Ascher, Amity-place, &c.

The above advertisement is clipped from the *Herald*.

"Dr. Ascher," alias "Rosensweig," of South Fifth-avenue, below Amity-street, claims to be a Russian, but his voice has the twang of a German Jew. He is very bulky in figure, about forty years of age, and is said to know more of saloon business than of medicine. His diploma is said to have cost $40. His house is a laree three-story and basement one, and is able to accommodate twelve patients. He does a large business. When called upon, he assures applicants: "These other fellows are all humpugsh; they bromish to do something vot thcy don't do. I poshitively do all operashuush widout any danger, and as sheap as anybody." The corpse-like faces to be seen peering through the bedroom blinds are enough to horrify the stoutest- hearted passersby.

The following are brief notes of some of the others who advertise the same business:

The *Police Gazette* says that Dr. Selden is the best physician for ladies in trouble. Thousands are relieved without accident. No. 241 Bleecker-street.

Dr. Selden is said to have "read medicine" for a period of at least six weeks, in Ohio. Fully aware of the effect of high-sounding professions and pretensions upon the unlettered populace, he was introduced to this City, some two or three years ago, as the late Demonstrator of Anatomy in a medical college in Washington, and, as such, proffered his medical services in the fœticide profession. Naturally of a migratory temperament and habit, doubtlessly strengthened and confirmed by a bold and unscrupulous practice, he has seldom remained long in any one locality and under the same name, his many neighborhood legacies in the form of unsettled debts constituting the philosophy of the frequent transmutations. Some of his aliases are, Dion, Leon, Hoi-Illius, the Arab, Clark, Powers, Evans, and Thompson.

The *Herald* also contains the following advertisement:

ATTENTION.—Twenty years' Prussian hospital experience. Private diseases always permanently cured without mercury. Consultation free. Dr. Franklin, Bleecker-street.

Dr. Franklin's real name is Jacoby, and formerly was a barber, who, until within three or four years past, conducted a shaving and hair-clipping saloon in Sixth-avenue.

This man, a German Jew, with no scientific and regular medical education, except what he has briefly gleaned from a confrère. He parades a diploma—price, $40.

The following are in the same business, and advertise more or less: Mme. VanBuskirk.— This woman's name is Gifford. She came from New-Bedford, Mass. Her reputation there was an equivocal one, to say the least. This bold, bad woman was not long since arraigned for malpractice, and notwithstanding her narrow escape from punishment, still pursues her infamous profession with indomitable will and energy.

Mme. Maxwell, alias Costello.—This woman, & graduate of Mme. Restell's when she was located in Chambers-street, notwithstanding her great age, still follows the iniquitous profession, and almost daily advertises that "she does not humbug ladies with medicine." Mme. Worcester, Charles-street.—This woman is a veteran also in crime, and as a nurse, constitutes the medium of communication between the doctor and his female patient, operating as a screen for both in case of legal trouble.

The mails go burdened with the circulars of such people, and come laden with money enclosures for "pills," "drops" and other vile humbugs. The best home firesides have been invaded by these advertisements, either in the newspapers or in letters. To what a frightful extent this outrage is rapidly increasing few can realize, The facts herein set forth are but a fraction of a greater mass that cannot be published with propriety. Certainly enough is here given to arouse the general public sentiment to the necessity of taking some decided and effectual action.

Ladies' Guide in Health and Disease: Girlhood, Maidenhood, Wifehood, Motherhood by John Harvey Kellogg (1882)

Introduction

In his preface, Dr. John Harvey Kellogg describes the need for this volume as "the very remarkable increase in the number and frequency of" diseases impacting women to the point that "a fashionable woman has her favorite gynecologist as well as her favorite milliner or dress-maker" (i). While most of the book centers on the information women need to maintain their health and to partner with their doctors, many sections read more like a conduct book warning against various social vices. In the chapter on "The Wife," the second section discusses the termination of pregnancy mostly from a moral and legal perspective. Kellogg also suggests a direct connection between abortion and gynecological cancers, which are discussed in Chap. 4.

The Wife: Criminal Abortion

The practice of abortion is one of the most revolting crimes which has ever become prevalent in any country at any period of the world's history. The pages of history are stained with the records of this most despicable of crimes. The records of civil laws of ancient nations show that this crime has been prevalent in all ages and among all nations. At some periods it has even been more prevalent than it is at the present. Strange as it may appear, there have in ancient times been found philosophers and great teachers, some of whom are respected event at the present day, who have justified this crime and recommended it as a means of limiting the growth of population. Aristotle not only did this, but even went so far as to insist that it was the duty of the State to enact laws enforcing the practice of abortion when the population had reached a certain state. The ancient Grecians and Romans had no law against this crime. Numerous historians represent the practice as almost universal in ancient times. History records that a niece of one of the Roman Emperors died in consequence of having committed the crime in obedience to the command of the emperor. The crime seems to have been looked upon by a large part of those nations who were guilty of it in ancient times very much as excesses in eating are regarded by the majority of persons at the present day, undoubtedly wrong, but so slightly criminal as to be easily condoned, and scarcely to be censured.

In modern times there have not been wanting apologists for this horrible crime; but on the whole it may be safely asserted that there is less tolerance for ante-natal murder at the present day than at any previous period of the world's history, so far as there is any record bearing on the subject. We do not attribute this improvement to any special increase in the moral sense of the people, but to the greater enlightenment which has resulted from the free discussion of the subject and the diffusion of knowledge respecting the wickedness of the act and the dangers to life and health attending it. It is only with the hope that we may be able to further the work of reform in this direction that we mention the revolting subject in these pages.

The prevalence of this crime even in this enlightened country, and that after all which has been said upon it by physicians and priests and clergymen, undoubtedly far surpasses the conception of any but those who have an opportunity for knowing the facts or an approximation to the truth. The crime is almost always a secret one, and hence no exact data respecting its prevalence can be obtained; but sufficient is known to indicate clearly that it is on the increase rather than otherwise, and to cause those who are interested in the welfare of the race to tremble at the future prospect.

It has become a notorious fact that the families of native Americans are getting to be so small on the average that the children hardly replace the parents. It has been stated on good authority that the increase of population is almost entirely due to immigration and the numerous families of the natives of foreign countries. In New England where families of eight and nine were formerly exceedingly common, it is now stated that the average number of persons to a family is scarcely more than three among the native born population. At this rate, it is evident that this monstrous vice threatens to exterminate the race if nothing is done to check its ravages. It is certainly high time that the public were thoroughly enlightened on the subject and a general and organized effort instituted against this enemy of the race which, to use the words of another employed in speaking of another vice, annually destroys more human beings than "war, pestilence, and famine combined."

Since the war by which the slaves of the South were liberated, the same appalling vice has become prevalent among them. With this exception, however, the crime is chiefly confined to the middle and higher classes of society. Professional abortionists who are, it is sad to know, too often women, ply their criminal trade in every large city of the land, and in almost every little hamlet as well. The newspapers still contain numerous advertisements which the initiated well understand. For almost any sum from $500 down to the paltry sum of $10 these fiends in human shape, the thugs of civilized lands, are ready at any time to undertake the destruction of a human being without the slightest compunction of conscience and with little danger of detection, so imperfect are the laws relating to the crime and so difficult the task of obtaining evidence sufficient to convict the criminal. The fact that jurymen as well as judges and attorneys are not infrequently indebted to the criminal for similar services, also has an important bearing on the results of the case in numerous instances. The impossibility of obtaining a conviction for the crime of abortion, no matter what may be the character of the evidence, is so notorious that persons who are well known as professional abortionists are allowed to ply their horrible trade year after year without being molested.

But the crime is not confined to professionals. Women sometimes become sufficiently skilled in the use of instruments for the purpose to be able to perform the operation upon themselves, and such women do not hesitate to instruct others in the art of destroying their unborn children. Thus the vile contagion spreads from one to another until in some instances a whole neighborhood becomes demoralized. It is not an uncommon thing for women to boast that they know too much to have children. Often these knowing ones may be seen leading around a solitary little one whose brothers and sisters have been all nipped in the bud by the cruel abortionist, or by the mother's own hand. Some little time ago a physician of intelligence who had observed somewhat closely, reported that in his neighborhood of several hundred families, there had been scarcely a child born in three or four years.

Every physician who has been a year in practice will testify that he has had already from one to twenty applications from women to aid them in accomplishing the murder of their helpless offspring. The majority of these cases are of married women whose only excuse is that they do not wish to endure the inconvenience and trouble of pregnancy and childbirth, or that they "do not want to have children," or that they "have children enough," or some other equally frivolous excuse. Often have we had women urge these and even more trifling arguments to induce us to comply with their request to assist them to secure an abortion.

Our first experience of this kind opened up to us a new phase of human nature. We had previously supposed that the reason why the crime was so prevalent was the ignorance of women with reference to its criminality and the possible, even probable consequences to themselves. We felt no doubt that to set before a woman the matter in its true light, would be sufficient to turn her from her purpose, and to institute are form in that particular case at least. Nothing could have surprised us more than to see our explanations and appeals received with the most unflinching coldness, and not allowed to have the least apparent weight in turning the woman from her purpose. No matter how great the crime nor how imminent the risk, she was willing and anxious to take the responsibility, and did not hesitate to state the fact, and to still persist in importuning us to assist her. She seemed lost to all sense of moral obligation, and was ready to do anything or to sacrifice anything to enable her to accomplish her object. So absorbed does a woman, intent on the commission of this crime, become in the accomplishment of her object, the most touching appeals are usually wholly unavailing. Some years ago a gentleman called at our private office, and after considerable preliminary explanation stated the fact that his wife was desirous of placing herself under our care as a patient for the purpose of securing the production of an abortion, it having occurred to her that the superior advantages afforded for treatment would enable her to escape the more surely from the dangers which she well knew to accompany the crime. We promptly gave him a negative answer and did not hesitate to supplement our refusal by a pretty full expression of our opinion of the operation both from a professional and a moral stand-point. He seemed really touched by our representations of the immorality of the act, and promised to return to his home in a neighboring city and induce his wife to visit us in the hope that she might be persuaded to look at the crime in its true light. We heard nothing more of the matter for several weeks, and the circumstance had almost passed from our mind when we were informed one day that a lady was waiting for us in the office, and on receiving her card, recognized her as the lady in question, whom we had been expecting. She at once stated her errand, saying that her husband had told her what we had said to him, but that she had come hoping nevertheless that she might be able to induce us to perform the operation for her, as she had no thought of giving it up, and should certainly employ someone else if we did not consent to do it. We promptly assured her that if the operation was performed at all, it must be done by someone else besides us, and at once began to lay before her some considerations calculated to divert her mind from her purpose. Our most earnest arguments and appeals seemed to have no weight with her, however, and at last we said to her, "Madam, you have had children before?" "Yes," she replied, "I have two beautiful children, aged three and five years." "Very well; you say that you do not feel capable of caring and rearing more than two children, and assign this as a reason why you are so anxious to destroy the child now developing within you. You are even willing not only to destroy the coming little one, but to incur the risk of losing your own life as well, or in all probability of becoming an invalid for life at least, to say nothing of the destruction of your peace of mind. Now I can suggest for your consideration a much more rational plan, one which will accomplish the same result, and which will be attended with little if any physical danger to yourself, and will be in no degree more criminal." She was eager to hear the plan I had to suggest, and expressed herself as very ready to adopt it if it would, as I said, accomplish the same result. We accordingly presented it to her as follows:—

"Since your chief reason for wishing to destroy your unborn child is your inability to care for more than the two children which you already have, a much better plan than that which you propose would be to take the life of one of the children already born, and thus save yourself the danger of an operation which is almost as likely to destroy your own life as that of your child. You could easily drop the little one into the river on some dark night, or could cut its throat or smother it, with little fear of detection, as no one would suspect you of such a crime, and then you could allow the present pregnancy to go on to full maturity and have no more children than you now have. The crime would be in no sense a greater one, and would not be so great in one sense, since if an abortion is produced, the result may virtually be suicide as well as murder. So far as the child is concerned, it is murder in either case, and of the most cowardly kind, since it is taking advantage of the weakness and helplessness of a human being unable to defend itself, an act which is seldom equaled in atrocity by the most heartless assassin or even the barbarian captor."

She weakened for a few moments, and we felt that possibly we might succeed in rescuing her from the commission of the crime which she had meditated; but it was only for a moment that she hesitated; she then rose and withdrew from our office with the assertion that if we would not do the operation she must find someone who would.

It would seem that such a view of the matter, so manifestly true and unanswerable as an argument, would arouse the conscience of any woman in whom still glowed a single spark of the instinct of motherhood; but unfortunately this is by no means the case. Too often the mind is so determinedly set upon the commission of the crime that even the thunders of Sinai would scarcely turn it from its purpose. Many times have we earnestly labored for hours with women who have applied to us for the performance of an operation or for medicine by which the same end might be accomplished, without other result than a very weak promise to consider the matter farther; and we knew too well that the consideration would all be in the opposite direction from what it should be. When a woman has so far smothered her womanly instincts as to wish to deliberately and in cold blood murder her innocent, unborn babe, even at an early period of its existence, she becomes desperate, and sometimes desperately wicked. Conscience seems to be asleep and the moral instincts benumbed.

Sometimes, however, we have been glad to know that the result of our efforts have been otherwise. Often, as we pass along the street, we meet a little fair-haired boy who does not know how narrowly his mother escaped the commission of the awful crime of murder, nor how earnestly we plead for his life when he was a helpless, yet undeveloped, and unfortunately, unwelcome child. Would to God that we could place before the mind of every woman in the land a picture of the evils of this awful crime, the sacrilege, the profanity, the worse than brutish cruelty of this crime against God, against the race, against nature, and against the perpetrator, a picture so vivid in coloring, so horrifying in its hideousness, that it would make an impression ineffaceable by any of the selfish and frivolous considerations usually urged as reasons justifying the act. Statistics and the experience of every physician of long practice show that abortion is many times more dangerous to the life of the mother under ordinary circumstances than pregnancy. The majority of those who are guilty of this crime, become invalids for life.

Criminal abortion is the cause to which thousands of women may trace a long line of ailments of a most obstinate and aggravating character. Many such cases have come under our care, and no class of diseases are so obstinate and often utterly intractable as this. After normal childbirth, the uterus and its appendages naturally undergo a change known as involution, by which the organ is rapidly restored to its natural and ordinary size and condition. After abortion, this change is very likely to be incomplete, leaving the uterus congested, enlarged, sensitive, and in a condition to invite the most serious disease. This is true even in the most favorable cases. Often the immediate results, as well as the more remote, are much more serious. Abortion is very likely to be followed by inflammations of various sorts, especially of the uterus, ovaries, and surrounding tissues, which if not immediately fatal, leave behind them results which render the woman a life-long sufferer, and frequently develop in later years into some form of malignant—disease. This is undoubtedly one of the most prolific causes of the increasing frequency of this most appalling and incurable of all human maladies, cancer.

One of the most frequent complications of abortion, and one which rarely occurs in natural childbirth, is blood poisoning from retention and decomposition of the placenta and membranes of the foetus. At the end of normal pregnancy, Nature prepares the way for the prompt separation of these attachments of the foetus, and thus obviates this danger; but in cases of abortion there has been no such preparation; indeed, the placenta is at this time becoming more and more firmly attached to the walls of the uterus, and consequently is likely to be retained to undergo gradual decomposition, thus involving the liability to blood poisoning, which will ruin the constitution for life if it does not at once terminate fatally.

Physicians alone are to any degree acquainted with the awful extent to which this crime prevails. Even they are not always able to get at the facts. Women who will commit this crime will resort to any means to conceal it from those whom they know regard it as such. Not long ago, on making an examination of a young unmarried woman, we were surprised to find a large tear of the neck of the womb which we could not doubt had been produced in this way, though she professed to know of nothing except a fall to which to attribute it.

A married woman who came under our care a few years ago for treatment for a uterine disease, stated that she had never borne a child, and adhered to the statement, although an examination disclosed a large tear in the neck of the womb which could not have been in any other way. Our confidence in the integrity of the patient for a time led us to think that the morbid condition might possibly be the result of the removal of a morbid growth from the uterus which she asserted had been done at a previous time; but we afterward learned that our first opinion was correct, the occasion for the tear having been a lapse from virtue when a girl,—a circumstance which had all her life been held a secret. The most horrible results often follow attempts at the performance of this crime which are unsuccessful. The instruments used frequently mutilate the innocent being against whose life these cruel efforts are directed, in a most terrible manner without accomplishing the desired result, so that the termination of the pregnancy often reveals a beautiful babe with a limb torn from its body, or frightfully disfigured in other ways, or a monster so deformed as to be scarcely recognizable as ever having had anything of a human shape. Cases have even occurred in which the head has actually been torn from the body without causing abortion or even preventing development of the remainder of the body. Nature sometimes endures all this violence rather than surrender her trust before the proper time for so doing; and every woman who subjects herself to an operation for the purpose of inducing abortion incurs the risk of becoming the unwilling mother of an eyeless or crippled child, or a headless monster.

Recent investigations have shown that there is still another result of criminal abortion which has been heretofore overlooked. Careful observations have developed the fact that the subsequent pregnancies are affected by an induced abortion not only as regards the liability to miscarriage, which is well known, but as regards the development of the foetus. Thousands of mothers have found that when they had repented of their criminal attempts to thwart the purposes of nature, and really desired children, the womb had either undergone such changes that pregnancy was impossible, or if it occurred, could not proceed to full development; or that if the development did continue to full term, the result was only a weak, puny creature, badly developed, and certain to be all its life-time a silent witness of the mother's criminal attempts.

This is a matter to be considered by mothers who desire to get rid of their unborn infants simply for their convenience; because they do not want to settle down to sober life just yet, or because they have planned a trip to Europe, or a summer at Saratoga. Are you willing, mother, to incur the risk not only of blighting the existence of the little innocent whom Nature has furnished you with instincts to protect, and to involve the liability of paying the penalty of your crime with your own life, but also to render almost certain the destruction of the prospects of the little ones who may come to you in future years, should you still be capable of becoming a mother?

One thing women ought to know. A skillful physician cannot be easily deceived as to the cause of an abortion. The symptoms of an abortion occurring spontaneously from ovarian disease, displacement, a fall or other accident, are different from those which accompany an instrumental abortion, and the difference will be readily detected by a physician of experience.

The time has fully come when there ought to be a general waking up on the part of all lovers of humanity, with reference to this devastating vice. Physicians and clergymen should "cry aloud and spare not." Laws are of no consequence, or at any rate are of little avail, since there are usually but two witnesses to the crime, both of whom are criminals, and both of course desirous of concealing their crimes. The professional abortionist is skilled in the art of concealment and evasion of justice. We have had some experience in attempting to bring these human fiends to justice, but not such as to encourage us in repeating the effort. The evidence may be clear and conclusive as possible, shrewd and unscrupulous lawyers will find some means for befogging the average jury to such an extent as to cause a disagreement if not an out and out acquittal.

The only hope for any better state of things than at present exists is in the education of the people. Women must be educated concerning themselves, and a wholesome respect for the sacredness of the reproductive function must be cultivated. Women must be informed of the perils which they incur in resorting to instrumental or medicinal means for producing abortion. Only a few weeks ago a young woman came to us for examination and treatment for dropsy. Her history disclosed the fact that she had taken a large dose of "tansy tea," as the result of which she sank into collapse and remained unconscious for many hours, her life being saved only by the greatest exertions. Since that time, she stated, she had been bloating, and had not menstruated. A few questions elicited the fact that the tansy was taken " to bring her around," as she said, menstruation not having occurred at the usual time, and the fear being entertained that she was pregnant. We at once understood the cause of the bloating, and the examination made apparent the correctness of our conclusions. The father soon arrived on the scene and made a most eloquent appeal to us to produce an abortion. We answered him in the usual way, and he was apparently satisfied; but his subsequent course was such as to lead us to suspect very strongly that he was determined not to rest until the desired end was accomplished. This case illustrates the fact that the mother's life may be greatly imperiled without any result so far as the foetus is concerned. All medicinal agents used for this purpose are powerful poisons, and quite as likely to produce the death of the mother as the expulsion of the foetus.

Every woman who commits or attempts to commit this horrible crime, and every husband who encourages it or even assents to its performance, ought to be treated as a criminal, and ostracized from society. So long as the act of abortion is looked upon as an offense so trifling as to be easily condoned, and hardly worthy of censure, its frequency will increase. Every pulpit in the land ought to send out in stirring and unmistakable tones, warnings against the gross immorality of this practice, drawing vivid pictures of its cruelty and unnaturalness, and pronouncing anathemas upon its perpetrators. The crime should he considered a just cause for church action to disfellowship, and the nature of the crime should not induce those who may have knowledge of it to keep it secret. The crime must be made odious, and the perpetrators condemned in unstinted terms.

Physicians must warn women of the physical as well as the moral calamities which follow in the wake of this inhuman practice, and the certainty of retribution in this life, as well as the next.

The Wife's Handbook by Henry Arthur Allbutt (1888)

Introduction

In this book, Dr. H. Arthur Allbutt follows many of the other guides to health for women in aiming "to save the lives and preserve the health of thousands of women, to rescue from death and disease children who may be born, to teach the young wife how to order her health during the most important period of her life, to remove from her mind the popular ignorance in which she may have been reared, and to enable her to learn truths concerning her duties as wife and mother." One of those topics was contraception, which Allbutt covers with a list of ten options for preventing pregnancy. This section led to the volume being deemed indecent and eventually cost Allbutt his medical license.

Chapter VII. How To Prevent Conception When Advised By The Doctor

(1) De. Giovanni Tari, a physician of Naples, was informed by a certain Italian priest that the poor women in Italy prevented conception from taking place, by sitting up in bed directly after connection, and coughing. The act of coughing expelled the semen (male fluid) from the vagina. Dr. Tari is of opinion that this simple method would answer in most cases. I do not, however, see how all the semen can be expelled, because

the vagina has ridges in it, and the semen lodges in the ridges; and coughing, however violent, could not entirely dislodge it. [4]

(2) The adoption of a certain order in sexual intercourse is often successful in preventing conception. Connection should be avoided from five days before the monthly flow till eight days after it. I am bound, however, to point out that this method fails in about five cases in every hundred. It is a method, notwithstanding, strongly recommended by Dr. William Hitchman, of Liverpool, who advocates it in every case.

(3) The " withdrawal" of the penis (male organ) before the ejection takes place is largely practised in France. This method (if withdrawal is complete before discharge takes place) is always successful. I believe, however, that the practice of withdrawal is hurtful to the nervous system in many persons, therefore I cannot strongly recommend this means of preventing conception. This method is, however, advocated by many eminent physicians.

(4) The use by the woman of an injection into the vagina immediately after connection is strongly recommended by many. The best solution to inject is one formed by adding a teaspoonful of alum to a pint of cold or tepid water. This solution must be injected thoroughly into the vagina by means of a Lambert's Improved Reverse Current Syphon Enema Syringe, fitted with vaginal tube containing vertical and reverse holes. This powerful syringe will wash out most completely every part of the vagina. Lambert's Enema Syringe can be obtained from E. Lambert and Son, 38—44 Mayfield Road, Kingsland, London, N. The vaginal tube is passed up as far as it will go into the vagina, and the solution is thus injected so as to thoroughly wash out the passage. About two pints of solution should be used. Dr. Palfrey's Powder (which consist of sulpho-carbolate of zinc and dried sulphate of zinc, of each one ounce, alum four ounces, in fine powder) may also be used with advantage according to the directions printed on the box containing Lambert's Syringe. The use, however, of the above method necessitates the woman rising from bed, and thus perhaps taking a chill. If, however, she uses an Irrigator (sold by most surgical instrument makers for 10s. 6d.) she can remain in bed. The Irrigator is a kind of can holding about two pints, which is hung against the wall by the woman's side of the bed, at the height of some four feet or more above the level of her head. This can has a long india rubber tube attached to a hole near its bottom, and at the

---

[4] Note in the original text: When a woman is advised by her doctor not to conceive on account of the state of her health, she had better consult him as to which of these methods of prevention would be best in her particular case.

mouth-piece end of the tube there is a little turn-tap. Before getting into bed the woman fills the can with a solution of alum and water, as recommended above, places a bed-pan and towel on a chair at the side of the bed; and after connection she has but to turn on her back and slip the bed-pan under her; then she inserts the mouth-piece of the india-rubber tube into the vagina as far as possible, turns the tap, and the alum solution flows in and out again without causing any wetting or trouble. The flow may be made either gentle or strong, according to the height at which the can is hung. I have know a great many cases, however, where injections as used above have failed in preventing conception. I believe, however, that if a quinine solution was used in place of an alum one, conception would be impossible. The strength of the quinine solution should be 20 grains to the pint of cold water. The objection would be the expense. If Messrs. Lambert would supply an Irrigator fitted with their vaginal tube containing both vertical and reverse tubes, I am persuaded fewer cases of failure would result from the use of injections. [5] Simple injections of cold water only often fail to prevent conception, and may even, in some cases, cause conception to take place by more thoroughly diluting the too thick semen. The thorough syringing-out of the vagina with vinegar and cold water (one part vinegar to six water), directly after connection, will in many cases prevent conception. It is a method, too, which has the advantage of being cheap.

(5) A very soft piece of sponge soaked in tepid water, or, better still, in a solution of quinine of the strength recommended as above, might be inserted into the vagina, high up, before having connection. In order to withdraw the sponge easily, there should be a piece of string or ribbon attached to it. This check to conception, especially when the sponge is soaked in quinine solution, is mostly successful, although I have known failure when the sponge has only been soaked in water. Davies, chemist, 101 and 103 Park Lane, Leeds, can supply properly prepared sponges for the purpose at 1s. each, or two for 1s. 9d.

(6) A very certain check is the " French Letter," which is a kind of sheath, made of thin india-rubber, worn by the husband. Its object is to prevent the semen from being discharged into the vagina. If the "French Letter" has the least hole in it some semen may escape, and conception take

---

[5] Note in the original text: Messrs. Lambert now manufacture such an irrigator.

place. Reliable "French Letters" may be bought at most respectable chemists and surgical instrument makers. [6]

(7) Dr. Mensinga, of Flensburg, has invented a preventive pessary, to be worn by the woman, which I believe will, when properly adjusted, be a real preventive of conception. This pessary is made in three sizes, and may be obtained from B. Vaughan, 33, Caledonian Road, Leeds. The pessary is in shape something like a round dish-cover, the dome portion of which is made of thin, smooth india-rubber, which will collapse with a touch. The rim surrounding the cover portion is made of a ring of thick rubber, which can be squeezed to any shape. The hollow portion of the pessary is intended to cover the neck and mouth of the womb during intercourse, so that no semen may penetrate into the womb. The pessary can, with a little practice, be inserted into the vagina by the woman herself. Of course, when it is in position the hollow portion of the cover looks upwards, and the rim expands and presses equally on all sides of the vagina, thus thoroughly preventing semen passing between. When the pessary is properly inserted there is nothing to interfere with free intercourse. Before removing the pessary in the morning, the woman would do wisely to syringe the vagina with tepid water, or with alum and water, or better still, with a weak quinine solution (ten grains to the pint), The price of each size of this pessary has lately been considerably reduced. In most cases the medium size is best. A Mensinga's Pessary is useful to wear as a support in cases of slight falling of the womb. It should not, however, be worn during the monthly period. My attention has been drawn to the Improved Check Pessary, manufactured by Messrs. E. Lambert and Son, 38—44 Mayfield Eoad, Kingsland, London. This pessary can be used by the woman "without inconvenience or knowledge of the husband." With care it will last a long time, and can be easily affixed so as to cover the mouth of the womb, and it can be removed without difficulty. It is on the same principle as Mensinga's Pessary, but has this advantage, it can be used either alone, or can be made more certain in action by putting, in the hollow part of it a compound composed of vaseline, cocoa-nut butter, and quinine. The pessaries are sold at 2s. 3d. each post free.

(8) Mr. W. J. Rendell, Chemist, 26 Great Bath Street, Earringdon Eoad, London, E.C., has invented some quinine pessaries which dissolve. They

---

[6] Note in original text: Dr. Henry Paterson's "Patent Circular Protectors," sold at 5s. per dozen by Constantine and Jackson, 9 and 10 Wych Street, Strand, London, W.C., are perhaps the best and safest form of "Letters" manufactured. Lambert's Malthus specialties are also well made and reliable. Davies, Leeds, is agent for the latter.

are sold at 2s. per dozen. One of these pessaries should be pushed high up into the vagina about a quarter of an hour before having connection, when the quinine contained in it will be partly dissolved out; and when the semen is discharged into the vagina during intercourse, the quinine, coming into contact with the active parts of the semen, destroys their activity at once, so preventing conception. There is nothing but quinine and cocoa-nut butter in these pessaries, consequently nothing to irritate either the woman's vagina or the male organ. It is but right to say that these pessaries are at present only on trial. Time will show whether they can be relied upon to prevent conception. My opinion is that they will do all their inventor claims for them.

(9) A kind of artificial sponge or vaginal Tampon, containing in its centre a friable capsule filled with slightly acidulated quinine solution, would, I believe, make a very good and cheap preventive. All that the woman would have to do before intercourse would be to take one of the Tampons, and squeeze it, which would break the capsule, setting free the solution, which would then permeate the whole sponge. She would then insert it into the vagina as far as possible. It would be better to have a string attached, so as to be able to withdraw it easily. If these Tampons were made in large numbers they would have a ready sale.

(10) The taking of arsenic and other drugs in small doses daily, to lessen male sexual vigor and thus produce impotence.

"Voluntary Motherhood" by Harriot Stanton Blatch (1891)

Introduction

In this speech, Harriot Stanton Blatch, suffragist and daughter of pioneering women's rights activist Elizabeth Cady Stanton, addresses the National Council of Women of the United States at an assembly in Washington, D.C. in February 1891. In addition to the end of forced maternity, she argues for education, financial independence, and access to divorce as essential to women's rights. This speech is part of a larger movement that promoted women's prerogative around marital abstinence, rather than contraception or abortion, as a way to ensure women could choose when to bear children.

"Voluntary Motherhood"

> The truth it, we are in the midst of such terrible error on the subject of woman and her veritable rights that it is frightful to think of.
> — Tolstoi's *Kreutzer Sonata*

The difficulty of approaching the subject of the relation of the sexes is tenfold, if the prerogatives of the dominant sex are challenged. It is because of its attack upon men that Tolstoi's "Kreutzer Sonata" has raised so much opposition. To decry this last publication of the Russian novelist as immoral is merely a little dust-throwing to blind women to the truths in the book, and it is to be hoped that neither this abase nor the author's own religious beliefs and Eastern philosophy will obscure for his readers the gospel set forth. True, Tolstoi is extreme; but humanity has been so misguided by the average man's thought, or rather passion, that it is scarcely ground for wonder that a sensitive thinker should regard as an ideal, entire continence.

Tolstoi aims to reach a solution of life for men; as to the feelings of women, he admits he is not informed. In this object he resembles most writers who deal with the relation of the sexes; for all look at this matter from the man's point of view, and seldom if ever from the side of the rights and duties of the mother and the interests of the child. Too weighty considerations are buffeted about according to the opinions open other subjects held by the persons handling them. The political economist of the Mill school tells the working-man that his trouble does not come from unequal distribution of wealth, but from his large family. The labor market is overstocked, and poverty results. The Malthusian, while foretelling terrible consequences if human increase is not limited, advocates various artificial checks, not to human license, but to race productivity. Many a socialist denies all these forebodings, and proclaims that even England now "has too small a population for a really high civilization."

Now, these contradictory theories resemble one another in one particular,—those who propound them think that economic considerations alone should settle this matter of population. In contrast to this, the man's commercial view of race production, stands the woman's intuition backed by reason. She asks, first, will the child be welcome? second, what will be its inheritance of physical, mental, and moral character? third, can the child be provided for in life? Every conscientious mother replies to the socialist and to the Malthusian that satisfactory answers must be given to the woman's first and second demands, and that with satisfactory answers to those questions the third consideration may safety be left to take care of itself.

In animal life, as soon as we get conscious motherhood, the strides is evolution become greater and more rapid.

Below the birds "the animal takes care of himself as soon as he begins to live. He has nothing to learn, and his career is a simple repetition the careers of countless ancestors." Among higher birds and mammals a great change takes place: the life of the creature becomes so varied and complex that habits cannot be fully organized in the nervous system before birth. The antenatal period is too short to allow of such development:. So we get a period of infancy, a time of plasticity, of teachableness. Of this time Fiske truly says, "The first appearance of infancy in the animal world heralded the new era which was to be crowned by the development of man." From this point in evolution the period of infancy lengthens, — indeed, this is the condition of progress. To reach a higher stage of development a longer time must be given to immaturity or growth, and that period will be one of greater or less dependence according as the adult being is of higher or lower species. What chiefly distinguishes the human being from the lower animals is the increase in the former of cerebral surface and organization, and the necessary accompaniment of this development, a lengthened period of infancy.

Now, this increased time of immaturity is a direct tax upon the mother in any species; so to her is due each step in evolution. Men talk of the sacredness of motherhood, but judging from their acts it is the last thing that is held sacred in the human species. Poets sing and philosophers reason about the holiness of the mother's sphere, but men in laws and customs have degraded the woman in her maternity. Motherhood is sacred,—that is, voluntary motherhood; but the woman who bears unwelcome children is outraging every duty she owes the race. The mothers of the human species should turn to the animals, and from the busy care takers, who are below them in most things, learn the simple truths of procreation. Let women but understand the part unenforced maternity has played in the evolution of animal life, and their reason will guide them to the true path of race development. Let them note that natural selection has carefully fostered the maternal instinct. The offspring of the fondest females in each animal species, having of course the most secure and prolonged infancy, are "naturally selected" to continue their kind. The female offspring gains by inheritance in philoprogenitiveness, and thus is built up the instinct which prepares the females of a higher species for a more developed altruism. Through countless ages mother-love has been evolved and been working out its mission; surely women should recognize the meaning of the instinct, and should refuse to prostitute their creative powers, and so jeopardize the progress of the human race. Upon the mothers roust rest in the last instance the development of any species.

In this work women need not hope for help from men. The sense of obligation to offspring, men possess but feebly; there has not been developed by animal evolution an instinct of paternity. They are not disinherited fathers; they are simply unevolved parents. There is no ground for wonder that this is so; for in but a few species among the lower animals is even a suggestion of paternal instinct found. The male bird often occupies itself with the hatching and feeding of the brood, and the lion is a pattern father; but usually we find no hint of paternal instinct in the male, and sometimes antagonism towards the young of the species. Evidently nature tried her hand on paternity, it did not fulfil the hopes she had of it, and she turned a cold shoulder upon its development. The paternal instinct is not a factor in evolution.

If, then, the law of natural selection is of weight, we should expect to find very little, if any, instinct of paternity in the male of the human species. Not only by such a priori reasoning is this conclusion reached, but a posteriori reasoning emphasizes the same troth. Men like to accumulate, and hand down their accumulations with their name. This is a method of securing some sort of immortality, and gives rise to the neglect of illegitimate children, the preference of male to female offspring, the law of primogeniture, and the selection, in case of male heirs failing, of a distant relation to inherit the property provided he will adopt the name of his benefactor. The masculine tendencies which have crystallized themselves in these customs bear no resemblance to paternal love. Area does not discriminate between her legitimate and illegitimate child; had mothers been instrumental in making legal codes there would not have been a law of entail.

But perhaps the strongest proof of the feebleness of philoprogenitiveness in men is the existence of their system of prostitution, with its accompanying thoughtlessness in which parenthood is risked, and the indifference with which rich fathers leave their children to a life of hardship, if not of crime. When Henry Ward Beecher made his famous assertion, in the Presidential campaign of '88, that if all the men who, like Grover Cleveland, had carried on illicit relations with women, voted for him, the Democratic candidate would sweep New York by an overwhelming majority, his words called forth no resentment. But goes such a statement, if it be a fact, imply a more vital truth? It means that but a handful of men could solemnly swear that they are certain no child of theirs is rotting out its life in some tenement or gutter. Could there be a more unanswerable argument against the existence of paternal feelings than the brief statement, that of the seventy thousand illegitimate children born each year in France, only five thousand are acknowledged by the fathers? And our very attitude towards men of the type of the other sixty thousand shows that we do not expect strong paternal feeling in men. No one feels that George Eliot drew an abnormal creature in Godfrey Cass. When he fails to acknowledge his child and leaves it with the despised weaver, the author does not describe his conduct as that of a brutal man. Again, no thoughtful person could fail to be struck in reading Darwin's Life and Letters, by the fact that the greatest student of heredity of our time, though himself the victim of an incurable and hereditary disease, never questioned his right to become the father of many children. And yet he was fully aware of the probability of ill health for his offspring; for in letters to friends he pours out his fears: "My dread is hereditary ill health. Even death is better for them." Is it only a woman's logic that would lead to the opposite conclusion: Better had they never been born? "Now, no one could say that Darwin was a bad man; on the contrary, if report speaks truly, we may look upon him as exceptionally good." The conclusion then forces itself upon us that even the best of men are lacking in that nice conscience which recognizes the sacredness of life responsibility of its creation. But humanity would suffer the minimum of evil from this cause, were not laws based upon the extraordinary assumption that, "by the law of nature and the law of God," the father is the sole guardian of the child, and the suicidal custom followed of giving the power of legislation and the social dominance, in all sex matters, into the hands of that half of the race which is unfitted by nature for any just comprehension of these questions.

Ever since the patriarchate was established, there has been a tendency to cramp the mother in her maternal rights; so we see no race improvement comparable with our advance in material science. Those who could improve humanity have been hindered by those who prefer to improve steam-engines. The sex which has been laboriously evolved by nature for the arduous work of race-building is handicapped; so more and more the best women turn from the work of motherhood and join the ranks of competitive labor, or seek in society and politics a field for the free play of their ambitions. And now certain of our thinkers forebode evil for a people whose women turn from the home to the frivolities of fashion and the excitement of the political arena. Their forebodings are not without foundation; but the remedy does not lie in depriving women of public freedom, but in according them absolute domestic liberty. The world must act, as well as talk, as if motherhood were important and sacred, before women will give full allegiance to that office. But so to act requires a complete right-about-face.

Frances Galton says, "It seems to me most essential to the well-being of future generations that the average standard of ability of the present time should be raised. We are in crying want of a greater fund of ability in all stations of life; for neither the classes of statesmen, philosophers, artisans, nor laborers are up to the modern complexity of their several professions. Our race is overweighted, and appears likely to be dragged into degeneracy by demands that exceed its powers." The need is that the race be lifted up. But how is a species raised? Always by lengthening the period of infancy. And at whose expense must this be done? At the mother's; more and more of her thought, more and more of her time must be given to the period of immaturity in her offspring; later and later should the child be brought into contact with the practical demands of life. This work requires as its first condition voluntary maternity; for the unwelcome child is mentally and physically below the average; and it is a direct drag upon the mother in the efficient performance of already assumed maternal duties. The evolution of humanity and enforced maternity are antagonistic.

A second condition of race-improvement is a broader education for women. It is amazing that the nineteenth century holds that any sort of education is good enough for girls. It indicates, too, how low an opinion we have of motherhood, that when a woman does receive superior training it is considered lost, unless she enters upon a competitive career. In a recent speech before a girls' school, Mr. Gladstone, commenting on the success women had achieved in education, said that as a result places of work would have to be thrown open to them; that "of course they could not be given the training, and be debarred from the use of that training." But surely is it not equally a matter of course that era if women were debarred from public life, they would not be debarred a very important use for all the knowledge of the universe in their sphere of race-builders? The fact is, few women and fewer men regard maternity in its true light; traced down to finalities, the birth of most human beings is a sexual accident. Of course, the person playing the chief rile in this game of haphazard is neither self-respecting nor respected; for a mother of chance is never held as holy, however much poets and philosophers, popes and bishops may declare the reverse.

A third condition of race progress is that women should divide with no other person authority over the child. When the work of race-building is left wholly to women, we may look for better results; for then the ambition of the best mothers will find a congenial field for action in their so-called "sphere." As the human being is always of more real value than the work, so to rear an astronomer is perchance a higher labor than to discover a comet. Who would not rather know the work of old Frau Goethe—viz., Goethe himself—than the child of his brain, Faust?

If nature has intended women for a special career, the way to defeat the object is to limit their responsibility and authority so completely that they turn to freer fields of work. May the time come when women, fully educated, will be left free to use their creative powers as a lever for raising humanity to a nobler type.

The first step towards making maternity voluntary is to secure for all women financial independence. There are those who think this can be done by women entering the world of competitive work. Now, there is no doubt that the female of the human race could win her way, if free of artificial hinderances. The female among the lower animals supports herself and her offspring; she is competent both as bread-winner and mother. Under present sex relations women have been enfeebled in two ways,—they have lost the mental training gained in bread-winning, and have been physically depleted by playing the double *rôle* of mother and mistress. But undoubtedly in freedom, women could again be self-supporting and efficient mothers, just as they were in the time of the matriarchate; but we may well doubt whether, in our dire need for the elevation of our species, it would be economy to make the mothers of the race enter the field of competition to gain their bread and cheese. However, if the choice lies between this and the financial dependence of one woman upon one man, then every well-wisher to the race must say, let the woman be self-supporting. But educated thought upon this subject will desire to make better terms with women, and the latter will finally make better terms with civilization. Undoubtedly the tendency at present is to seek independence by undertaking competitive work, rather than to demand that work done in the home shall be recognized and command money return. Just where this tendency is to lead is not plain; but if with self-support should come an increasing neglect of maternal duties, the result will be race decadence; but if self-support leads women to the conditions, in some co-operative form, of life in the time of the Mutterrecht, human improvement may be carried to a high point of perfection. But the field of race production is so fundamental in its importance, so broad in its possibilities, it opens an arena so wide for the play of the loftiest ambitions and of the most varied talents, that time and leisure to be secured, on honorable terms, to those cultivating this field, seems but justice the most meagre and wisdom the most evident.

The solution most often offered for our social difficulties is divorce. But it is a solution which does not touch the real source of the trouble, and its agitation diverts attention from more vital questions. It is because divorce merely shifts the disease from one home to another, because it in no way lessens our trouble—the financial dependence of women, and enforced maternity—that the carrying of legislation upon the lines of easier dissolution of the marriage contract proves but a barren victory. Any one visiting the States of the American Union where the freest divorce laws have been passed, will be forced to the conclusion that in Indiana and in Illinois people suffer from the same social evils as in England, for there, as here, no solution of the knotty problem of the money independence of women has been attempted, and the child of the West as seldom as in Europe receives its birthright of a hearty welcome to the world. Divorce does not overcome these two difficulties, difficulties which, until they are met and overcome, will destroy peace in domestic relations and progress in race development. As public opinion grows upon our two great needs, legislation will probably take more the line of securing to the woman her fair share of the family income, and giving her absolute right to her children.

What the final relation of man and woman may be it is futile to prophesy; but we may be sure, if there is an ideal relation, it is to be reached by honesty, not by pretence. As a race we talk much of monogamy, and practise it very little. Monogamy implies one marriage, and no more. And that means no prostitution, no divorce, no second marriage. A second sex-relation is just as promiscuous, physiologically speaking, whether the first partner is literally buried in the graveyard or only figuratively so in the far West of America. But yet every Christian church sanctions second marriage, most civilized states grant divorce for some cause, and in every nation society winks at prostitution. It would be becoming in us, then, to claim to be no more than agnostics in the philosophy of the true relation of the sexes. But while we hesitate to foretell finalities, we must take cognizance of the undeniable fact that each day is adding to the number of thoughtful men and women who see the discrepancy between our theories and human needs and practices; each day the birth-rate of girls is rising in England upon that of boys, and already the number of women exceeds that of men by one million, and yet each day adds to the number of free, self-supporting women, women, too, who have lost none of their strong maternal instinct. We need not stop to prophesy the sex-relation of the future; we can only hope that an enlightened humanity may see that we must be true

To higher allegiance, higher than our lore,

and that we could have no more inspiring religious motto than the words of Froebel, —

Let us live for our children.

"The Welcome Child" by Lady Henry Somerset (1895)

Introduction

In this essay, Lady Isabella Somerset advocates against compulsory motherhood, arguing that forced maternity prevents the progress of women's rights. She bases her position on Christian beliefs, which aligned with her role in the temperance movement. This was published in *The Arena*, an American social reform magazine that also advocated for birth control.

"The Welcome Child" (*The Arena*, March 1895)

I suppose that to all connected with reform movements the consciousness comes with overwhelming force that we attack too late the evils we desire to remedy. The set of brain is fixed, the trend of the life bent one way; and in vain we endeavor to retrace the lines drawn by the centuries. Questions dealing with the best interests of the race with which the ancients were familiar have been overlooked in our modern life. Nothing is more startling than to find the most modern theories standing out grim and stern from classic pages—milestones that measure their civilization and our stagnation.

Coming down to later times, it is interesting to recall the arguments of those who oppose the woman movement of our day on the ground that it will unfit the sex for its special duty, and then to realize what was the attitude taken by women and approved by men not a hundred years ago. For we read in the fiction of that period (and it is a true portraiture of the social life) of women being bled in order to look delicate. In a volume of "Advice to Ladies" the author says, "They must not seem robust, as that will diminish their attractiveness to men, who prefer the weak, frail women"! Maria Edgeworth's stories are full of allusions to the thin shoes in which in summer and winter women were wont to walk; other writers allude to the damp dresses that were worn in order to obtain the lines and folds that were to suit the classic garb of the First Empire. To these follies we are undoubtedly indebted for the seeds of that lung disease which has held in its clutches victims innumerable in England and America.

Only lately has the pendulum swung back, and it is perhaps the dawning of socialistic and therefore truly Christian principles, that has brought with it the renewed consciousness that every man and woman lives not an individual life but one that makes for the upbuilding or the destruction of the race itself Slowly but surely the realization of this truth has brought us to understand that the study of child life in all its aspects is vital to the welfare of the world.

There is no question to-day as to the importance of heredity. The light of science has revealed to us the depths and heights of this question. Frances Power Cobbe, one of the truest friends that woman has had in this century, commences her intensely interesting autobiography with the sentence, "I was well born!" Nothing would be more significant than this avowal. She does not make it in any conventional, but in the truest scientific sense: I was born under propitious, happy, right circumstances. It is the keynote to her joyous life—a life which she sums up by saying, "To me it has been so well worth living, I would gladly live it over again."

If I were asked by the devotees of older creeds to state what I mean, or rather what I think they mean, by original sin, I should say: The unwelcome child is its completed definition. I believe original sin began there; for how many blighted, blasted, bewildered lives may this not account? And the millennium will set in when every child is welcome. Let us remember the number of children that are at this moment awakening into this world whose mothers greet them with a sigh, and hold out their arms to take them with a sob instead of a kiss, wishing that the little baby face turned up to theirs had never seen the light; yet they crowd in, these little unwelcome strangers, upon the weary workers of the world, the women who bend over their tasks until they lie down under the great agony of maternity, and know that, when it is over, weak and wan they must take up their labor again with another mouth to feed and less strength to gain the wherewithal. Through those dreary months before the final tragedy, that child has been environed with the consciousness that it was not wanted; gloomy anticipation has robbed the little one of joy and hope, and so once more a being comes into existence with a life blighted, a nature narrowed and cramped, affections chilled, before it has seen the sun in the heavens or drawn the breath of life. And this happens not only in the garret and cellar, but in homes of opulence and ease. The unwritten tragedy of woman's life is there.

It is all told in the fact that by our sinful, short-sighted ignorance we have trained man to believe that he dominates woman. We have perverted passages in the Bible, and built up a creed as far from the laws of God as the poles are asunder. Economic independence, social and political independence, are of vast import to women; but there is a deeper lesson and a harder one to teach— the personal independence of woman; and only when both man and woman have learned that the most sacred of all functions given to woman must be exercised by her free will alone, can children be born into the world who have in them the joyous desire to live, who claim that sweetest privilege of childhood, the certainty that they can expand in the sunshine of the love which is their due. Whoever doubts this has only to study the laws of God written in the life of the animal world, and he will find that the whole creation in a natural state is founded on the principle of the mother's right to choose when she will become a mother. This is the chief corner-stone of that holy temple we are to build—our character.

We trace the prenatal influence in a thousand ways; indeed I believe it would be impossible to examine any marked or developed characteristic without finding some solution for it in the laws that govern such influence. Nothing is more striking than to study the history of our prominent men. There is a tongue in America that is gifted with a greater power of prose poetry than perhaps any other in our day; none speaks in more beautiful rhythm; and although the matter of its discourse is to us often painful, many of us believe that some of its work has possibly been beneficial in awakening men and women from the deadening influence of the men-made creeds which have so often taken the place of the gospel teaching of true brotherhood. But all will agree that the despairing materialism of this great orator, that deliberate crushing of the wingéd spirit in man that naturally ascends to things unseen as the sparks fly upward, that absolute want of the skyey nature that turns to God because there alone it finds an echo for the divine in its own heart, is one of the great losses of the century.

It will be of interest to know the following facts, which are from the lips of the man himself to a confidential friend. He said that his mother, who was most impressionable, recoiled from the Calvinistic doctrines taught by his father, who was a minister, and during the prenatal period of his life his mother went on a visit to the home of a relative where she found the writings of Voltaire. She had never read infidel literature, but her mind was naturally given to doubt. In her present nervous state the books had a fascination for her and she read them with intense interest. When the boy was born he had a fine poetic nature and one to which restraint was odious, and as he developed he was from the first a pronounced unbeliever in the divine revelation. It is also of interest to learn, that when a cousin of this same gifted man, who is a woman of rare intellect and a philanthropist, told him some years ago of her Christian faith which, though deep and strong, was free from Calvinism and extreme doctrinal views, he said, while the tears coursed down his cheeks, "I would give all I have, cousin, if I could believe as you do, but I cannot." From these two incidents it is apparent that heredity had a decided influence on the career of the man whose writings have done more than any other author of his time to unsettle the faith of the people of this country in the eternal verities.

Dr. Norman Kerr has clearly demonstrated the heredity of inebriety as an established physiological axiom, and to every one who has studied the subject this fact has probably come home with terrible emphasis. I remember on one occasion the nurse who had charge of a child, one of whose parents had died of alcoholism, telling me that when the little boy was but three years old she had the greatest difficulty in restraining him from stealing down to the dinner table not only in the dining room but in the servants' apartment, to drain every glass in order to get a few drops of the drug for which he had inherited so strong a craving. And this is but an example among the many that, have come under my personal observation.

Flaxman, the great limner, had a mother who was so desirous of creating the beautiful that she procured the most exquisite studies of Greek art and ranged them round her in order that her imagination might be steeped in their beautiful forms.

I might indefinitely multiply instances as illustrations of this law. It is not the exception but the rule. The world's mothers are the most fateful beings that it contains, and well will it be for the world when they ponder more than they do now over the responsibility of such knowledge; when their surroundings, their knowledge of art and literature, of science and government, shall be such that they can endow their little ones; can make those months that follow nature's great annunciation a holy retreat into the most beautiful surroundings that the world can yield in form and color, thought and utterance. These may seem truisms repeated again and again, but I feel that if we realized them more profoundly women would be helped in a hundred ways and protected where now they are exposed. The frictions of family life would be avoided, and a peace would reign round them like the sacred silence of some hallowed place. This will be the culmination of all we hope for from the coming brotherhood of man in society and the state.

There is a point of difference between England and America that I would like to touch upon, and I do so very apologetically because in all the delicate consideration that can be shown to women, the younger country is ahead of us; but there has grown up in America an artificially imposed silence upon all questions relating to maternity, until that holy thing has become a matter almost of shame. Will not the women try to break this down? It seems to me life will be truer and nobler the more we recognize that there is no indelicacy in the climax and coronation of creative power, but rather that it is the highest glory to the race.

It has been held by mothers who are in positions of ease that in the early years of a child, responsibility is dormant; that to get a trustworthy nurse who keeps a child in health and ministers to its wants is all that is really needed; but I am hoping to see an entire revolution in the position of the woman taken in that capacity, and instead of some half educated, well-meaning but ignorant nurse, I believe the day will come when no woman will be considered too highly educated or too refined to mould the early impressions of the youngest child, and that mothers will see that in order to secure the services of such refined and cultured ladies they must make a revolution in the accepted ideas of the position of nurse in the houses of the rich. There ought to be no situation so honorable, no friend so trusted, as the one who from the earliest moment of the child's awakening intelligence undertakes to guide the thought and form the character at a time when such formative influence is vital to future well-being.

The trouble is that we commence too late; we allow a child's mind to become a garden of weeds, and then before we can plant we see that we have to uproot that which has been sown during the most fruitful years; and, therefore, time is lost in undoing which is invaluable for cultivation. The games, the rhymes, the songs, the associations, of the nursery, should all have a decided color, should all help to bend the young mind in the right direction, and the impressions made at a time when they leave ineffaceable traces should be drawn with the deliberate intention that they shall thus potently affect the character.

The sorrows of childhood are not so near the surface as they are supposed to be. "A boy's will is the wind's will, and the thoughts of youth are long, long thoughts." How many children chafe under the sense of injustice that the treatment of their difficulties brings to them! I knew a child who, because she was outspoken as to the doubts that arose in her mind—perplexities that have bowed many a thoughtful head in every age—was spoken of in her family as a moral pariah, kept apart from all the other members of the household alone upstairs in her room; mentally tortured into a submission which was only given because there seemed no alternative, but which left a mind bewildered between the sense of her extreme wickedness and its revolt against the injustice which she could not reconcile with any ethical standard or religious principle. Many a sorrow eats into a child's heart that it has not the strength to express or the courage to share with its elders; but I think that if instead of posing as infallible—a role which at best breaks down very soon—we were to speak more freely of our difficulties to the young, we should find out the beautiful law which binds us together, and which makes mutual confidence the most delightful feature of home life.

A friend of mine asked a little girl, six years old, to tell her what she really thought about grown-up people, and what were the differences between older people and young people; and as the child spoke, this friend wrote down exactly what she said, without any change of words or suggestions from her of any kind.

"In the first place," said the child, "they are bigger; and then they don't like sweets—not very often; and next they don't like to climb trees; and next they don't like to ride donkeys so much, because they like to do other things. They like to write books, and they like to go to meetings, and also they don't like to be always with children for it takes them from doing these things. Another difference is, they don't like to pretend because they want to know what is really going to happen. I have seen them get angry, so I know they are not always good. Sometimes they tell children to do what is not right; they tell us not to ride on donkeys because they might get kicked, but the children don't mind that, they rather like it. They are a great deal older; some are twice as old as others. You must be twenty-one to be grown up, and after that you keep on being so. Here's a way in which they are both exactly opposite to each other. Grown people think that children are naughty and children think that grown-up people are naughty. There's another difference: they know how to swim—that is, some do, but some children do. They live for money; some, not all, spend it for useful things, which children think are not useful because they don't like them; therefore they think the money is wasted. They think when a person gets langouste [a sort of French fish], they think the money is wasted on that because they don't like it. Some live to give things away, and there's one person I know that nearly almost lives for children, and that is grandma. I don't think there would be another one like grandma. They have long dresses and trousers. They generally, that is, sometimes, care more for their friends than for children, but this particular person that I am talking about doesn't. They do their hair differently; they screw it up, but men have it cut short but they have beards. Some grown ups are nice, and some children; but this particular person, grandma, is nicer than any child. I really can't explain any more."

We are apt to overlook the extreme nervousness that often renders life a perfect misery to a little child. This nervousness is often treated as cowardice, and the elders endeavor to overcome it either by ridicule or by forcing the child to do that which brings abject misery to its life. But were we wiser, we should remember that childishness is not folly; it is only the inability to understand of what to be afraid and what to dread; a child's mind can grasp an argument as well as an adult's if that argument be brought before it with tender consideration.

I do not believe we ought to underrate the power of discipline but rather to emphasize it, because this will be the truest help to self-discipline by and by. Mrs. Booth, the mother of the Salvation Army, speaks in her autobiography of the way she conquered once and forever the will of her baby son when he was still in the cradle. The child wanted to get out of his little cot, when she intended he should lie still, and for over two hours that mother sat by his side to gain her point. How many of us would have lifted up the crying child because we could not bear to withstand his crying any longer, and so have missed a golden opportunity. Not so that devoted mother; she loved her little one too well. After that day she never had to do anything but express her determination, and his obedience was perfect. That boy grew up to be a character whom to know is to admire, in its calm, conscientious self-restraint.

Above all else I would entreat that a child's illusions (if they are illusions) should not be rudely destroyed. There is, no doubt, in a child's mind a natural reverence—a worship of the beautiful, a belief in the great and good; that is the divine untouched by contact with the human. Children believe in the goodness of others until they have had reason to doubt it; they believe that the world is beautiful until they have been shown the sadness, the misery or the sin; and I think that many a conversation would be guarded and many a light and perhaps cynical remark from older lips would be hushed if a more reverent understanding were arrived at as to the effect of such talk on a child's mind. Why not leave as long as possible unimpaired that beautiful faith of youth and foster, as far as in us lies, the belief that all on which the child eyes rest is what it seems? But so often motives are ascribed to others hastily, and criticisms are passed that awaken children all too early to a sense that however much good may be apparent, underneath may lie the rottenness which they have not discovered. Let us leave children their faith in humanity, their faith in goodness, their faith in divinity; for too often on the one hand we cultivate it dogmatically and destroy it conversationally.

Edouard Rod in his beautiful book, "Le Sens de la Vie," puts this thought in one passage that I think contains the idea I fain would impress. He describes his visit to the Pantheon and tells how his mind had revolted against the accepted ideas of a conventional Christianity, and how the hatred which such revolt had caused had been succeeded by a profound indifference. At the time of the securalization of the Pantheon, when Paris had deposed God in order to replace Him by Victor Hugo, by chance he entered that temple. Some of the municipal councillors were there, talking) discussing—politicians of all sorts, their hats upon their heads, their cigars in their mouths, proud to chase away by the fumes of their tobacco any lingering incense of devotion that might still hover about the building. They laughed, gesticulated, insolent in their desire to mark their disrespect for any sacred memories. In a corner, however, he says, one altar had remained that had not yet been removed, and there an old peasant woman, her head bound in the black kerchief, in her blue apron and her shabby dress of coarse material, prayed fervently as she knelt. She had brought two little tapers, and their light scintillated and cast meagre shadows around her under the great vaulted roof. The author says that as he gazed upon her bent figure he wondered what burden she had come to lay there; what remorse, perhaps, what confidence, was she addressing so silently yet so fervently to Him, who, she believed, understood and pardoned? And when the last altar would be laid low, which of all these political place mongers would be able to give her the means of assuaging her pain? And in an instant he said he perceived that to take from her that which was highest and best was to rob her of what he could never replace; and thus overcome by a profound reverence he knelt, feeling that the divine communion in her with the great Unseen found at any rate an echo in the best of all that he possessed in his own nature.

And so I believe that if with children, instead of showing them, too often through sheer thoughtlessness, the seamy side of life, we built up in them that reverence for humanity, that expansion towards what is great and good, if we permitted them to breathe the atmosphere only of that rarefied air that is to be found on moral heights, they would learn to live to see the best in all, and face the evil of the world by and by only in order to remedy it by their deeds, but most of all by their inspiration and their character.

"The Case of Dr. Collins" (1898)

Introduction

This article brings together the concerns around puerperal fever from Chap. 2 of this book and surgical abortion, as it details a legal case against Dr. William Maunsell Collins, an Irish doctor practicing in London whose patient died from an infection. Collins had previously had his name removed from the medical register in 1892 but continued practicing. For periodical coverage of such a case, the essay explores the social more than the sensational aspects, which aligns with the magazine that published it.

The Case of Dr. Collins (*The Speaker*, 9 July 1898)

The French newspapers have been gloating over the latest London scandal. It is a nasty thing to gloat over, but we cannot say that our Parisian friends are all together without excuse. So they find it proved that a crime against morality, and the family, which some of us have been disposed to regard as peculiarly French, has been systematically perpetrated in the center of fashionable London. A lady whose husband had made a big fortune in the City found herself pregnant at the beginning of a London season. She had no just excuse for shirking the duties of maternity. Everything which wealth could do would have alleviated her pain; neither she nor her husband had any reason for wishing to restrict the number of their offspring. There was no motive for concealment, as when unhappy woman who has been wronged, seeks to conceal her shame. On the contrary, one would have supposed to that both Mr. And Mrs. Uzielli would have rejoiced at the prospect of having a third child. Nor was there any suggestion that Mrs. Uzielli had so suffered in health during previous pregnancies as to have any excuse on that account for avoiding becoming a mother. Her only motive was, perhaps, the most trumpery, which ever suggested abortion: the desire not to spoil a London season. She had recently become a lady of fashion, and feared that "society" might forget her if her one summer, she did not entertain. Under these circumstances, she went to Dr. Collins, and to her death.

There is nothing to suggest that Mrs. Uzielli was a very callous woman, who was likely to run any risk to attain her end. On the contrary, she seems to have been of a nervous disposition, and not liking and affection. She would not have submitted to be the instrument of crime and less crime have been very easy. At Dr. Colin's establishment in Cadogan place. Everything was his easy and simple as possible. A surgeon of great skill, he had retired from the position of surgeon to one of the regiments of guards, in order to take up a practice, mainly among women. And then came to him, and he cured them cleverly. He was a man of easy and accommodating temper, and found himself oppressed by women who desires to save themselves the trouble of becoming mothers. There are probably very few young doctors in the west of London, who do not receive slip similar solicitation. As a rule, they have sufficient strength of mind to decline; but Dr. Collins liked good living, and did not like to refuse so he did when he was asked. It became generally known that any woman who desired to have her offspring destroyed had only to go to Dr. Collins to have the operation performed skillfully and safely for a moderate fee. And Mrs. Uzielli's case it was about the price of a new ball dress. Was murder ever more simple?

This sort of thing has been going on for a long time. It may, indeed, seem strange that the police had never been able to previously bring home to Dr. Collins, the crime which everyone knew he made his living by practicing. But the crime is not a difficult one to conceal one practiced by a clutter surgeon. It ought to be scarcely possible for the deaf to intervene when abortion is procured, and an early stage of pregnancy, with the exercise of proper care. Every operation is dangerous: a cut in the figure may lead to blood poisoning. Any interference with the womb by an unskillful person may cause death, as the records of our criminal, courts, abundantly testify. But the operation is not an unsafe, one, as operations go. When it is successful, detection is practically impossible, for every person concern has every motive for concealment. When death supervene, Dr. Collins was able at first to give a false certificate. Unless the relations of the dead woman interfered, parentheses as they were very unlikely to do) the corner with hear nothing about the matter. Some years ago, Dr. Collins lost the power of giving certificates. He was convicted of forgery, and they'll buy some strange bit of leniency. He was not sent to gaol, he was struck off the medical register. His clientele, however, did not deserve him. He retains some general practice, and in one case for Andrew

Clark, ignorant of his identity, was called in to consult with him. Sir Andrew Clark was very angry when he found out, but there are many other doctors, who are less particular. Usually some doctor was found to give a death certificate if the patient died. Probably, to do Dr. Collins justice, he was not so negligent as to let many patients die. In one case, where a widow, with grown-up daughters had lost her life in the endeavor to avoid shame, he was very nearly found out, but the poor woman had not given away the secret, and there was no satisfactory evidence to convict him of illegal practices. Even in the Uzielli case he was only discovered by what might have seemed to him very bad luck. He used an unclean instrument, which means that he had become careless. The lady did not it first to take proper care of herself. She gave him away by hysterical exclamations. The nurses who he obtained we're not at all the sort of person she might have deserve the job. The husband was not in the secret, and called in an independent medical man. Dr. Collins himself was so ill advised as to give evidence of the inquest, and to tell a story there, which at once left credibility and involved in fatal admissions. And thus, almost a succession of accidents, his career of crime came to an end.

The extraordinary thing is that under the circumstances, the jury should've recommended him to mercy. They knew, as the writer to the verdict shows, that this was not an isolated case. There was no possible suggestion of sympathy with human suffering to palliate the breach of the law. It was a crime perpetrated purely as a matter of business by a man who made a business of crime. We can only suppose if there was some jury man who was so impressed by Mr. Gill's able defence of the prisoner that he refused to join in the verdict, unless it was combined with a recommendation to mercy. All we can say is the Dr. Collins was very fortunate in being defended by Mr. Gill. Many doctors and midwives have been sentenced to death, who had much less excuse, and, without urging that the death penalty ought to be enforced, in such cases, seven years penal, servitude is but a late punishment with a practice criminal is it last convicted of a crime difficult to detect.

Manual of Health for Women: Plain Advice in Sickness and Health by Peter J. Latz (1906)

Introduction

In the preface to the volume, Dr. Peter J. Latz explains his belief that women should understand the diseases common among them enough to live a healthy life and to consult her doctor when she needs treatment. His larger purpose is on the ability of women to procreate, as "a sickly mother cannot give birth to healthy, vigorous children" (7). His approach to contraception in this volume, however, centers on his social and moral views, rather than medical advice. This indicates the kind of message women interested in controlling their fertility received from many popular guides to health.

b. Voluntary Sterility, or the Wilful Prevention of Conception

Children are not a curse, but a blessing, and although it cannot be denied that the rearing and educating of children involves burdens and cares, sacrifices of money, labor and time, yet the best qualities in man are developed when he is forced to battle energetically for his family's welfare. Then he learns to exert himself, to be modest in his wants, to check egotism, and cultivate true self denial. The patience, forbearance, condescension and love required to rear children leave their impression on the parents. Thoughtfulness, prudence, and a resourceful spirit are indispensable and at the same time these sacrifices shape the character of the educator. Hence in all justice it may be said that parents not only educate their children, but also children their parents, and thereby the moral development of mankind is materially influenced. This reason alone is sufficient to condemn those who laud the small family, or advise married people to remain childless.

In defense of these immoral teachings the advocates of "small families" point to the precepts of certain economists, who would have us believe that poverty is a result of over-population and that, therefore, restriction of propagation is a means of increasing the wealth, welfare and happiness of the working classes.

We cannot dwell on the fallacy of these theories, but desire to say that they have been disproven by eminent thinkers and scientists. In reality egotism, love of pleasure and the world, has much more to do with the small family, consisting of husband, wife and one or two children, so prevalent today, than the belief in the truth of the theories of Malthus.

Every artificial means that serves to prevent conception, whether it aims at the destruction or removal of the seminal fluid, or whether it consists in so-called preventives or in the interruption of the conjugal act, etc., is unnatural, immoral, damnable, and injurious to health.

For married people to prevent conception is nothing but conjugal onanism, and a wife that consents to it permits herself to be used as the vile tool of unnatural lust; a decent woman would feel deeply insulted at any such proposal, and the man who could propose such an abomination to his wife has little or no esteem of a woman's true greatness and knows nothing of her great power of endurance, patience and suffering.

Now, what are the dangers connected with artificial sterility? Whosoever believes that these preventives are quite harmless, is greatly mistaken. All neuropathists agree that preventive intercourse in marriage ruins the nervous system. Besides, other morbid changes are observed in the vital organs. Nutrition suffers. A continued intercourse of this nature will cause disorders in the female organs, especially the womb. Nature, moreover, punishes the violation of her laws by a diminution of mental powers, particularly by a weakening of the memory. Onanism shows its evil effects much more and much sooner in women than in men.

If, in conclusion, we are asked: Are there means which a physician might recommend to prevent conception, where such prevention would be justified—a means morally licit and physically harmless? we reply: It is well known that the greatest probability of conception obtains when intercourse follows immediately upon the cessation of the menses. Later this probability decreases from day to day until finally there is a time when conception becomes improbable. According to the best experience this time is the third week after the beginning of menstruation. Hence married people have only to follow a certain rule in their marital intercourse to prevent too frequent conceptions.

It is evident that intercourse regulated in this manner has nothing in common with artificial sterility and, consequently, is also free from evil consequences. Although conception is not impossible in the third week after the menses, yet it is less probable than shortly before or after menstruation. Thus the physiologist Racibowski has found that of one hundred women no more than six or seven conceive at that time. In the last days before the beginning of another menstruation the probability of conception again increases. Hence where it is advisable to limit the progeny, intercourse should not take place within the two weeks after menstruation and the three or four days preceding it.

Where there are serious reasons for the prevention of conception, married people by mutual agreement, should abstain from intercourse for a while, which will not be extraordinarily difficult if they only possess the firm will to put their sensuality under the rule of reason.

It is the duty of physicians to call the attention of men and women to the immorality of artificial sterility and its sad consequences. Whatever is unnatural in sexual intercourse brings about its own peculiar punishment. Were it possible to stop conjugal onanism, general debility and nervousness would largely disappear.

"Waste" by Harvey Granville-Barker (1907)

Introduction

In this play, the protagonist Henry Trebell is an ambitious politician who has an affair with the married Amy O'Connell. In the second act, Trebell is convincing Amy to have an abortion. Then, in the third, Dr. Wedgecroft explains he initially refused to terminate Amy's pregnancy but then cared for her when she was sick after an abortion from another practitioner. In the fourth act, Trebell reflects on Amy's death with his sister Frances. The play was originally refused a license and could only be performed privately.

Excerpt from The Second Act

Trebell *follows him to the door which he shuts. Then he turns to face* Amy, *who is tearing up the paper she wrote on.*
Trebell. What is it?
Amy. [*Her steady voice breaking, her carefully calculated control giving way.*] Oh Henry ... Henry!
Trebell. Are you in trouble?
Amy. You'll hate me, but ... oh, it's brutal of you to have been away so long.
Trebell. Is it with your husband?
Amy. Perhaps. Oh, come nearer to me ... do.
Trebell. [*Coming nearer without haste or excitement.*] Well? [*Her eyes are closed.*] My dear girl, I'm too busy for love-making now. If there are any facts to be faced, let me have them ... quite quickly.
She looks up at him for a moment; then speaks swiftly and sharply as one speaks of disaster.
Amy. There's a danger of my having a child ... your child ... some time in April. That's all.
Trebell. [*A sceptic who has seen a vision.*] Oh ... it's impossible.
Amy. [*Flashing at him, revengefully.*] Why?
Trebell. [*Brought to his mundane self*] Well ... are you sure?
Amy. [*In sudden agony.*] D'you think I want it to be true? D'you think I—? You don't know what it is to have a thing happening in spite of you.
Trebell. [*His face set in thought.*] Where have you been since we met?
Amy. Not to Ireland ... I haven't seen Justin[7] for a year.
Trebell. All the easier for you not to see him for another year.
Amy. That wasn't what you meant.

---

[7] Her husband, Justin O'Connell.

Trebell. It wasn't ... but never mind.
They are silent for a moment ... miles apart ... Then she speaks dully.
Amy. We do hate each other ... don't we!
Trebell. Nonsense. Let's think of what matters.
Amy. [*Aimlessly.*] I went to a man at Dover ... picked him out of the directory ... didn't give my own name ... pretended I was off abroad. He was a kind old thing ... said it was all most satisfactory. Oh, my God!
Trebell. [*He goes to bend over her kindly.*] Yes, you've had a torturing month or two. That's been wrong, I'm sorry.
Amy. Even now I have to keep telling myself that it's so ... otherwise I couldn't understand it. Any more than one really believes one will ever die ... one doesn't believe that, you know.
Trebell. [*On the edge of a sensation that is new to him.*] I am told that a man begins to feel unimportant from this moment forward. Perhaps it's true.
Amy. What has it to do with you anyhow? We don't belong to each other. How long were we together that night? Half an hour! You didn't seem to care a bit until after you'd kissed me and ... this is an absurd consequence.
Trebell. Nature's a tyrant.
Amy. Oh, it's my punishment ... I see that well enough ... for thinking myself so clever ... forgetting my duty and religion ... not going to confession, I mean. [*Then hysterically.*] God can make you believe in Him when he likes, can't he?
Trebell. [*With comfortable strength.*] My dear girl, this needs your pluck. [*And he sits by her.*] All we have to do is to prevent it being found out.
Amy. Yes ... the scandal would smash you, wouldn't it?
Trebell. There isn't going to be any scandal.
Amy. No ... if we're careful. You'll tell me what to do, won't you? Oh, it's a relief to be able to talk about it.
Trebell. For one thing, you must take care of yourself and stop worrying.
It soothes her to feel that he is concerned; but it is not enough to be soothed.
Amy. Yes, I wouldn't like to have been the means of smashing you, Henry ... especially as you don't care for me.
Trebell. I intend to care for you.
Amy. Love me, I mean. I wish you did ... a little; then perhaps I shouldn't feel so degraded.
Trebell. [*A shade impatiently, a shade contemptuously*] I can say I love you if that'll make things easier.
Amy. [*More helpless than ever.*] If you'd said it at first I should be taking it for granted ... though it wouldn't be any more true, I daresay, than now ... when I should know you weren't telling the truth.
Trebell. Then I'd do without so much confusion.
Amy. Don't be so heartless.
Trebell. [*As he leaves her.*] We seem to be attaching importance to such different things.

Amy. [*Shrill even at a momentary desertion.*] What do you mean? I want affection now just as I want food. I can't do without it ... I can't reason things out as you can. D'you think I haven't tried? [*Then in sudden rebellion.*] Oh, the physical curse of being a woman ... no better than any savage in this condition ... worse off than an animal. It's unfair.

Trebell. Never mind ... you're here now to hand me half the responsibility, aren't you?

Amy. As if I could! If I have to lie through the night simply shaking with bodily fear much longer ... I believe I shall go mad.

This aspect of the matter is meaningless to him. He returns to the practical issue.

Trebell. There's nobody that need be suspecting, is there?

Amy. My maid sees I'm ill and worried and makes remarks ... only to me so far. Don't I look a wreck? I nearly ran away when I saw Dr. Wedgecroft ... some of these men are so clever.

Trebell. [*Calculating.*] Someone will have to be trusted.

Amy. [*Burrowing into her little tortured self again.*] And I ought to feel as if I had done Justin a great wrong ... but I don't. I hate you now; now and then. I was being myself. You've brought me down. I feel worthless.

The last word strikes him. He stares at her.

Trebell. Do you?

Amy. [*Pleadingly.*] There's only one thing I'd like you to tell me, Henry ... it isn't much. That night we were together ... it was for a moment different to everything that has ever been in your life before, wasn't it?

Trebell. [*Collecting himself as if to explain to a child.*] I must make you understand ... I must get you to realise that for a little time to come you're above the law ... above even the shortcomings and contradictions of a man's affection.

Amy. But let us have one beautiful memory to share.

Trebell. [*Determined she shall face the cold logic of her position.*] Listen. I look back on that night as one looks back on a fit of drunkenness.

Amy. [*Neither understanding nor wishing to; only shocked and hurt.*] You beast.

Trebell. [*With bitter sarcasm.*] No, don't say that. Won't it comfort you to think of drunkenness as a beautiful thing? There are precedents enough ... classic ones.

Amy. You mean I might have been any other woman.

Trebell. [*Quite inexorable.*] Wouldn't any other woman have served the purpose ... and is it less of a purpose because we didn't know we had it? Does my unworthiness then ... if you like to call it so ... make you unworthy now? I must make you see that it doesn't.

Amy. [*Petulantly hammering at her idée fixe.*] But you didn't love me ... and you don't love me.

Trebell. [*Keeping his patience.*] No ... only within the last five minutes have I really taken the smallest interest in you. And now I believe I'm half jealous. Can you understand that? You've been talking a lot of nonsense about your emotions and your immortal soul. Don't you see it's only now that you've become a person of some importance to the world ... and why?

Amy. [*Losing her patience, childishly.*] What do you mean by the World? You don't seem to have any personal feelings at all. It's horrible you should have thought of me like that. There has been no other man than you that I would have let come anywhere near me ... not for more than a year.

He realises that she will never understand.

Trebell. My dear girl, I'm sorry to be brutal. Does it matter so much to you that I should have wished to be the father of your child?

Amy. [*Ungracious but pacified by his change of tone.*] It doesn't matter now.

Trebell. [*Friendly still.*] On principle I don't make promises. But I think I can promise you that if you keep your head and will keep your health, this shall all be made as easy for you as if everyone could know. And let's think what the child may mean to you ... just the fact of his birth. Nothing to me, of course! Perhaps that accounts for the touch of jealousy. I've forfeited my rights because I hadn't honourable intentions. You can't forfeit yours. Even if you never see him and he has to grow up among strangers ... just to have had a child must make a difference to you. Of course, it may be a girl. I wonder.

As he wanders on so optimistically she stares at him and her face changes. She realises...

Amy. Do you expect me to go through with this? Henry! ... I'd sooner kill myself.

There is silence between them. He looks at her as one looks at some unnatural thing. Then after a moment he speaks, very coldly.

Trebell. Oh ... indeed. Don't get foolish ideas into your head. You've no choice now ... no reasonable choice.

Amy. [*Driven to bay; her last friend an enemy.*] I won't go through with it.

Trebell. It hasn't been so much the fear of scandal then—

Amy. That wouldn't break my heart. You'd marry me, wouldn't you? We could go away somewhere. I could be very fond of you, Henry.

Trebell. [*Marvelling at these tangents.*] Marry you! I should murder you in a week.

This sounds only brutal to her; she lets herself be shamed.

Amy. You've no more use for me than the use you've made of me.

Trebell. [*Logical again.*] Won't you realise that there's a third party to our discussion ... that I'm of no importance beside him and you of very little. Think of the child.

Amy *blazes into desperate rebellion.*

Amy. There's no child because I haven't chosen there shall be and there shan't be because I don't choose. You'd have me first your plaything and then Nature's, would you?

Trebell. [*A little abashed.*] Come now, you knew what you were about.

Amy. [*Thinking of those moments.*] Did I? I found myself wanting you, belonging to you suddenly. I didn't stop to think and explain. But are we never to be happy and irresponsible ... never for a moment?

Trebell. Well … one can't pick and choose consequences.
Amy. Your choices in life have made you what you want to be, haven't they? Leave me mine.
Trebell. But it's too late to argue like that.
Amy. If it is, I'd better jump into the Thames. I've thought of it.
He considers how best to make a last effort to bring her to her senses. He sits by her.
Trebell. Amy … if you were my wife—
Amy. [*Unresponsive to him now.*] I was Justin's wife, and I went away from him sooner than bear him children. Had I the right to choose or had I not?
Trebell. [*Taking another path.*] Shall I tell you something I believe? If we were left to choose, we should stand for ever deciding whether to start with the right foot or the left. We blunder into the best things in life. Then comes the test … have we faith enough to go on … to go through with the unknown thing?
Amy. [*So bored by these metaphysics.*] Faith in what?
Trebell. Our vitality. I don't give a fig for beauty, happiness, or brains. All I ask of myself is … can I pay Fate on demand?
Amy. Yes … in imagination. But I've got physical facts to face.
But he has her attention now and pursues the advantage.
Trebell. Very well then … let the meaning of them go. Look forward simply to a troublesome illness. In a little while you can go abroad quietly and wait patiently. We're not fools and we needn't find fools to trust in. Then come back to England…
Amy. And forget. That seems simple enough, doesn't it?
Trebell. If you don't want the child let it be mine … not yours.
Amy. [*Wondering suddenly at this bond between them.*] Yours! What would you do with it?
Trebell. [*Matter-of-fact.*] Provide for it, of course.
Amy. Never see it, perhaps.
Trebell. Perhaps not. If there were anything to be gained … for the child. I'll see that he has his chance as a human being.
Amy. How hopeful! [*Now her voice drops. She is looking back, perhaps at a past self.*] If you loved me … perhaps I might learn to love the thought of your child.
Trebell. [*As if half his life depended on her answer.*] Is that true?
Amy. [*Irritably.*] Why are you picking me to pieces? I think that is true. If you had been loving me for a long, long time—[*The agony rushes back on her.*] But now I'm only afraid. You might have some pity for me … I'm so afraid.
Trebell. [*Touched.*] Indeed … indeed, I'll take what share of this I can.
She shrinks from him unforgivingly.
Amy. No, let me alone. I'm nothing to you. I'm a sick beast in danger of my life, that's all … cancerous!
He is roused for the first time, roused to horror and protest.
Trebell. Oh, you unhappy woman! … if life is like death to you…

Amy. [*Turning on him.*] Don't lecture me! If you're so clever put a stop to this horror. Or you might at least say you're sorry.
Trebell. Sorry! [*The bell on the table rings jarringly.*] Cantelupe!
He goes to the telephone. She gets up cold and collected, steadied merely by the unexpected sound.
Amy. I mustn't keep you from governing the country. I'm sure you'll do it very well.
Trebell. [*At the telephone.*] Yes, bring him up, of course ... isn't Mr. Kent there? [*then to her.*] I may be ten minutes with him or half an hour. Wait and we'll come to a conclusion.
Kent *comes in, an open letter in his hand.*
Kent. This note, sir. Had I better go round myself and see him?
Trebell. [*As he takes the note.*] Cantelupe's come.
Kent. [*Glancing at the telephone.*] Oh, has he!
Trebell. [*As he reads.*] Yes I think you had.
Kent. Evans was very serious.
He goes back into his room. Amy *moves swiftly to where* Trebell *is standing and whispers.*
Amy. Won't you tell me whom to go to?
Trebell. No.
Amy. Oh, really ... what unpractical sentimental children you men are! You and your consciences ... you and your laws. You drive us to distraction and sometimes to death by your stupidities. Poor women—!

Excerpt from The Third Act

Cantelupe. Didn't you say she came to you first of all?
Wedgecroft. I met her one morning at Trebell's.
Farrant. Actually *at* Trebell's!
Wedgecroft. The day he came back from abroad.
Farrant. Oh! No one seems to have noticed them together much at any time. My wife ... No matter!
Wedgecroft. She tackled me as a doctor with one part of her trouble ... added she'd been with O'Connell in Ireland, which of course it turns out wasn't true ... asked me to help her. I had to say I couldn't.
Horsham. [*Echoing rather than querying.*] You couldn't.
Farrant. [*Shocked.*] My dear Horsham!
Wedgecroft. Well, if she'd told me the truth!... No, anyhow I couldn't. I'm sure there was no excuse. One can't run these risks.
Farrant. Quite right, quite right.
Wedgecroft. There are men who do on one pretext or another.
Farrant. [*Not too shocked to be curious.*] Are there really?

Wedgecroft. Oh yes, men well known … in other directions. I could give you four addresses … but of course I wasn't going to give her one. Though there again … if she'd told me the whole truth!… My God, women are such fools! And they prefer quackery … look at the decent doctors they simply turn into charlatans. Though, there again, that all comes of letting a trade work mysteriously under the thumb of a benighted oligarchy … which is beside the question. But one day I'll make you sit up on the subject of the Medical Council, Horsham.

Horsham *assumes an impenetrable air of statesmanship.*

Horsham. I know. Very interesting … very important … very difficult to alter the status quo.

Wedgecroft. Then the poor little liar said she'd go off to an appointment with her dressmaker; and I heard nothing more till she sent for me a week later, and I found her almost too ill to speak. Even then she didn't tell me the truth! So, when O'Connell arrived, of course I spoke to him quite openly and all he told me in reply was that it wouldn't have been his child.

Farrant. Poor devil!

Wedgecroft. O'Connell?

Farrant. Yes, of course.

Wedgecroft. I wonder. Perhaps she didn't realize he'd been sent for … or felt then she was dying and didn't care … or lost her head. I don't know.

Farrant. Such a pretty little woman!

Wedgecroft. If I could have made him out and dealt with him, of course, I shouldn't have come to you. Farrant's known him even longer than I have.

Farrant. I was with him at Harrow.

Wedgecroft. So I went to Farrant first.

…

O'Connell. I am Justin O'Connell.

Trebell. I guess that.

O'Connell. There's a dead woman between us, Mr. Trebell.

A tremor sweeps over Trebell; *then he speaks simply.*

Trebell. I wish she had not died.

O'Connell. I am called upon by your friends to save you from the consequences of her death. What have you to say about that?

Trebell. I have been wondering what sort of expression the last of your care for her would find … but not much. My wonder is at the power over me that has been given to something I despised.

Only O'Connell *grasps his meaning. But he, stirred for the first time and to his very depths, drives it home.*

O'Connell. Yes…. If I wanted revenge I have it. She was a worthless woman. First my life and now yours! Dead because she was afraid to bear your child, isn't she?

Trebell. [*In agony.*] I'd have helped that if I could.

O'Connell. Not the shame ... not the wrong she had done me ... but just fear—fear of the burden of her woman-hood. And because of her my children are bastards and cannot inherit my name. And I must live in sin against my church, as—God help me—I can't against my nature. What are men to do when this is how women use the freedom we have given them? Is the curse of barrenness to be nothing to a man? And that's the death in life to which you gentlemen with your fine civilisation are bringing us. I think we are brothers in misfortune, Mr. Trebell.

Trebell. [*Far from responding.*] Not at all, sir. If you wanted children you did the next best thing when she left you. My own problem is neither so simple nor is it yet anyone's business but my own. I apologise for alluding to it.

Excerpt from The Fourth Act

Frances *comes in quickly, evidently in search of her brother. Though she has not been crying, her eyes are wide with grief.*
Frances. Oh, Henry ... I'm so glad you're still up. [*She notices* Wedgecroft.] How d'you do, Doctor?
Trebell. [*Doubling his mask of indifference.*] Meistersinger's over early.
Frances. Is it?
Trebell. Not much past twelve yet.
Frances. [*The little gibe lost on her.*] It was Tristan to-night. I'm quite upset. I heard just as I was coming away ... Amy O'Connell's dead. [*Both men hold their breath.* Trebell *is the first to find control of his and give the cue.*]
Trebell. Yes ... Wedgecroft has just told me.
Frances. She was only taken ill last week ... it's so extraordinary. [*She remembers the doctor.*] Oh ... have you been attending her?
Wedgecroft. Yes.
Frances. I hear there's to be an inquest.
Wedgecroft. Yes.
Frances. But what has been the matter?
Trebell. [*Sharply forestalling any answer.*] You'll know to-morrow.
Frances. [*The little snub almost bewildering her.*] Anything private? I mean...
Trebell. No ... I'll tell you. Don't make Gilbert repeat a story twice.... He's tired with a good day's work.
Wedgecroft. Yes ... I'll be getting away.
Frances *never heeds this flash of a further meaning between the two men.*
Frances. And I meant to have gone to see her to-day. Was the end very sudden? Did her husband arrive in time?
Wedgecroft. Yes.
Frances. They didn't get on ... he'll be frightfully upset.
Trebell *resists a hideous temptation to laugh.*

Wedgecroft. Good night, Trebell.
Trebell. Good night, Gilbert. Many thanks.
...
Frances. Henry ... this is dreadful about that poor little woman.
Trebell. An unwelcome baby was arriving. She got some quack to kill her.
These exact words are like a blow in the face to her, from which, being a woman of brave common sense, she does not shrink.
Trebell. What do you say to that?
She walks away from him, thinking painfully.
Frances. She had never had a child. There's the common-place thing to say.... Ungrateful little fool! But...
Trebell. If you had been in her place?
Frances. [*Subtly.*] I have never made the mistake of marrying. She grew frightened, I suppose. Not just physically frightened. How can a man understand?
Trebell. The fear of life ... do you think it was ... which is the beginning of all evil?
Frances. A woman must choose what her interpretation of life is to be ... as a man must too in his way ... as you and I have chosen, Henry.
Trebell. [*Asking from real interest in her.*] Was yours a deliberate choice and do you never regret it?
Frances. [*Very simply and clearly.*] Perhaps one does nothing quite deliberately and for a definite reason. My state has its compensations ... if one doesn't value them too highly. I've travelled in thought over all this question. You mustn't blame a woman for wishing not to bear children. But ... well, if one doesn't like the fruit one mustn't cultivate the flower. And I suppose that saying condemns poor Amy ... condemned her to death ... [*Then her face hardens as she concentrates her meaning.*] and brands most men as ... let's unsentimentally call it illogical, doesn't it?
...
Frances. I don't think I shall sleep to-night. Poor Amy O'Connell!
Trebell. [*Curiously.*] Are you afraid of death?
Frances. [*With humorous stoicism.*] It will be the end of me, perhaps.
...
Frances. Henry, it's a foolish idea ... I suppose I have it because I hardly slept for thinking of her. Your trouble is nothing to do with Amy O'Connell, is it?
Trebell. [*His voice strangled in his throat.*] Her child should have been my child too.
Frances. [*Her eyes open, the whole landscape of her mind suddenly clear.*] Oh, I ... no, I didn't think so ... but...
Trebell. [*Dealing his second blow as remorselessly as dealt to him.*] Also I'm not joining the new Cabinet, my dear sister.

Frances. [*Her thoughts rushing now to the present—the future.*] Not! Because of…? Do people know? Will they…? You didn't…?
…
Frances. [*Lifting her voice; some tone returning to it.*] Unconsciously … I've known for years that this sort of thing might happen to you.
Trebell. Why?
Frances. Power over men and women and contempt for them! Do you think they don't take their revenge sooner or later?
Trebell. Much good may it do them!
Frances. Human nature turns against you … by instinct … in self-defence.
Trebell. And my own human-nature!
Frances. [*Shocked into great pity, by his half articulate pain.*] Yes … you must have loved her, Henry … in some odd way. I'm sorry for you both.
Trebell. I'm hating her now … as a man can only hate his own silliest vices.
Frances. [*Flashing into defence.*] That's wrong of you. If you thought of her only as a pretty little fool… Bearing your child … all her womanly life belonged to you … and for that time there was no other sort of life in her. So she became what you thought her.
Trebell. That's not true.
Frances. It's true enough … it's true of men towards women. You can't think of them through generations as one thing and then suddenly find them another.
Trebell. [*Hammering at his fixed idea.*] She should have brought that child into the world.
Frances. You didn't love her enough!
Trebell. I didn't love her at all.
Frances. Then why should she value your gift?
Trebell. For its own sake.
Frances. [*Turning away.*] It's hopeless … you don't understand.
Trebell. [*Helpless; almost like a deserted child.*] I've been trying to … all through the night.

"A Sunday Morning Tragedy" by Thomas Hardy (1909)

Introduction

In this ballad set in the 1860s, Thomas Hardy presents the narrative of a mother whose beautiful daughter has become pregnant by her lover who refuses to marry her. The mother brews an abortifacient potion, which kills her daughter. The poem uses relatively simple language, though the dialect may be unfamiliar.

A Sunday Morning Tragedy (*circa* 186–)

I bore a daughter flower-fair,
In Pydel Vale, alas for me;
I joyed to mother one so rare,
But dead and gone I now would be.

Men looked and loved her as she grew,
And she was won, alas for me;
She told me nothing, but I knew,
And saw that sorrow was to be.

I knew that one had made her thrall,
A thrall to him, alas for me;
And then, at last, she told me all,
And wondered what her end would be.

She owned that she had loved too well,
Had loved too well, unhappy she,
And bore a secret time would tell,
Though in her shroud she'd sooner be.

I plodded to her sweetheart's door
In Pydel Vale, alas for me:
I pleaded with him, pleaded sore,
To save her from her misery.

He frowned, and swore he could not wed,
Seven times he swore it could not be;
"Poverty's worse than shame," he said,
Till all my hope went out of me.

"I've packed my traps to sail the main"—
Roughly he spake, alas did he—
"Wessex beholds me not again,
'Tis worse than any jail would be!"

—There was a shepherd whom I knew,
A subtle man, alas for me:
I sought him all the pastures through,
Though better I had ceased to be.

I traced him by his lantern light,
And gave him hint, alas for me,
Of how she found her in the plight
That is so scorned in Christendie.

"Is there an herb…?" I asked. "Or none?"
Yes, thus I asked him desperately.
"—There is," he said; "a certain one…"
Would he had sworn that none knew he!

"To-morrow I will walk your way,"
He hinted low, alas for me.—
Fieldwards I gazed throughout next day;
Now fields I never more would see!

The sunset-shine, as curfew strook,
As curfew strook beyond the lea,
Lit his white smock and gleaming crook,
While slowly he drew near to me.

He pulled from underneath his smock
The herb I sought, my curse to be—
"At times I use it in my flock,"
He said, and hope waxed strong in me.

"'Tis meant to balk ill-motherings"—
(Ill-motherings! Why should they be?)—
"If not, would God have sent such things?"
So spoke the shepherd unto me.

That night I watched the poppling brew,
With bended back and hand on knee:
I stirred it till the dawnlight grew,
And the wind whiffled wailfully.

"This scandal shall be slain," said I,
"That lours upon her innocency:
I'll give all whispering tongues the lie;"—
But worse than whispers was to be.

"Here's physic for untimely fruit,"
I said to her, alas for me,
Early that morn in fond salute;
And in my grave I now would be.

—Next Sunday came, with sweet church chimes
In Pydel Vale, alas for me:
I went into her room betimes;
No more may such a Sunday be!

"Mother, instead of rescue nigh,"
She faintly breathed, alas for me,

"I feel as I were like to die,
And underground soon, soon should be."

From church that noon the people walked
In twos and threes, alas for me,
Showed their new raiment—smiled and talked,
Though sackcloth-clad I longed to be.

Came to my door her lover's friends,
And cheerly cried, alas for me,
"Right glad are we he makes amends,
For never a sweeter bride can be."

My mouth dried, as 'twere scorched within,
Dried at their words, alas for me:
More and more neighbours crowded in,
(O why should mothers ever be!)

"Ha-ha! Such well-kept news!" laughed they,
Yes—so they laughed, alas for me.
"Whose banns were called in church to-day?"—
Christ, how I wished my soul could flee!

"Where is she? O the stealthy miss,"
Still bantered they, alas for me,
"To keep a wedding close as this…"
Ay, Fortune worked thus wantonly!

"But you are pale—you did not know?"
They archly asked, alas for me,
I stammered, "Yes—some days-ago,"
While coffined clay I wished to be.

"'Twas done to please her, we surmise?"
(They spoke quite lightly in their glee)
"Done by him as a fond surprise?"
I thought their words would madden me.

Her lover entered. "Where's my bird?—
My bird—my flower—my picotee?
First time of asking, soon the third!"
Ah, in my grave I well may be.

To me he whispered: "Since your call—"
So spoke he then, alas for me—
"I've felt for her, and righted all."
—I think of it to agony.

"She's faint to-day—tired—nothing more—"
Thus did I lie, alas for me…
I called her at her chamber door
As one who scarce had strength to be.

No voice replied. I went within—
O women! scourged the worst are we…
I shrieked. The others hastened in
And saw the stroke there dealt on me.

There she lay—silent, breathless, dead,
Stone dead she lay—wronged, sinless she!—
Ghost-white the cheeks once rosy-red:
Death had took her. Death took not me.

I kissed her colding face and hair,
I kissed her corpse—the bride to be!—
My punishment I cannot bear,
But pray God *not* to pity me.
January 1904.

Gloria Gray—Love Pirate by Pearl Doles Bell (1914)

Introduction

This novel tells the story of Gloria Gray, a young woman working as a secretary whose affair with her boss Marvin Cunningham results in an unplanned pregnancy. In the chapter excerpted here, Gloria is in the hospital undergoing surgery and treatment to complete her abortion and heal her after abortifacient pills she bought from an unlicensed provider caused complications.

Chapter XXVI. A Four Leaf Clover.

It was late in September when I awoke one day with the odor of chloroform strong in my nostrils. At first only dim outlines of the furniture in the room met my half conscious eyes, and then as the details began to fit into the outlines and the unfamiliar pieces of furniture became more clear to my eyes, my brain threw off its stupor and became curiously alert.

The room was in semi-darkness and a close, sickening odor of chloroform hung about it like an evil vapor. The wall opposite was white enameled as were the articles of furniture that came within my range of vision.

Suddenly I became conscious of the presence of two spirits or ghosts, one on either side of my bed, which apparently was standing in the center of the room. One of the ghosts, a tall white-coated thing with a white cap on its head, was holding its fingers on some one's wrist, and a watch lay in the palm of its other hand.

The hand that drooped from the wrist the ghost was holding, was relaxed and white like the hand of one who is dead. It fascinated me and I was watching it curiously when the ghost moved the wrist slightly and the slender white fingers of the lifeless hand were turned more directly toward me.

There were two rings glistening on one of the fingers, that I recognized at once as belonging to me. I felt no surprise that some one else was wearing my rings, only a detached wonder and curiosity. Suddenly the ghost laid the hand that wore my rings down upon the bed beside me. My brain rebelled a little at that and I tried to lift my head to see if they had dared put a dead person in bed with me merely because that person had in some way got possession of my rings.

My head refused to lift and for the first time I became conscious of the awful noise about my ears. I tried again to lift my head but without success. It was wedged in between two big boiler factories and the blows of the hammers hurt and jarred me frightfully.

"It is all right, nurse; her pulse is nearly normal. You may tell those of her relatives who are below, that she will live." The voice came from several blocks away and the noise of the hammers made it almost impossible for me to hear, but I was aware that one of the white-clad figures immediately left the room.

A few moments later mother and Peggy entered. At the door mother broke from Peggy's supporting arm and ran to my bed with incoherent cries of joy.

"Oh, my little girl! My little Gloria! She will live! Oh, dear God, thou art good, good!"

She was kneeling beside the bed and I knew that she was crying as was Peggy who came over and kissed my forehead, and left a hot tear on it that burned like fire into the cold dampness of my skin.

"Don't cry, dears. I am all right. Can't you see I am all right?" I said this to reassure them but to my surprise no sound issued from my mouth; the words were inaudible. I tried to speak but my lips were dumb.

I wanted to put my hand out to mother but I couldn't find it and I was just getting sorely puzzled when the ghost led mother and Peggy gently from the room.

When mother first learned that I was to be operated upon she argued with me for hours and then later with the doctors, her main point being that she could not understand why girls, unmarried girls, needed to be operated upon in the present generation, when such a thing was unheard of when she was young. But dear little mother; she hadn't much time to argue, for they hurried me off to a hospital on the West Side and it was not "an hour too soon," the doctors later informed me.

I had been taking treatments from a downtown physician who was none too reputable, and the day I was taken to the hospital I had gone home at noon with a chill. Fifteen minutes after I had arrived at home one of the city's prominent surgeons called, whispering to me at his first opportunity that Mr. Cunningham had sent him.

I do not know what he told mother was the cause of my illness, nor what sort of an operation would have to be performed, but I do know he did not tell her the truth and that the maid was told that I had appendicitis.

"It is serious?" I asked with lips that had become dry and feverish, as he sat by me in the ambulance on the way to the hospital.

"Yes," he said gently.

"And he—he sent you to care for me?"

"Yes. And he asked me to tell you that for your own sake he could not be near you now, but that he would neither eat nor sleep until the danger was past."

"You are his friend? You have known him long?" I asked.

"Yes, we have been friends a great many years. His is the grandest character I have ever known."

"Thank you," I said, unconsciously accepting his words as a tribute or compliment to some one belonging to me.

At the hospital when mother and Peggy had kissed me good-bye and had gone sobbing from the room, and just as the long cart which was to carry me to the operating room was pushed up beside my bed, a nurse entered and handed me an envelope, saying that a gentleman had just asked that it be given to me. I glanced at the surgeon inquiringly as the nurse withdrew to the far end of the room.

"Yes, it is likely from him. Shall I open it for you?"

I nodded weakly.

He tore the end of the envelope hastily and there fell upon my breast a withered four-leaved clover. Tears rushed to my eyes as I recognized the mute message that wished me luck.

"It is one I gave him a year ago and which he has carried since in the case of his watch. It is supposed to bring luck, you know. He kept it, not because of any superstition," I hastened to add, "but because I had picked it and given it to him."

I did not blush as I said this for somehow this doctor friend of his who shared our secret seemed to understand it all so thoroughly, although I was sure Mr. Cunningham had told him only that which was necessary for him to know.

The dry little clover lay in my palm, a mute little message of cheer from the one person in all the world who dared not enter my sick room.

The man for whom I was that moment was suffering, I knew, even more than I, dared not show as much anxiety about my condition as the veriest stranger might, lest my reputation suffer as a consequence.

"It is not fair," I cried, pressing the dry little clover to my lips. "The world and her conventions are wrong! Wrong! Wrong!"

"Calm yourself, child. It may all come right in time—your troubles, I mean."

I shook my head wearily, and then pulling at the edge of the white cap that had been drawn over my head, I pushed the little clover up under it and left it to nestle against the hair that he loved, during my journey along the uncertain shore of the darkness.

Harper's Weekly Series on The Control of Births by Mary Alden Hopkins (1915)

Introduction

In this series, popular American magazine *Harper's Weekly* presents the complicated issue of birth control, balancing the views of different sides as well as legal, religious, and social aspects. The four pieces included here are the brief teaser for the series, the first article giving an overview of the topic, an interview with Anthony Comstock, and views from Dr. William Robinson. Other articles in the series explore infant mortality, family planning and poverty, trends in birth rates in America and around the world, perspectives from the Catholic Church, child labor, and views from various doctors.

"The Control of Births" (*Harper's Weekly,* 3 April 1915)

Birth control is one of a number of subjects which are discussed in Europe from the scientific point of view, but which are treated in this country as if mere mention were a crime. Recently "The Call" and "The New Republic" and perhaps other publications have touched upon the subject. We think they have done wisely. Whatever the arguments on both sides, it is only fair that they should be put before the people. It is perfectly well known that the well-to-do classes, who ought to have the most children, do control births, and the poor lack the knowledge to make choice possible. *Harper's Weekly* does not at present express an opinion. The subject is complicated and profound. We shall have for our purpose the presentation of the facts and of opposing arguments. We start with the promise that eugenic subjects in general should be discussed rationally not emotionally. This particular topic touches the family and the nation. A distinguished judge once said to us that, if he were free to enforce or not enforce the laws existing in his district about preventive appliances, he would punish all druggists who sold such appliances within two blocks of Fifth Avenue and encourage those who sold them in the slums. On the other hand, many observers, Colonel Roosevelt for instance, believe that any interference whatever with the size of families is not only wicked, in a sort of abstract way, but definitely harmful to the community and to the family.

The person whom we have selected to open the discussion in *Harper's Weekly* with a series of articles is Mary Alden Hopkins, whose solid and scholarly work is known. She has worked as an employee in commercial laundries, hotels, white goods and other factories and in mercantile establishments. She has done field work for the Consumers League, the National Child Labor Committee, the Massachusetts Minimum Wage Commission and other organizations. Her special interest has been in the poorer classes of women and children. The writings she has already done for *Harper's Weekly* are sufficient to convince us that her presentation of this case will show grasp of the facts and an impartial, scientific spirit.

"The Control of Births" (*Harper's Weekly*, 10 April 1915)

"Is there no way to prevent those who are born into this world from becoming sickly both physically and mentally? It seems almost impossible as long as the riches provided by this world are accessible to a part of the living only. The resources for prevention or cure are inaccessible to many—sometimes even to a majority. *That is why it has become an indispensable suggestion that only a certain number of babies should be born into the world."*

These words were spoken by Dr. Abraham Jacobi, the dean of American physicians, sometimes called "the well-beloved doctor," in his presidential address in 1912 to the American Medical Association.

"As long as not infrequently even the well-to-do limit the number of their off- spring, the advice to the poor—or to those to whom the raising of a large family is more than merely difficult—to limit the number of children, even the healthy ones, is perhaps more than merely excusable."

The experience of a long life, the wisdom of a brilliant mind, the dignity of a high position give weight to the slow and serious words that followed:

"I often hear that an American family has had ten children but only three or four survived. Before the former succumbed, they were a source of expense, poverty and morbidity to the few survivors. *For the interest of the latter and the health of the community at large, they had better not have been born.*"

This public statement, made by the president of the American Medical Association, marks dramatically the change in our attitude toward the question of limiting families. Today men of high standing, scientists of international reputation, physicians, psychologists, political economists, sociologists and literati advocate birth control as a counter-move against poverty and disease. They consider it an effective weapon against infant mortality and prostitution. So wide-spread is interest in the subject that one American scientist receives literally thousands of letters from general practitioners asking for reliable information.

...

The advocates of birth control: in America recommend two measures: first, the repeal or amendment of both the federal and the state laws prohibiting the giving of information concerning family limitation; and, secondly, after their repeal, the dissemination of scientific knowledge.

Our present laws confuse the issue by classing—in a shockingly ignorant fashion—contraception, abortion, and pornography, in the same category. The group is treated in the New York State Penal Code under the astonishing title of "Indecent Articles." The eye of the law distinguishes no difference between the books of August Forel, a scientist revered in laboratories all over the world, and the obscene penny postcard sold by some slinking vendor.

Our federal law forbids the sending by mail or express any formula, method, or suggestion for the prevention of conception. The maximum penalty is five years imprisonment and five thousand dollars fine. Decoy letters, relating piteous stories, stating that the husbands are epileptic or slightly insane and appealing for help are constantly sent to physicians by spies. If the physician gives the information asked, his letter is complete evidence against him in court. One well-known doctor states that he receives such letters by the hundreds every year.

Offenders are sometimes punished with incredible severity, Dr. G. Alfred Elliott, of Kansas, was fined ten thousand dollars and sentenced to ten years in the penitentiary at Leavenworth, for having given this information, without pay, to a woman spy who begged it under false pretenses. He received double the maximum sentence and double the maximum fine because he replied to a second decoy letter following the first from the same woman. Dr. Elliott was released from the penitentiary after serving seven years.

The state codes forbid the giving of this information orally as well as in writing.

A physician is allowed no discretion in the matter. There are cases where pregnancy means almost certain death to the woman. In cases of Bright's disease, tuberculosis, and pelvic malformation, it is fraught with the gravest danger. Yet a doctor telling such a woman how to avoid pregnancy is liable to imprisonment.

The penalties vary in the different states. They usually have a maximum of one year and a thousand dollars. Sometimes it seems as if a judge thought he proved his personal rectitude by being extremely shocked at the offense, yet the more general tendency is toward light sentences. In Portland, Oregon, a judge listened with attention to the defendant's exposition of the principles of birth control, expressed his interest, and said that, in conformity with the law, he would be obliged to impose a fine, but he should make it light. In Chicago, recently, a judge fined a defendant in such a case—one cent.

The European laws on this subject are in striking contrast to ours. They treat contraception and abortion as two separate matters. The laws against abortion are strict. The laws concerning contraception are directed against distasteful advertising but not against private advice or public propaganda. In England the applicant must state in writing over his or her signature that he or she is married or about to be married. In Holland formulas and methods may be supplied privately but must not be publicly advertised. In Germany there is no law on the matter but sentiment is strongly opposed to advertising. In Switzerland it is forbidden to advertise or circularize. In Norway and Sweden advertising is not expected. Italy and France have no law on the subject. In Russia advertising in the newspapers is common. Everywhere in Europe contraceptives are for sale at pharmacies.

In America the friends of the movement suggest different policies. No legislation has yet been attempted. Without doubt during the next few years bills will be introduced into some of the state legislatures. Some people wish simply to repeal the law forbidding the giving of formulas, methods and suggestions of contraception. They believe that the matter will naturally fall into the hands of doctors and pharmacists and further supervision than that furnished in all matters pertaining to health will be unnecessary. Others desire the amendment of the laws in such a manner that information can be given to married people only. Others would have it given to adults and not to minors. Some think it should be given by licensed practitioners in consultation. Others would trust district nurses also. Still others would add hospitals, clinics and dispensaries. One foresees considerable controversy, perhaps not without its instructive value.

The effect of the present laws is deplorable. They silence the scientist but do not shut the mouth of the ignorant midwife. The reputable physician does not like to risk imprisonment; the conscienceless quack will take a chance. Safe, harmless and rational contraceptives exist, and fraudulent devices are covertly advertised and circulated by commercial concerns. The limitation of families is very commonly practiced on a basis of old wives' misinformation.

The distinction between anti-conception and abortion must be held clearly in mind. The newspapers at present contain references to the attempt in European countries to alter or set aside the stringent regulations governing abortions, on account of the wholesale rape which is said to have followed the progress of the huge devastating armies. That is an entirely separate affair. The long-standing controversy as to whether or not abortion is as dangerous has been commonly held, is also the question. The birth control movement is antagonistic to the general practice of abortion. The Hungarian senate, a few years ago, declared that the limitation of families by prevention of conception was absolutely necessary in order to check the wide-spread evil of attempted abortion.

The control of birth is held by its partisans to be the next step in the progress of civilization. Civilization advances just as fast as mankind obtains the mastery over environment. To quote a common illustration, electricity became a servant as soon as its governing laws were discovered. Tribes exist that do not yet know how to use fire. Floods and earthquakes are still our tyrants. Every time we take a force out of the wild domain of nature and place it in the regulated domain of science we have made the world better to live in. It now seems to many people that the time has come to take childbirth out of the realm of chance, that the birth of human beings is too important to be left to irresponsible nature.

The limitationists hold that this change will benefit the individual family and revolutionize industrial conditions. In the family it will lower the rate of infant mortality and increase the health of the mother. A small family of children can have proper food and warm clothing where double the number would suffer from malnutrition and go always ragged. They can have medical attention when sick if clinics and hospitals are not swamped as at present. With small families children may not be forced so soon into the factories, but can remain in school till they get their education. In brief, small families among the very poor will raise the standard of living.

What it may do in the world of industry is indicated by the *geburtstreik* (birth strike) which the more radical element of the Social Democrat Party in

Germany were demanding before the war as a revolutionary weapon against militarism and capitalism. The radical and the conservative branches of the party argued the question vehemently. Whenever "Birth Strike" was the subject announced for a meeting, the hall was jammed with working men and women. They came directly from their work, to get seats, bringing their suppers with them. Women were in the majority.

The argument of the supporters of the movement was that when the proletariat ceased to produce the over-supply of laborers who kept wages down, industrial conditions would improve. The argument of the opponents was that the only hope of the proletariat lay in producing so huge a number that they would overwhelm the ruling class by their immense number of fighters.

It is noteworthy that just at this time Dr. Grotjah, Professor of Hygiene in the University of Berlin, published a book containing all sides of the question and giving specific information concerning the limitation of offspring. That book, written by a scientist of unquestioned standing, can go all over the continent of Europe, but it cannot come into America.

The war is a setback to the birth control movement in Europe. The necessity of rapidly breeding a large number of males to replace those destroyed is recognized by the governments. Women are urged in the name of patriotism to marry hastily soldiers on the eve of departure to the front. A strong sentiment seems to exist, however, that this is not the ideal of marriage and that this is not the fine, high manner of bringing human beings into the world. For the first time in history women dare criticize that model Spartan mother. Thinking women face, with a new awe-struck apprehension, their responsibility for the lives they have bade to be.

"Birth Control and Public Morals: An Interview with Anthony Comstock" (*Harper's Weekly*, 22 May 1915)

"Have read your articles. Self-control and obedience to Nature's laws, you seem to overlook. Let men and women live a life above the level of the beasts. I see nothing in either of your articles along these lines. Existing laws are an imperative necessity in order to prevent the downfall of youths of both sex," wrote Mr. Anthony Comstock, secretary of the New York Society for the Suppression of Vice, replying to my request for an interview on the subject of Birth Control.

During the interview which he kindly allowed me, he reiterated the absolute necessity of drastic laws.

"To repeal the present laws would be a crime against society," he said, "and especially a crime against young women."

Although the name Anthony Comstock is known all over the country and over of the civilized world, comparatively few people know for exactly what Mr. Comstock stands and what he has accomplished. It has been the policy of those who oppose his work to speak flippantly of it and to minimize its results. The Society for the Suppression of Vice was formed to support Mr. Comstock, from the beginning he has been its driving force, and it is giving him only the credit which is due him to say that the tremendous accomplishments of the society in its fight against vicious publications for the last forty years have been in reality the accomplishments of Mr. Comstock.

Up to 1914, Mr. Comstock had caused to be arraigned in state and federal courts 3697 persons, of whom 2740 were either convicted or pleaded guilty. On these were imposed fines to the extent of $237,134.30 and imprisonments to the length of 565 years, 11 months, and 20 days.

To this remarkable record of activity can be added since that date 176 arrests and 141 convictions.

The story of how Mr. Comstock began his unusual profession is as interesting as the story of any of the famous captains of industry. He has, if one may borrow a stage term, "created" his unique position.

"My attention was first drawn to the publication of vile books forty-three years ago when I was a clerk here in New York City," said Mr. Comstock.

"There was in existence at that time a kind of circulating library where my fellow clerks went, made a deposit, and received the vilest of literature, and after reading it, received back the deposit or took other books. 1 saw young men being debauched by this pernicious influence.

"On March 2nd, 1872, I brought about the arrest of seven persons dealing in obscene books, pictures, and articles. found that there were 169 books some of which had been in circulation since before I was born and which were publicly advertised and sold in connection with articles for producing abortion, prevention of conception, articles to aid seductions, and for indiscreet and immoral use. I had four publishers dealing in these arrested and the plates for 167 of these book destroyed. The other two books dropped out of sight. I have not seen a copy of one of them for forty years."

From this time he devoted his attention to this work, although it was, as he once said, like standing at the mouth of a sewer. Several times men whom he has arrested, have later tried to kill him. There were no laws covering this ostracised business at that time. In March, 1873, Mr. Comstock secured the passage of stringent federal laws closing the mails and the ports to this atrocious business. Two days afterwards, upon the request of certain Senators, Mr.

Comstock was appointed Special Agent of the Post Office Department to enforce these laws. He now holds the position of Post Office Inspector. The federal law at present stands is as follows:

United States Criminal Code, Section 211.

(Act of March 4th, 1909, Chapter 321, Section 211, United States Statutes at Large, vol.35, part 1, page 1088 et seq.)

> Every obscene, lewd, or lascivious and every filthy book, pamphlet, picture, paper, letter, writing, print, or other publication of an indecent character, and every article or thing designated, adapted or intended for preventing conception or procuring abortion, or for any indecent or immoral use; and every article, instrument, substance, drugs, medicine, or thing which is advertised or described in a manner calculated to lead another to use or apply it for preventing conception or producing abortion, or for any indecent or immoral purpose; and every written or printed card, circular, book, pamphlet, advertisement or notice or any kind giving information, directly, or indirectly, where or how, or by what means any of the hereinbefore mentioned matters, articles or things may be obtained or made, or where or by whom any act or operation of any kind for the procuring or producing of abortion will be done or performed, or how or by what means conception may be prevented or abortion produced, whether sealed or unsealed; and every letter, packet or package or other mail matter containing any filthy, vile or indecent thing, device or substance; and every paper, writing, advertisement or representation that any article, instrument, substance, drug, medicine or thing may, or can be used or applied for preventing conception or producing abortion, or for any indecent or immoral purpose; and every description calculated to induce or incite a person to so use or apply any such article, instrument, substance, drug, medicine or thing, is hereby declared to be non-mailable matter, and shall not be conveyed in the mails or delivered from any post office or by any letter carrier. Whosoever shall knowingly deposit or cause to be deposited for mailing or delivery, anything declared by this section to be non-mailable, or shall knowingly take, or cause the same to be taken, from the mails for the purpose of circulating or disposing thereof, or of aiding in the circulation or disposition of the same, shall be fined not more than $5000, or imprisoned not more than five years, or both.

Anyone who has the patience to read through this carefully drawn law will see that it covers—well, everything. The detailed accuracy with which it is constructed partly explains Mr. Comstock's almost uniform success in securing convictions. One possible loophole suggested itself to me.

"Does it not," I asked, "allow the judge considerable leeway in deciding whether or not a book or a picture, is immoral?"

"No," replied Mr. Comstock, "the highest courts in Great Britain and the United States, have laid down the test in all such matters. What he has to decide is *whether or not in might arouse in young and inexperienced minds, lewd or libidinous thoughts.*"

In these words lies the motive of Mr. Comstock's work—the protection of children under twenty-one. If at times his ban seems to some to be too sweepingly applied it is because his faith looks forward to a time when there shall be in all the world not one object to awaken sensuous thoughts in the minds of young people. He expressed this sense of the terrible danger in which young people stand and his society's duty toward them in his fortieth annual report:

> …we first of all return thanks to Almighty God, the giver of every good and perfect gift, for the opportunities of service for Him in defense of the morals of the more than forty-two million youths and children twenty-one years of age, or under, in the United States of America. His blessings upon our efforts during the past year call for profound thanksgiving to Almighty God and for grateful and loyal service in the future. This Society in a peculiar manner is permitted to stand at a vital and strategic point where the foes to moral purity seek to concentrate their most deadly forces against the integrity of the rising generation. We have been assigned by the Great Commander to constantly face some of the most insidious and deadly forces for evil that Satan is persistently aligning against the integrity of the children of the present age.

And in a letter read at the fortieth anniversary he expresses himself thus:

There are three points of special importance to be emphasized:

1. Every child is a character-builder.
2. In the heart of every child there is a chamber of imagery, memory's storehouse, the commissary department in which is received, stored up and held in reserve every good or evil influence for future requisition.
3. "Be not deceived, God is not mocked. For whatsoever a man soweth that he shall also reap." "Keep thy heart with all diligence, for out of it are the issues of life."

> The three great crime-breeders of today are intemperance, gambling, and evil reading. The devil is sowing his seed for his future harvest. There is no foe so much to be dreaded as that which perverts the imagination, sears the conscience, hardens the heart, and damns the soul.
>
> If you allow the devil to decorate the Chamber of Imagery in your heart with licentious and sensual things, you will find that he has practically thrown a noose about your neck and will forever after exert himself to draw you away

from the "Lamb of God which taketh away sins of the world." You have practically put rope on memory's bell and placed the other end of the rope in the devil's hands, and, though you may will out your mind, the memory of some vile story or picture that you may have looked upon, be assured that even in your most solitary moments the devil will ring memory's bell and call up the hateful thing to turn your thoughts away from God and undermine all aspirations for holy things.

Let me emphasize one fact, supported by my nearly forty-two years of public life in fighting this particular foe. My experience leads me to the conviction that once these matters enter through the eye and ear into the chamber of imagery in the heart of the child, nothing but the grace of God can ever erase or blot it out. Finally, brethren, "let us not be weary in well doing, for in due season we shall reap if we faint not." Raise over each of your heads the banner of the Lord Jesus Christ. Look to Him as your Commander and Leader.

I was somewhat confused at first that Mr. Comstock should class contraceptives with pornographic objects which debauch children's fancies, for I knew that the European scientists who advocate their use have no desire at all to debauch children. When I asked Mr. Comstock about this, he replied—with scant patience of "theorizers'" who do not know human nature:

"If you open the door to anything, the filth will all pour in and the degradation of youth will follow."

The federal law, which we have quoted, covers only matter sent by post. This would leave large unguarded fields were it not for the state laws. The year following the passage of the federal law, Mr. Comstock obtained the passage of drastic laws in several states, and later in all states. The New York state law reads as follows:

Section 1142 of the Penal Law:

A person who sells, lends, gives away, or in any manner exhibits or offers to sell, lend or give away, or has in his possession with intent to sell, lend or give away, or advertises, or offers for sale, loan or distribution, any instrument or article, or any recipe, drug or medicine for the prevention of conception or for causing unlawful abortion, or purporting to be for the prevention of conception, or for causing unlawful abortion, or advertises, or holds out representations that it can be so used or applied, or any such description as will be calculated to lead another to so use or apply any such article, recipe, drug, medicine or instrument, or who writes or prints, or causes to be written or printed a card, circular, pamphlet, advertisement or notice of any kind, or gives information orally, stating when, where, how, of whom, or by what means such an instrument, article, recipe, drug or medicine can be purchased or obtained, or who manufactures any such instrument, article recipe, drug or medicine, is guilty of a misdemeanor, and shall be liable to the same penalties as provided in section eleven hundred and forty-one of this chapter.

This punishment is a sentence of not less than ten days nor more than one year's imprisonment or a fine not less than fifty dollars or both fine and imprisonment for each offense.

"Do not these laws handicap physicians?" I asked, remembering that this criticism is sometimes made.

"They do not," replied Mr. Comstock emphatically. "No reputable physician has ever been prosecuted under these laws. Have you ever known of one?" I had not, and he continued, "Only infamous doctors who advertise or send their foul matter by mail. A reputable doctor may tell his patient in his office what is necessary, and a druggist may sell on a doctor's written prescription drugs which he would not be allowed to sell otherwise."

This criticism of the laws interfering with doctors is so continuously made that I asked again:

"Do the laws never thwart the doctor's work; in cases, for instance, where pregnancy would endanger a woman's life?"

Mr. Comstock replied with the strongest emphasis:

"A doctor is allowed to bring on an abortion in cases where a woman's life is in danger. And is there anything in these laws that forbids a doctor's telling a woman that pregnancy must not occur for a certain length of time or at all? Can they not use self-control? Or must they sink to the level of the beasts?"

"But," I protested, repeating an argument often brought forward, although I felt as if my persistence was somewhat placing me in the ranks of those who desire evil rather than good, "If the parents lack that self-control, the punishment falls upon the child."

"It does not," replied Mr. Comstock. "The punishment falls upon the parents. When a man and woman marry they are responsible for their children. You can't reform a family in any of these superficial ways. You have to go deep down into their minds and souls. The prevention of conception would work the greatest demoralization. God has set certain natural barriers. If you turn loose the passions and break down the fear you bring worse disaster than the war. It would debase sacred things, break down the health of women and disseminate a greater curse than the plagues and diseases of Europe."

"Is Contraception Immoral?" (*Harper's Weekly*, 19 June 1915)

In the seventeenth century the intellectual battles of the world raged about religion. Men and women who tried to change the accepted ideals were considered the enemies of society. To persecute and kill them was a holy work to the glory of God and the good of mankind.

During the closing years of the nineteenth century and the present years of the twentieth century the intellectual battles of the world rage about sex. Although our breadth of outlook has somewhat widened, we still suspect men and women who are trying to change the sex ideals of being dangerous persons. Although state killing has gone out of fashion except for murderers, we still have imprisonment for those whose views differ from ours, suppression of publications, and that most subtle of all persecutions, slander and calumny.

We put our fingers in our ears when we first heard demands for sex instruction; we felt that the sterilization of insane criminals wasn't proper; we were afraid that the successful treatment of venereal diseases would increase "immorality." Now we are almost hysterically nervous lest contraception be brought out from that black ignorance which covers most sexual matters. Some of us say emphatically that if men and women knew how to prevent conception by any means except the abrogation of sex life, then the unmarried would abandon chastity, the married would cease to have children, and humanity would descend to the level of beasts.

It seems only fair to hear what the regulationists have to say about personal morality under the limitation of offspring system which they advocate. Morality is the spiritual and physical well-being of the individual and the community. If contraception advances well-being it is good; if it lessens well-being it is bad. Mr. Comstock, in a previous article, voiced the emotions of those who believe that contraception is an immoral action. I have asked Dr. Robinson to explain why the regulationists hold that it is a moral action.

Everyone who reads these articles knows the name of Anthony Comstock. Not so many have heard of Dr. Robinson. He is, perhaps, more honored and quoted abroad than in his own country. It is only within recent years that our prudery has forgiven him for having specialized in the field of sexual diseases and for holding ideas in advance of general opinion. For twenty years he has preached, "Fewer and Better Babies." One may judge from his list of offices and titles, how much. or, how little weight to place, upon his words: President of the American Society of Medical Sociology, President of the Northern Medical Society, Ex-president of the Berlin Anglo-American Medical Society,

Fellow of the New York Academy of Medicine, Member of American Medical Editors' Association, American Medical Association, New York State Medical. Society, Medical Society of the County of New York, American Urological Association, etc. He is editor of *The American Journal of Urology, Venereal and Sexual Diseases*, editor of *The Critic and Guide* and the author of many medical books. Some of his views I quote from his recent volume *The Limitation of Offspring* and some he has told me himself.

"The chief thing that distinguishes the human being from other animals is his intellect," says Dr. Robinson. "It is by the aid of the intellect alone that we have been fighting and conquering Nature, wresting from her and unraveling her secrets, balking her at every step when it becomes necessary for our welfare. The human intellect has given us remedies which, while permitting men and women to marry at the proper age and to live a normal sex life as Nature intended, still help them to control the number of their children. And try as I may, I cannot see what there is wrong in people who cannot afford to have many children using means which will prevent them from having many, which will help them to have just as many as they wish to have and can afford to have, and just at such times as they wish to have them."

"The limitation of children to the number who can be supported is the sign of a high morality," Dr. Robinson holds, and his following remarks may be taken as his reply to the beasts-of-the-field argument. "The animals and the people nearest them have no such responsibility; they breed unrestrictedly, leaving nature or God to take care of their off-spring or to kill it off as they may see fit. But thinking parents from their sense of responsibility refuse to bring into the world too large a number."

Dr Robinson does not look upon an undesired child as the just punishment dealt out to parents who will not live celibate lives in marriage. He considers children too valuable to be wasted on the discipline of parents. Besides, Dr. Robinson is not enthusiastically in favor of sexless marriages. He thinks they are not healthful.

When Dr. Robinson talks he never uses the word "sin" or "vile" or any other of those accusing terms with which we so often discuss sex. He employs clean definite medical terms that indicate exactly the thought behind. Indeed I doubt if he recognizes the essential sinfulness of man. Phenomena is divided for him into what is healthy and sane and what is mentally aberrant and physically sick. His problem is to restore to the normal the deviations which he meets. He is perhaps a subtler diagnostician of sexual warping than persons more seriously shocked by its existence. His attitude of the curer rather than the avenger, comes out most clearly in his reply to the accusation that a knowledge of contraception will break down the chastity of unmarried women.

In the vast majority of cases, he thinks, a girl's chastity is not determined by her fear of pregnancy. It is the result of her general bringing up, her general and religious education, the custom of the country, hereditary influence, and the general monogamous tendency of the female. The fear of consequences can be removed without being followed by a general breakdown of virtue. This may seem too optimistic to some people, Of the smaller number whose conduct would be altered he speaks thus:

"And if some women are bound to have illicit relations, is it not better that they should know the use of a harmless preventative than that they should become pregnant, disgracing and ostracizing themselves, and their families, or that they should subject themselves to the degradation and risks of an abortion, or failing this take carbolic acid or bichloride, jump into the river or throw themselves under the wheels of a running train? I may be wrong, my views may be strabismic, but I cannot help believing that I am kinder and humaner than those cruel bigots who demand that any woman who has indulged in illicit relations should expiate her "crime" by death or by all the humiliation, ostracism and suffering which are now imposed upon the mother of an illegitimate child."

Like all regulationists Dr. Robinson makes a clear distinction between contraception and abortion. In the twenty years of his practice he has never deviated. One child whom he calls Beatrice, twenty years old, came to Dr, Robinson when she was pregnant, without the slightest doubt that he would help her.

"She knew me and knew that I was kind, and she hoped that I would help her out of her misery," Dr. Robinson tells her story. "But she did not know how cruel the kind can sometimes be, how selfish the good often are. When I as gently as I could, but none the less positively, refused her, I saw that had I hit her on the head with a sledge-hammer I could not have hurt her more. She looked stunned. She did not say much. She did not make any threats of suicide, she gave me one reproachful look with her tear-filled eyes and left.

"And the next morning they carried her mangled little body from under the elevated train into the hospital. She gave my name and wanted to see me. It was hard for me to go and see her, but I could not refuse her dying wish, and came. She had sustained severe internal injuries, and one could see that she had but a few hours to live. But she was fully conscious. She asked me to hold her hand, And then she said, 'Forgive me. Good-bye.' And I went. But were I to live a hundred years more, I should not forget her liquid, veiled eyes. I see them now, just as if she stood before me."

In the name of all the unhappy pregnant women who have left his office with their last hope destroyed, who have gone out to violent death, who have drowned themselves in the river, hanged themselves, drunk carbolic acid, paris green, corrosive sublimate, or heads of matches soaked in water—in the name of these many women, he begs that the knowledge of contraception be no longer withheld. Dr. Robinson does not believe that the well-being of the community rests upon the humiliation of Beatrice.

After twenty years of practice, chiefly in venereal diseases and sexual disorders, he firmly believes in the goodness of human nature. He is familiar with the diseases that follow debauchery, and the sexual deviations that accompany a starved emotional life. He has seen mothers despair that their children are born and men weep that they can have no offspring. He has found men and women wantonly spreading horrible infection. He knows the untold stories that lie behind the suicide headlines in the morning paper. Yet through twenty years of close companionship with suffering, misery and death, he has seen also joy and health. Those whom others would call wicked he sees as crippled souls struggling toward happiness.

Over and over he reiterates that it is not through fear of consequences that we are decent; that those who lead rational lives do so because they want to and not because they are afraid. This same statement he applies to the protest that the use of contraceptives will lead to excesses in married life.

"And then," he adds, "we must not forget that there is no royal short road to prevention. Every efficient method demands a little care, a little trouble, a little expense. And this alone will act as a check."

It is perhaps natural that a man with so sturdy a faith in the fathers and mothers of the race should resent the charge that they would not have any children if they knew how to help it. He thinks it absurd to argue that if a man doesn't want ten children he doesn't want five or that a woman who balks at her eighth pregnancy would balk at her third. He finds in his practice that they are as set on having the first half of the family as they are opposed to the second half. Childless men and women are willing to undergo the most tedious treatment to become able to have children. "When I see to what interminable trouble and expense some men and women go in order to have children: when I see what tortures and risks, endangering her very life—a prospective mother will undergo in order to have a living child, I have no fear that the use of preventatives will result in the dying out of the human race."

Summer by Edith Wharton (1917)

Introduction

In this novel, Edith Wharton presents the story of Charity Royall a young women living in a small New England town after she was adopted by the town lawyer Mr. Royall from an impoverished community on the local mountain. Charity meets and falls in love with Lucius Harney, with whom she becomes pregnant. When she learns that Harney is engaged to Annabel Balch, Charity debates how to handle the pregnancy, considering a quick marriage to someone to cover the pregnancy, terminating the pregnancy with local abortionist Dr. Merkle, or returning up the mountain away from the town's society to have her child.

Excerpt from Chapter VII

She continued to crouch on the steps, holding her breath and stiffening herself into complete immobility. One motion of her hand, one tap on the pane, and she could picture the sudden change in his face. In every pulse of her rigid body she was aware of the welcome his eyes and lips would give her; but something kept her from moving. It was not the fear of any sanction, human or heavenly; she had never in her life been afraid. It was simply that she had suddenly understood what would happen if she went in. It was the thing that did happen between young men and girls, and that North Dormer ignored in public and snickered over on the sly. It was what Miss Hatchard was still ignorant of, but every girl of Charity's class knew about before she left school. It was what had happened to Ally Hawes's sister Julia, and had ended in her going to Nettleton, and in people's never mentioning her name.

It did not, of course, always end so sensationally; nor, perhaps, on the whole, so untragically. Charity had always suspected that the shunned Julia's fate might have its compensations. There were others, worse endings that the village knew of, mean, miserable, unconfessed; other lives that went on drearily, without visible change, in the same cramped setting of hypocrisy. But these were not the reasons that held her back. Since the day before, she had known exactly what she would feel if Harney should take her in his arms: the melting of palm into palm and mouth on mouth, and the long flame burning her from head to foot. But mixed with this feeling was another: the wondering pride in his liking for her, the startled softness that his sympathy had put into her heart. Sometimes, when her youth flushed up in her, she had imagined yielding like other girls to furtive caresses in the twilight; but she could not so cheapen herself to Harney. She did not know why he was going; but since he was going she felt she must do nothing to deface the image of her that he carried away. If he wanted her he must seek her: he must not be surprised into taking her as girls like Julia Hawes were taken…

Excerpt from Chapter IX

"Don't you ever feel like going down to Nettleton for a day?" she asked.

Ally shook her head without looking up. "No, I always remember that awful time I went down with Julia—to that doctor's."

"Oh, Ally——"

"I can't help it. The house is on the corner of Wing Street and Lake Avenue. The trolley from the station goes right by it, and the day the minister took us down to see those pictures I recognized it right off, and couldn't seem to see anything else. There's a big black sign with gold letters all across the front—'Private Consultations.' She came as near as anything to dying…"

"Poor Julia!" Charity sighed from the height of her purity and her security. She had a friend whom she trusted and who respected her. She was going with him to spend the next day—the Fourth of July—at Nettleton. Whose business was it but hers, and what was the harm? The pity of it was that girls like Julia did not know how to choose, and to keep bad fellows at a distance…. Charity slipped down from the bed, and stretched out her hands.

"Is it sewed? Let me try it on again." She put the hat on, and smiled at her image. The thought of Julia had vanished…

…

Charity looked up and saw on the corner a brick house with a conspicuous black and gold sign across its front. "Dr. Merkle; Private Consultations at all hours. Lady Attendants," she read; and suddenly she remembered Ally Hawes's words: "The house was at the corner of Wing Street and Lake Avenue… there's a big black sign across the front…" Through all the heat and the rapture a shiver of cold ran over her.

Excerpts from Chapter XV

She took a sheet of letter paper from Mr. Royall's office, and sitting by the kitchen lamp, one night after Verena had gone to bed, began her first letter to Harney. It was very short:

I want you should marry Annabel Balch if you promised to. I think maybe you were afraid I'd feel too bad about it. I feel I'd rather you acted right. Your loving CHARITY.

She posted the letter early the next morning, and for a few days her heart felt strangely light. Then she began to wonder why she received no answer.

One day as she sat alone in the library pondering these things the walls of books began to spin around her, and the rosewood desk to rock under her elbows. The dizziness was followed by a wave of nausea like that she had felt on the day of the exercises in the Town Hall. But the Town Hall had been crowded and stiflingly hot, and the library was empty, and so chilly that she had kept on her jacket. Five minutes before she had felt perfectly well; and now it seemed as if she were going to die. The bit of lace at which she still languidly worked dropped from her fingers, and the steel crochet hook clattered to the floor. She pressed her temples hard between her damp hands, steadying herself against the desk while the wave of sickness swept over her. Little by little it subsided, and after a few minutes she stood up, shaken and terrified, groped for her hat, and stumbled out into the air. But the whole sunlit autumn whirled, reeled and roared around her as she dragged herself along the interminable length of the road home.

...

Two days later, she descended from the train at Nettleton, and walked out of the station into the dusty square. The brief interval of cold weather was over, and the day was as soft, and almost as hot, as when she and Harney had emerged on the same scene on the Fourth of July. In the square the same broken-down hacks and carry-alls stood drawn up in a despondent line, and the lank horses with fly-nets over their withers swayed their heads drearily to and fro. She recognized the staring signs over the eating-houses and billiard saloons, and the long lines of wires on lofty poles tapering down the main street to the park at its other end. Taking the way the wires pointed, she went on hastily, with bent head, till she reached a wide transverse street with a brick building at the corner. She crossed this street and glanced furtively up at the front of the brick building; then she returned, and entered a door opening on a flight of steep brass-rimmed stairs. On the second landing she rang a bell, and a mulatto girl with a bushy head and a frilled apron let her into a hall where a stuffed fox on his hind legs proffered a brass card-tray to visitors. At the back of the hall was a glazed door marked: "Office." After waiting a few minutes in a handsomely furnished room, with plush sofas surmounted by large gold-framed photographs of showy young women, Charity was shown into the office...

When she came out of the glazed door Dr. Merkle followed, and led her into another room, smaller, and still more crowded with plush and gold frames. Dr. Merkle was a plump woman with small bright eyes, an immense mass of black hair coming down low on her forehead, and unnaturally white and even teeth. She wore a rich black dress, with gold chains and charms hanging from her bosom. Her hands were large and smooth, and quick in all their movements; and she smelt of musk and carbolic acid.

She smiled on Charity with all her faultless teeth. "Sit down, my dear. Wouldn't you like a little drop of something to pick you up?... No.... Well, just lay back a minute then.... There's nothing to be done just yet; but in about a month, if you'll step round again... I could take you right into my own house for two or three days, and there wouldn't be a mite of trouble. Mercy me! The next time you'll know better'n to fret like this..."

Charity gazed at her with widening eyes. This woman with the false hair, the false teeth, the false murderous smile—what was she offering her but immunity from some unthinkable crime? Charity, till then, had been conscious only of a vague self-disgust and a frightening physical distress; now, of a sudden, there came to her the grave surprise of motherhood. She had come to this dreadful place because she knew of no other way of making sure that she was not mistaken about her state; and the woman had taken her for a miserable creature like Julia.... The thought was so horrible that she sprang up, white and shaking, one of her great rushes of anger sweeping over her.

Dr. Merkle, still smiling, also rose. "Why do you run off in such a hurry? You can stretch out right here on my sofa..." She paused, and her smile grew more motherly. "Afterwards—if there's been any talk at home, and you want to get away for a while... I have a lady friend in Boston who's looking for a companion... you're the very one to suit her, my dear..."

Charity had reached the door. "I don't want to stay. I don't want to come back here," she stammered, her hand on the knob; but with a swift movement, Dr. Merkle edged her from the threshold.

"Oh, very well. Five dollars, please."

Charity looked helplessly at the doctor's tight lips and rigid face. Her last savings had gone in repaying Ally for the cost of Miss Balch's ruined blouse, and she had had to borrow four dollars from her friend to pay for her railway ticket and cover the doctor's fee. It had never occurred to her that medical advice could cost more than two dollars.

"I didn't know... I haven't got that much..." she faltered, bursting into tears.

Dr. Merkle gave a short laugh which did not show her teeth, and inquired with concision if Charity supposed she ran the establishment for her own amusement? She leaned her firm shoulders against the door as she spoke, like a grim gaoler making terms with her captive.

"You say you'll come round and settle later? I've heard that pretty often too. Give me your address, and if you can't pay me I'll send the bill to your folks… What? I can't understand what you say…. That don't suit you either? My, you're pretty particular for a girl that ain't got enough to settle her own bills…" She paused, and fixed her eyes on the brooch with a blue stone that Charity had pinned to her blouse.

"Ain't you ashamed to talk that way to a lady that's got to earn her living, when you go about with jewellery like that on you?… It ain't in my line, and I do it only as a favour… but if you're a mind to leave that brooch as a pledge, I don't say no…. Yes, of course, you can get it back when you bring me my money…"

On the way home, she felt an immense and unexpected quietude. It had been horrible to have to leave Harney's gift in the woman's hands, but even at that price the news she brought away had not been too dearly bought. She sat with half-closed eyes as the train rushed through the familiar landscape; and now the memories of her former journey, instead of flying before her like dead leaves, seemed to be ripening in her blood like sleeping grain. She would never again know what it was to feel herself alone. Everything seemed to have grown suddenly clear and simple. She no longer had any difficulty in picturing herself as Harney's wife now that she was the mother of his child; and compared to her sovereign right Annabel Balch's claim seemed no more than a girl's sentimental fancy.

…

Face to face with his admission of the fact, she sat staring at the letter. A cold tremor ran over her, and the hard sobs struggled up into her throat and shook her from head to foot. For a while she was caught and tossed on great waves of anguish that left her hardly conscious of anything but the blind struggle against their assaults. Then, little by little, she began to relive, with a dreadful poignancy, each separate stage of her poor romance. Foolish things she had said came back to her, gay answers Harney had made, his first kiss in the darkness between the fireworks, their choosing the blue brooch together, the way he had teased her about the letters she had dropped in her flight from the evangelist. All these memories, and a thousand others, hummed through her brain till his nearness grew so vivid that she felt his fingers in her hair, and his warm breath on her cheek as he bent her head back like a flower. These things were hers; they had passed into her blood, and become a part of her, they were building the child in her womb; it was impossible to tear asunder strands of life so interwoven.

…

Harney had written that she had made it easier for him, and she was glad it was so; she did not want to make things hard. She knew she had it in her power to do that; she held his fate in her hands. All she had to do was to tell him the truth; but that was the very fact that held her back.... Distinctly and pitilessly there rose before her the fate of the girl who was married "to make things right." She had seen too many village love-stories end in that way. Poor Rose Coles's miserable marriage was of the number; and what good had come of it for her or for Halston Skeff? They had hated each other from the day the minister married them; and whenever old Mrs. Skeff had a fancy to humiliate her daughter-in-law she had only to say: "Who'd ever think the baby's only two? And for a seven months' child—ain't it a wonder what a size he is?" North Dormer had treasures of indulgence for brands in the burning, but only derision for those who succeeded in getting snatched from it; and Charity had always understood Julia Hawes's refusal to be snatched...

Only—was there no alternative but Julia's? Her soul recoiled from the vision of the white-faced woman among the plush sofas and gilt frames. In the established order of things as she knew them she saw no place for her individual adventure...

She sat in her chair without undressing till faint grey streaks began to divide the black slats of the shutters. Then she stood up and pushed them open, letting in the light. The coming of a new day brought a sharper consciousness of ineluctable reality, and with it a sense of the need of action. She looked at herself in the glass, and saw her face, white in the autumn dawn, with pinched cheeks and dark-ringed eyes, and all the marks of her state that she herself would never have noticed, but that Dr. Merkle's diagnosis had made plain to her. She could not hope that those signs would escape the watchful village; even before her figure lost its shape she knew her face would betray her.

Excerpt from Chapter XVII

What mother would not want to save her child from such a life? Charity thought of the future of her own child, and tears welled into her aching eyes, and ran down over her face. If she had been less exhausted, less burdened with his weight, she would have sprung up then and there and fled away...

The grim hours of the night dragged themselves slowly by, and at last the sky paled and dawn threw a cold blue beam into the room. She lay in her corner staring at the dirty floor, the clothes-line hung with decaying rags, the old woman huddled against the cold stove, and the light gradually spreading across the wintry world, and bringing with it a new day in which she would have to live, to choose, to act, to make herself a place among these people—or to go back to the life she had left. A mortal lassitude weighed on her. There were moments when she felt that all she asked was to go on lying there unnoticed; then her mind revolted at the thought of becoming one of the miserable herd from which she sprang, and it seemed as though, to save her child from such a fate, she would find strength to travel any distance, and bear any burden life might put on her.

Vague thoughts of Nettleton flitted through her mind. She said to herself that she would find some quiet place where she could bear her child, and give it to decent people to keep; and then she would go out like Julia Hawes and earn its living and hers. She knew that girls of that kind sometimes made enough to have their children nicely cared for; and every other consideration disappeared in the vision of her baby, cleaned and combed and rosy, and hidden away somewhere where she could run in and kiss it, and bring it pretty things to wear. Anything, anything was better than to add another life to the nest of misery on the Mountain…

Excerpt from Chapter XVIII

A few minutes later Charity went out, too. She had watched to see in what direction he was going, and she took the opposite way and walked quickly down the main street to the brick building on the corner of Lake Avenue. There she paused to look cautiously up and down the thoroughfare, and then climbed the brass-bound stairs to Dr. Merkle's door. The same bushy-headed mulatto girl admitted her, and after the same interval of waiting in the red plush parlor she was once more summoned to Dr. Merkle's office. The doctor received her without surprise, and led her into the inner plush sanctuary.

"I thought you'd be back, but you've come a mite too soon: I told you to be patient and not fret," she observed, after a pause of penetrating scrutiny.

Charity drew the money from her breast. "I've come to get my blue brooch," she said, flushing.

"Your brooch?" Dr. Merkle appeared not to remember. "My, yes—I get so many things of that kind. Well, my dear, you'll have to wait while I get it out of the safe. I don't leave valuables like that laying round like the noospaper."

She disappeared for a moment, and returned with a bit of twisted-up tissue paper from which she unwrapped the brooch.

Charity, as she looked at it, felt a stir of warmth at her heart. She held out an eager hand.

"Have you got the change?" she asked a little breathlessly, laying one of the twenty-dollar bills on the table.

"Change? What'd I want to have change for? I only see two twenties there," Dr. Merkle answered brightly.

Charity paused, disconcerted. "I thought… you said it was five dollars a visit…"

"For YOU, as a favour—I did. But how about the responsibility and the insurance? I don't s'pose you ever thought of that? This pin's worth a hundred dollars easy. If it had got lost or stole, where'd I been when you come to claim it?"

Charity remained silent, puzzled and half-convinced by the argument, and Dr. Merkle promptly followed up her advantage. "I didn't ask you for your brooch, my dear. I'd a good deal ruther folks paid me my regular charge than have 'em put me to all this trouble."

She paused, and Charity, seized with a desperate longing to escape, rose to her feet and held out one of the bills.

"Will you take that?" she asked.

"No, I won't take that, my dear; but I'll take it with its mate, and hand you over a signed receipt if you don't trust me."

"Oh, but I can't—it's all I've got," Charity exclaimed.

Dr. Merkle looked up at her pleasantly from the plush sofa. "It seems you got married yesterday, up to the 'Piscopal church; I heard all about the wedding from the minister's chore-man. It would be a pity, wouldn't it, to let Mr. Royall know you had an account running here? I just put it to you as your own mother might."

Anger flamed up in Charity, and for an instant she thought of abandoning the brooch and letting Dr. Merkle do her worst. But how could she leave her only treasure with that evil woman? She wanted it for her baby: she meant it, in some mysterious way, to be a link between Harney's child and its unknown father. Trembling and hating herself while she did it, she laid Mr. Royall's money on the table, and catching up the brooch fled out of the room and the house…

In the street she stood still, dazed by this last adventure. But the brooch lay in her bosom like a talisman, and she felt a secret lightness of heart. It gave her strength, after a moment, to walk on slowly in the direction of the post office, and go in through the swinging doors. At one of the windows she bought a sheet of letter-paper, an envelope and a stamp; then she sat down at a table and dipped the rusty post office pen in ink. She had come there possessed with a fear which had haunted her ever since she had felt Mr. Royall's ring on her finger: the fear that Harney might, after all, free himself and come back to her. It was a possibility which had never occurred to her during the dreadful hours after she had received his letter; only when the decisive step she had taken made longing turn to apprehension did such a contingency seem conceivable. She addressed the envelope, and on the sheet of paper she wrote:

I'm married to Mr. Royall. I'll always remember you. CHARITY.

The last words were not in the least what she had meant to write; they had flowed from her pen irresistibly. She had not had the strength to complete her sacrifice; but, after all, what did it matter? Now that there was no chance of ever seeing Harney again, why should she not tell him the truth?

The Crisis: A Record of the Darker Races (October 1922)

Introduction

This issue of *The Crisis*, a monthly periodical edited by W. E. B. DuBois, focused on children and includes two pieces on fertility control. First in one section of his opening editorial, DuBois discusses the value of birth control as it pertains to the Black community, focusing on infant mortality and the health of women. Then, in a two-stanza poem by Georgia Douglas Johnson, the speaker directly addresses the children she refuses to have about the cruel world from which she is protecting them.

Excerpt from "Opinion" by W. E. B. DuBois, Birth

Yesterday I saw a young man and woman and their three children. And I was told: Four of their children are dead. I said: "That is a crime! It is not simply a misfortune—it is a deliberate crime which deserves condign punishment." No woman can bear seven children in ten years and preserve her own health and theirs. No man who asks or permits this deserves to be a husband or father.

Birth control is science and sense applied to the bringing of children into the world, and of all who need it we Negroes are first. We in America are becoming sharply divided into the mass who have endless children and the class who through long postponement of marriage have few or none. The first result is a terrible infant mortality: of every 10,000 colored children born 1,356 die in the first year, while only 821 die among whites. The second result is the senseless putting off of marriage until middle life because of the fear that marriage must necessarily mean many children.

Parents owe their children, first of all, health and strength. Few women can bear more than two or three children and retain strength for the other interests of life. And there are other interests for women as for men and only reactionary barbarians deny this. Even this small number of children should come into the world at intervals which will allow for the physical, economic and spiritual recovery of the parents. Housework is still a desperately hard and exacting occupation. It can and should be simplified and lightened by the laundry, the bakery, the restaurant, and the vacuum cleaner; but with all that it remains a job calling for strength, time and training. Social intercourse, which is largely in the hands of wives, is a matter of thought, effort and delicate adjustment. The education of children in the home calls for intelligence, study and leisure. To add to all this the physical pain and strain of child birth is to give a woman as much as she can possibly endure once in three, four or five years.

"Motherhood" by Georgia Douglas Johnson

> Don't knock on my door, little child,
> I cannot let you in;
> You know not what a world this is,
> Of cruelty and sin.
> Wait in the still eternity
> Until I come to you.
> The world is cruel, cruel, child,
> I cannot let you through.
>
> Don't knock at my heart, little one,
> I cannot bear the pain
> Of turning deaf ears to your call,
> Time and time again.
> You do not know the monster men
> Inhabiting the earth.
> Be still, be still, my precious child,
> I cannot give you birth.

The Beautiful and the Damned by F. Scott Fitzgerald (1922)

Introduction

This novel presents the story of a flapper couple, Anthony and Gloria, who plan to have their first child on their third anniversary, suggesting that they are employing some form of birth control. However, Gloria appears to be pregnant just a year into marriage, which leads to the discussion between the couple in the excerpt provided here. The text never explicitly says abortion, so as their conversation progresses, both character vaguely say "it" which could refer to a baby or an abortion. Interestingly the character Anthony's full name is Anthony Comstock Patch, which his grandfather chose in admiration for the namesake of the Comstock Act that banned distribution of any texts about vice. The real-life Comstock is referenced in other texts in this chapter, including on Madame Restell's arrest and an interview in the *Harper's Weekly* series on birth control.

Book II, Chapter II, Nietzschean Incident

Gloria's independence, like all sincere and profound qualities, had begun unconsciously, but, once brought to her attention by Anthony's fascinated discovery of it, it assumed more nearly the proportions of a formal code. From her conversation it might be assumed that all her energy and vitality went into a violent affirmation of the negative principle "Never give a damn."

"Not for anything or anybody," she said, "except myself and, by implication, for Anthony. That's the rule of all life and if it weren't I'd be that way anyhow. Nobody'd do anything for me if it didn't gratify them to, and I'd do as little for them."

She was on the front porch of the nicest lady in Marietta when she said this, and as she finished she gave a curious little cry and sank in a dead faint to the porch floor.

The lady brought her to and drove her home in her car. It had occurred to the estimable Gloria that she was probably with child.

She lay upon the long lounge down-stairs. Day was slipping warmly out the window, touching the late roses on the porch pillars.

"All I think of ever is that I love you," she wailed. "I value my body because you think it's beautiful. And this body of mine—of yours—to have it grow ugly and shapeless? It's simply intolerable. Oh, Anthony, I'm not afraid of the pain."

He consoled her desperately—but in vain. She continued:

"And then afterward I might have wide hips and be pale, with all my freshness gone and no radiance in my hair."

He paced the floor with his hands in his pockets, asking:

"Is it certain?"

"I don't know anything. I've always hated obstetrics, or whatever you call them. I thought I'd have a child some time. But not now."

"Well, for God's sake don't lie there and go to pieces."

Her sobs lapsed. She drew down a merciful silence from the twilight which filled the room. "Turn on the lights," she pleaded. "These days seem so short—June seemed—to—have—longer days when I was a little girl."

The lights snapped on and it was as though blue drapes of softest silk had been dropped behind the windows and the door. Her pallor, her immobility, without grief now, or joy, awoke his sympathy.

"Do you want me to have it?" she asked listlessly.

"I'm indifferent. That is, I'm neutral. If you have it I'll probably be glad. If you don't—well, that's all right too."

"I wish you'd make up your mind one way or the other!"

"Suppose you make up *your* mind."

She looked at him contemptuously, scorning to answer.

"You'd think you'd been singled out of all the women in the world for this crowning indignity."

"What if I do!" she cried angrily. "It isn't an indignity for them. It's their one excuse for living. It's the one thing they're good for. It *is* an indignity for *me*."

"See here, Gloria, I'm with you whatever you do, but for God's sake be a sport about it."

"Oh, don't *fuss* at me!" she wailed.

They exchanged a mute look of no particular significance but of much stress. Then Anthony took a book from the shelf and dropped into a chair.

Half an hour later her voice came out of the intense stillness that pervaded the room and hung like incense on the air.

"I'll drive over and see Constance Merriam to-morrow."

"All right. And I'll go to Tarrytown and see Grampa."

"—You see," she added, "it isn't that I'm afraid—of this or anything else. I'm being true to me, you know."

"I know," he agreed.

"Mr. Durant" by Dorothy Parker (1924)

Introduction

In this short story by Dorothy Parker, a married businessman's affair with a younger secretary in his office results in an unwanted pregnancy. The responses of the titular character to his mistress Rose's pregnancy, a woman on the bus, and a stray dog at home with his family reveal his views on women. "Mr. Durant" was originally published in first year of *The American Mercury*, which featured work from some of the most famous writers in its early years.

"Mr. Durant" (*The American Mercury*, September 1924)

Not for some ten days had Mr. Durant known any such ease of mind. He gave himself up to it, wrapped himself, warm and soft, as in a new and an expensive cloak. God, for Whom Mr. Durant entertained a good-humored affection, was in His heaven, and all was again well with Mr. Durant's world.

Curious how this renewed peace sharpened his enjoyment of the accustomed things about him. He looked back at the rubber works, which he had just left for the day, and nodded approvingly at the solid red pile, at the six neat stories rising impressively into the darkness. You would go far, he thought, before you would find a more up-and-coming outfit, and there welled in him a pleasing, proprietary sense of being a part of it.

He gazed amiably down Center Street, noting how restfully the lights glowed. Even the wet, dented pavement, spotted with thick puddles, fed his pleasure by reflecting the discreet radiance above it. And to complete his comfort, the car for which he was waiting, admirably on time, swung into view far down the track. He thought, with a sort of jovial tenderness, of what it would bear him to; of his dinner—it was fish-chowder night—of his children, of his wife, in the order named. Then he turned his kindly attention to the girl who stood near him, obviously awaiting the Center Street car, too. He was delighted to feel a sharp interest in her. He regarded it as being distinctly creditable to himself that he could take a healthy notice of such matters once more. Twenty years younger—that's what he felt.

Rather shabby, she was, in her rough coat with its shagginess rubbed off here and there. But there was a something in the way her cheaply smart turban was jammed over her eyes, in the way her thin young figure moved under the loose coat. Mr. Durant pointed his tongue, and moved it delicately along his cool, smooth upper lip.

The car approached, clanged to a stop before them. Mr. Durant stepped gallantly aside to let the girl get in first. He did not help her to enter, but the solicitous way in which he superintended the process gave all the effect of his having actually assisted her.

Her tight little skirt slipped up over her thin, pretty legs as she took the high step. There was a run in one of her flimsy silk stockings. She was doubtless unconscious of it; it was well back toward the seam, extending, probably from her garter, half-way down the calf. Mr. Durant had an odd desire to catch his thumb-nail in the present end of the run, and to draw it on down until the dim line of the dropped stitches reached to the top of her low shoe. An indulgent smile at his whimsy played about his mouth, broadening to a grin of affable evening greeting for the conductor, as he entered the car and paid his fare.

The girl sat down somewhere far up at the front. Mr. Durant found a desirable seat toward the rear, and craned his neck to see her. He could catch a glimpse of a fold of her turban and a bit of her brightly rouged cheek, but only at a cost of holding his head in a strained, and presently painful, position. So, warmed by the assurance that there would always be others, he let her go, and settled himself restfully. He had a ride of twenty minutes or so before him. He allowed his head to fall gently back, to let his eyelids droop, and gave himself to his thoughts. Now that the thing was comfortably over and done with, he could think of it easily, almost laughingly. Last week, now, and even part of the week before, he had had to try with all his strength to force it back every time it wrenched itself into his mind. It had positively affected his sleep. Even though he was shielded by his newly acquired amused attitude, Mr. Durant felt indignation flood within him when he recalled those restless nights.

He had met Rose for the first time about three months before. She had been sent up to his office to take some letters for him. Mr. Durant was assistant manager of the rubber company's credit department; his wife was wont to refer to him as one of the officers of the company, and, though she often spoke thus of him to people in his presence, he never troubled to go more fully into detail about his position. He rated a room, a desk, and a telephone to himself; but not a stenographer. When he wanted to give dictation or to have some letters typewritten, he telephoned around to the various other offices until he found a girl who was not busy with her own work. That was how Rose had come to him.

She was not a pretty girl. Distinctly, no. But there was a rather sweet fragility about her, and an almost desperate timidity that Mr. Durant had once found engaging, but that he now thought of with a prickling irritation. She was twenty, and the glamour of youth was around her. When she bent over her work, her back showing white through her sleazy blouse, her clean hair coiled smoothly on her thin neck, her straight, childish legs crossed at the knee to support her pad, she had an undeniable appeal.

But not pretty—no. Her hair wasn't the kind that went up well, her eyelashes and lips were too pale, she hadn't much knack about choosing and wearing her cheap clothes. Mr. Durant, in reviewing the thing, felt a surprise that she should ever have attracted him. But it was a tolerant surprise, not an impatient one. Already he looked back on himself as being just a big boy in the whole affair.

It did not occur to him to feel even a flicker of astonishment that Rose should have responded so eagerly to him, an immovably married man of forty-nine. He never thought of himself in that way. He used to tell Rose, laughingly, that he was old enough to be her father, but neither of them ever really believed it. He regarded her affection for him as the most natural thing in the world—there she was, coming from a much smaller town, never the sort of girl to have had admirers; naturally, she was dazzled at the attentions of a man who, as Mr. Durant put it, was approaching the prime. He had been charmed with the idea of there having been no other men in her life; but lately, far from feeling flattered at being the first and only one, he had come to regard it as her having taken a sly advantage of him, to put him in that position.

It had all been surprisingly easy. Mr. Durant knew it would be almost from the first time he saw her. That did not lessen its interest in his eyes. Obstacles discouraged him, rather than led him on. Elimination of bother was the main thing.

Rose was not a coquettish girl. She had that curious directness that some very timid people possess. There were her scruples, of course, but Mr. Durant readily reasoned them away. Not that he was a master of technique, either. He had had some experiences, probably a third as many as he habitually thought of himself as having been through, but none that taught him much of the delicate shadings of wooing. But then, Rose's simplicity asked exceedingly little.

She was never one to demand much of him, anyway. She never thought of stirring up any trouble between him and his wife, never besought him to leave his family and go away with her, even for a day. Mr. Durant valued her for that. It did away with a lot of probable fussing.

It was amazing how free they were, how little lying there was to do. They stayed in the office after hours—Mr. Durant found many letters that must be dictated. No one thought anything of that. Rose was busy most of the day, and it was only considerate that Mr. Durant should not break in on her employer's time, only natural that he should want as good a stenographer as she was to attend to his correspondence.

Rose's only relative, a married sister, lived in another town. The girl roomed with an acquaintance named Ruby, also employed at the rubber works, and Ruby, who was much taken up with her own affairs of the emotions, never appeared to think it strange if Rose was late to dinner, or missed the meal entirely. Mr. Durant readily explained to his wife that he was detained by a rush of business. It only increased his importance, to her, and spurred her on to devising especially pleasing dishes, and solicitously keeping them hot for his return. Sometimes, important in their guilt, Rose and he put out the light in the little office and locked the door, to trick the other employees into thinking that they had long ago gone home. But no one ever so much as rattled the doorknob, seeking admission.

It was all so simple that Mr. Durant never thought of it as anything outside the usual order of things. His interest in Rose did not blunt his appreciation of chance attractive legs or provocative glances It was an entanglement of the most restful, comfortable nature. It even held a sort of homelike quality, for him.

And then everything had to go and get spoiled. "Wouldn't you know?" Mr. Durant asked himself, with deep bitterness.

Ten days before, Rose had come weeping to his office. She had the sense to wait till after hours, for a wonder, but anybody might have walked in and seen her blubbering there; Mr. Durant felt it to be due only to the efficient management of his personal God that no one had. She wept, as he sweepingly put it, all over the place. The color left her cheeks and collected damply in her nose, and rims of vivid pink grew around her pale eyelashes. Even her hair became affected; it came away from the pins, and stray ends of it wandered limply over her neck. Mr. Durant hated to look at her, could not bring himself to touch her.

All his energies were expended in urging her for God's sake to keep quiet; he did not ask her what was the matter. But it came out, between bursts of unpleasant-sounding sobs. She was "in trouble." Neither then nor in the succeeding days did she and Mr. Durant ever use any less delicate phrase to describe her condition. Even in their thoughts, they referred to it that way.

She had suspected it, she said, for some time, but she hadn't wanted to bother him about it until she was absolutely sure. "Didn't want to bother me!" thought Mr. Durant.

Naturally, he was furious. Innocence is a desirable thing, a dainty thing, an appealing thing, in its place; but carried too far, it is merely ridiculous. Mr. Durant wished to God that he had never seen Rose. He explained this desire to her.

But that was no way to get things done. As he had often jovially remarked to his friends, he knew "a thing or two." Cases like this could be what people of the world called "fixed up"—New York society women, he understood, thought virtually nothing of it. This case could be fixed up, too. He got Rose to go home, telling her not to worry, he would see that everything was all right. The main thing was to get her out of sight, with that nose and those eyes.

But knowing a thing or two and putting the knowledge into practice turned out to be vastly different things. Mr. Durant did not know whom to seek for information. He pictured himself inquiring of his intimates if they could tell him of "someone that this girl he had heard about could go to." He could hear his voice uttering the words, could hear the nervous laugh that would accompany them, the terrible flatness of them as they left his bps. To confide m one person would be confiding in at least one too many. It was a progressing town, but still small enough for gossip to travel like a typhoon. Not that he thought for a moment that his wife would believe any such thing, if it reached her; but where would be the sense in troubling her?

Mr. Durant grew pale and jumpy over the thing as the days went by. His wife worried herself into one of her sick spells over his petulant refusals of second helpings. There daily arose in him an increasing anger that he should be drawn into conniving to find a way to break the law of his country—probably the law of every country in the world. Certainly of every decent, Christian place.

It was Ruby, finally, who got them out of it. When Rose confessed to him that she had broken down and told Ruby, his rage leaped higher than any words. Ruby was secretary to the vice-president of the rubber company. It would be pretty, wouldn't it, if she let it out? He had lain wide-eyed beside his wife all that night through. He shuddered at the thought of chance meetings with Ruby in the hall.

But Ruby had made it delightfully simple, when they did meet. There were no reproachful looks, no cold turnings away of the head. She had given him her usual smiling "good-morning," and added a little upward glance, mischievous, understanding, with just the least hint of admiration in it. There was a sense of intimacy, of a shared secret binding them cozily together. A fine girl, that Ruby!

Ruby had managed it all without any fuss. Mr. Durant was not directly concerned in the planning. He heard of it only through Rose, on the infrequent occasions when he had had to see her. Ruby knew, through some indistinct friends of hers, of "a woman." It would be twenty-five dollars. Mr. Durant had gallantly insisted upon giving Rose the money. She had started to sniffle about taking it, but he had finally prevailed. Not that he couldn't have used the twenty-five very nicely himself, just then, with Junior's teeth, and all!

Well, it was all over now. The invaluable Ruby had gone with Rose to "the woman"; had that very afternoon taken her to the station and put her on a train for her sister's. She had even thought of wiring the sister beforehand that Rose had had influenza and must have a rest.

Mr. Durant had urged Rose to look on it as just a little vacation. He promised, moreover, to put in a good word for her whenever she wanted her job back. But Rose had gone pink about the nose again at the thought. She had sobbed her rasping sobs, then had raised her face from her stringy handkerchief and said, with an entirely foreign firmness, that she never wanted to see the rubber works or Ruby or Mr. Durant again. He had laughed indulgently, had made himself pat her thin back. In his relief at the outcome of things, he could be generous to the pettish.

He chuckled inaudibly, as he reviewed that last scene. "I suppose she thought she'd make me sore, saying she was never coming back," he told himself. "I suppose I was supposed to get down on my knees and coax her."

It was fine to dwell on the surety that it was all done with. Mr. Durant had somewhere picked up a phrase that seemed ideally suited to the occasion. It was to him an admirably dashing expression. There was something stylish about it; it was the sort of thing you would expect to hear used by men who wore spats and swung canes without self-consciousness. He employed it now, with satisfaction.

"Well, that's that," he said to himself. He was not sure that he didn't say it aloud.

The car slowed, and the girl in the rough coat came down toward the door. She was jolted against Mr. Durant—he would have sworn she did it purposely—uttered a word of laughing apology, gave him what he interpreted as an inviting glance. He half rose to follow her, then sank back again. After all, it was a wet night, and his corner was five blocks farther on. Again there came over him the cozy assurance that there would always be others.

In high humor, he left the car at his street, and walked in the direction of his house. It was a mean night, but the insinuating cold and the black rain only made more graphic his picture of the warm, bright house, the great dish of steaming fish chowder, the well-behaved children and wife that awaited him. He walked rather slowly to make them seem all the better for the wait, humming a little on his way down the neat sidewalk, past the solid, reputably shabby houses.

Two girls ran past him, holding their hands over their heads to protect their hats from the wet. He enjoyed the click of their heels on the pavement, their little bursts of breathless laughter, their arms upraised in a position that brought out all the neat lines of their bodies. He knew who they were—they lived three doors down from him, in the house with the lamp-post in front of it. He had often lingeringly noticed their fresh prettiness. He hurried, so that he might see them run up the steps, their narrow skirts sliding up over their legs. His mind went back to the girl with the run in her stocking, and amusing thoughts filled him as he entered his own house.

His children rushed, clamoring, to meet him, as he unlocked the door. There was something exciting going on, for Junior and Charlotte were usually too careful-mannered to cause people discomfort by rushing and babbling. They were nice, sensible children, good at their lessons, and punctilious about brushing their teeth, speaking the truth, and avoiding playmates who used bad words. Junior would be the very picture of his father, when they got the bands off his teeth, and little Charlotte strongly resembled her mother. Friends often commented on what a nice arrangement it was.

Mr. Durant smiled good-naturedly through their racket, carefully hanging up his coat and hat. There was even pleasure for him in the arrangement of his apparel on the cool, shiny knob of the hatrack. Everything was pleasant, tonight. Even the children's noise couldn't irritate him.

Eventually he discovered the cause of the commotion. It was a little stray dog that had come to the back door. They were out in the kitchen helping Freda, and Charlotte thought she heard something scratching, and Freda said nonsense, but Charlotte went to the door, anyway, and there was this little dog, trying to get in out of the wet. Mother helped them give it a bath, and Freda fed it, and now it was in the living-room. Oh, Father, couldn't they keep it, please, couldn't they, couldn't they, please, Father, couldn't they? It didn't have any collar on it—so you see it didn't belong to anybody. Mother said all right, if he said so, and Freda liked it fine.

Mr. Durant still smiled his gentle smile. "We'll see," he said.

The children looked disappointed, but not despondent. They would have liked more enthusiasm, but "we'll see," they knew by experience, meant a leaning in the right direction.

Mr. Durant proceeded to the living-room, to inspect the visitor. It was not a beauty. All too obviously, it was the living souvenir of a mother who had never been able to say no. It was a rather stocky little beast with shaggy white hair and occasional, rakishly placed patches of black. There was a suggestion of Sealyham terrier about it, but that was almost blotted out by hosts of reminiscences of other breeds. It looked, on the whole, like a composite photograph of Popular Dogs. But you could tell at a glance that it had a way with it. Scepters have been tossed aside for that.

It lay, now, by the fire, waving its tragically long tail wistfully, its eyes pleading with Mr. Durant to give it a fair trial. The children had told it to lie down there, and so it did not move. That was something it could do toward repaying them.

Mr. Durant warmed to it. He did not dislike dogs, and he somewhat fancied the picture of himself as a soft-hearted fellow who extended shelter to friendless animals. He bent, and held out a hand to it.

"Well, sir," he said, genially. "Come here, good fellow."

The dog ran to him, wriggling ecstatically. It covered his cold hand with joyous, though respectful kisses, then laid its warm, heavy head on his palm. "You are beyond a doubt the greatest man in America," it told him with its eyes.

Mr. Durant enjoyed appreciation and gratitude. He patted the dog graciously.

"Well, sir, tow'd you like to board with us?" he said. "I guess you can plan to settle down." Charlotte squeezed Junior's arm wildly. Neither of them, though, thought it best to crowd their good fortune by making any immediate comment on it.

Mrs. Durant entered from the kitchen, flushed with her final attentions to the chowder. There was a worried line between her eyes. Part of the worry was due to the dinner, and part to the disturbing entrance of the little dog into the family life. Anything not previously included in her day's schedule threw Mrs. Durant into a state resembling that of one convalescing from shell-shock. Her hands jerked nervously, beginning gestures that they never finished.

Relief smoothed her face when she saw her husband patting the dog. The children, always at ease with her, broke their silence and jumped about her, shrieking that father said it might stay.

"There, now—didn't I tell you what a dear, good father you had?" she said in the tone parents employ when they have happened to guess right. "That's fine. Father. With that big yard and all, I think we'll make out all right. She really seems to be an awfully good little——"

Mr. Durant's hand stopped sharply in its patting motions, as if the dog's neck had become red-hot to his touch. He rose, and looked at his wife as at a stranger who had suddenly begun to behave wildly.

"She?" he said. He maintained the look and repeated the word. "She?"

Mrs. Durant's hands jerked.

"Well—" she began, as if about to plunge into a recital of extenuating circumstances. "Well—yes," she concluded.

The children and the dog looked nervously at Mr. Durant, feeling something was gone wrong. Charlotte whimpered wordlessly.

"Quiet!" said her father, turning suddenly upon her. "I said it could stay, didn't I? Did you ever know Father to break a promise?"

Charlotte politely murmured, "No, Father," but conviction was not hers. She was a philosophical child, though, and she decided to leave the whole issue to God, occasionally jogging Him up a bit with prayer.

Mr. Durant frowned at his wife, and jerked his head backward. This indicated that he wished to have a few words with her, for adults only, in the privacy of the little room across the hall, known as "Father's den."

He had directed the decoration of his den, had seen that it had been made a truly masculine room. Red paper covered its walls, up to the wooden rack on which were displayed ornamental steins, of domestic manufacture. Empty pipe-racks—Mr. Durant smoked cigars—were nailed against the red paper at frequent intervals. On one wall was an indifferent reproduction of a drawing of a young woman with wings like a vampire bat, and on another, a water-colored photograph of "September Mom," the tints running a bit beyond the edges of the figure as if the artist's emotions had rendered his hand unsteady. Over the table was carefully flung a tanned and fringed hide with the profile of an unknown Indian maiden painted on it, and the rocking-chair held a leather pillow bearing the picture, done by pyrography, of a girl in a fencing costume which set off her distressingly dated figure.

Mr. Durant's books were lined up behind the glass of the bookcase. They were all tall, thick books, brightly bound, and they justified his pride in their showing. They were mostly accounts of favorites of the French court, with a few volumes on odd personal habits of various monarchs, and the adventures of former Russian monks. Mrs. Durant, who never had time to get around to reading, regarded them with awe, and thought of her husband as one of the country's leading bibliophiles. There were books, too, in the living-room, but those she had inherited or been given. She had arranged a few on the living-room table; they looked as if they had been placed there by the Gideons.

Mr. Durant thought of himself as an indefatigable collector and an insatiable reader. But he was always disappointed in his books, after he had sent for them. They were never so good as the advertisements had led him to believe.

Into his den Mr. Durant preceded his wife, and faced her, still frowning. His calm was not shattered, but it was punctured. Something annoying always had to go and come up. Wouldn't you know?

"Now you know perfectly well, Fan, we can't have that dog around," he told her. He used the low voice reserved for underwear and bathroom articles and kindred shady topics. There was all the kindness in his tones that one has for a backward child, but a Gibraltar-like firmness was behind it. "You must be crazy to even think we could for a minute. Why, I wouldn't give a she-dog house-room, not for any amount of money. It's disgusting, that's what it is."

"Well, but, Father——" began Mrs. Durant, her hands again going off into their convulsions.

"Disgusting," he repeated. "You have a female around, and you know what happens. All the males in the neighborhood will be running after her. First thing you know, she'd be having puppies—and the way they look after they've had them, and all! That would be nice for the children to see, wouldn't it? I should think you'd think of the children, Fan. No, sir, there'll be nothing like that around here, not while I know it. Disgusting!"

"But the children," she said. "They'll be just simply——?"

"Now you just leave all that to me," he reassured her. "I told them the dog could stay, and I've never broken a promise yet, have I? Here's what I'll do — I'll wait till they're asleep, and then I'll just take this little dog and put it out. Then, in the morning, you can tell them it ran away during the night, see?"

She nodded. Her husband patted her shoulder, in its crapy-smelling black silk. His peace with the world was once more intact, restored by this simple solution of the little difficulty. Again his mind wrapped itself in the knowledge that everything was all fixed, all ready for a nice, fresh start. His arm was still about his wife's shoulder as they went on in to dinner.

"Hills Like White Elephants" by Ernest Hemingway (1927)

Introduction

This short story is one of the most widely analyzed literary representations of abortion, though the narration does not explicitly say the term. The story is a single scene featuring a woman named Jig (called the girl) and an American (called the man) while they wait for a train to Madrid. Some of the notable features include the many symbolic elements, the simple style, and the dialogue which comprises most of the text.

Hills Like White Elephants (*transition*, August 1927)

The hills across the valley of the Ebro were long and white. On this side there was no shade and no trees and the station was between two lines of rails in the sun. Close against the side of the station there was the warm shadow of the building and a curtain, made of strings of bamboo beads, hung across the open door into the bar, to keep out flies. The American and the girl with him sat at a table in the shade, outside the building. It was very hot and the express from Barcelona would come in forty minutes. It stopped at this junction for two minutes and went on to Madrid.

"What should we drink?" the girl asked. She had taken off her hat and put it on the table.

"It's pretty hot," the man said.

"Let's drink beer."

"*Dos cervezas*," the man said into the curtain.

"Big ones?" a woman asked from the doorway.

"Yes. Two big ones."

The woman brought two glasses of beer and two felt pads. She put the felt pads and the beer glasses on the table and looked at the man and the girl. The girl was looking off at the line of hills. They were white in the sun and the country was brown and dry.

"They look like white elephants," she said.

"I've never seen one," the man drank his beer.

"No, you wouldn't have."

"I might have," the man said. "Just because you say I wouldn't have doesn't prove anything."

The girl looked at the bead curtain. "They've painted something on it," she said. "What does it say?"

"Anis del Toro. It's a drink."

"Could we try it?"

The man called "Listen" through the curtain. The woman came out from the bar.

"Four reales."

"We want two Anis del Toro."

"With water?"

"Do you want it with water?"

"I don't know," the girl said. "Is it good with water?"

"It's all right."

"You want them with water?" asked the woman.

"Yes, with water."

"It tastes like licorice," the girl said and put the glass down.

"That's the way with everything."

"Yes," said the girl. "Everything tastes of licorice. Especially all the things you've waited so long for, like absinthe."

"Oh, cut it out."

"You started it," the girl said. "I was being amused. I was having a fine time."

"Well, let's try and have a fine time."

"All right. I was trying. I said the mountains looked like white elephants. Wasn't that bright?"

"That was bright."

"I wanted to try this new drink. That's all we do, isn't it—look at things and try new drinks?"

"I guess so."

The girl looked across at the hills.

"They're lovely hills," she said. "They don't really look like white elephants. I just meant the coloring of their skin through the trees."

"Should we have another drink?"

"All right."

The warm wind blew the bead curtain against the table. "The beer's nice and cool," the man said.

"It's lovely," the girl said.

"It's really an awfully simple operation, Jig," the man said. "It's not really an operation at all."

The girl looked at the ground the table legs rested on.

"I know you wouldn't mind it, Jig. It's really not anything. It's just to let the air in."

The girl did not say anything.

"I'll go with you and I'll stay with you all the time. They just let the air in and then it's all perfectly natural."

"Then what will we do afterward?"

"We'll be fine afterward. Just like we were before."

"What makes you think so?"

"That's the only thing that bothers us. It's the only thing that's made us unhappy."

The girl looked at the bead curtain, put her hand out, and took hold of two of the strings of beads.

"And you think then we'll be all right and be happy."

"I know we will. You don't have to be afraid. I've known lots of people that have done it."

"So have I," said the girl. "And afterward they were all so happy."

"Well," the man said, "if you don't want to you don't have to. I wouldn't have you do it if you didn't want to. But I know it's perfectly simple."

"And you really want to?"

"I think it's the best thing to do. But I don't want you to do it if you don't really want to."

"And if I do it you'll be happy and things will be like they were and you'll love me?"

"I love you now. You know I love you."

"I know. But if I do it, then it will be nice again if I say things are like white elephants, and you'll like it?"

"I'll love it. I love it now but I just can't think about it. You know how I get when I worry."

"If I do it you won't ever worry?"

"I won't worry about that because it's perfectly simple."

"Then I'll do it. Because I don't care about me."

"What do you mean?"

"I don't care about me."

"Well, I care about you."

"Oh, yes. But I don't care about me. And I'll do it and then everything will be fine."

"I don't want you to do it if you feel that way."

The girl stood up and walked to the end of the station. Across, on the other side, were fields of grain and trees along the banks of the Ebro. Far away, beyond the river, were mountains. The shadow of a cloud moved across the field of grain and she saw the river through the trees.

"And we could have all this," she said. "And we could have everything and every day we make it more impossible."

"What did you say?"

"I said we could have everything."

"We can have everything."

"No, we can't."

"We can have the whole world."

"No, we can't."

"We can go everywhere."

"No, we can't. It isn't ours any more."

"It's ours."

"No, it isn't. And once they take it away, you never get it back."

"But they haven't taken it away."

"We'll wait and see."

"Come on back in the shade," he said. "You mustn't feel that way."

"I don't feel any way," the girl said. "I just know things."

"I don't want you to do anything that you don't want to do ——"

"Nor that isn't good for me," she said. "I know. Could we have another beer?"

"All right. But you've got to realize ——"

"I realize," the girl said. "Can't we maybe stop talking?"

They sat down at the table and the girl looked across at the hills on the dry side of the valley and the man looked at her and at the table.

"You've got to realize," he said, "that I don't want you to do it if you don't want to. I'm perfectly willing to go through with it if it means anything to you."

"Doesn't it mean anything to you? We could get along."

"Of course it does. But I don't want anybody but you. I don't want any one else. And I know it's perfectly simple."

"Yes, you know it's perfectly simple."

"It's all right for you to say that, but I do know it."

"Would you do something for me now?"

"I'd do anything for you."

"Would you please please please please please please please stop talking?"

He did not say anything but looked at the bags against the wall of the station. There were labels on them from all the hotels where they had spent nights.

"But I don't want you to," he said, "I don't care anything about it."

"I'll scream," the girl said.

The woman came out through the curtains with two glasses of beer and put them down on the damp felt pads. "The train comes in five minutes," she said.

"What did she say?" asked the girl.

"That the train is coming in five minutes."

The girl smiled brightly at the woman, to thank her.

"I'd better take the bags over to the other side of the station," the man said. She smiled at him.

"All right. Then come back and we'll finish the beer."

He picked up the two heavy bags and carried them around the station to the other tracks. He looked up the tracks but could not see the train. Coming back, he walked through the barroom, where people waiting for the train were drinking. He drank an Anis at the bar and looked at the people. They were all waiting reasonably for the train. He went out through the bead curtain. She was sitting at the table and smiled at him.

"Do you feel better?" he asked.

"I feel fine," she said. "There's nothing wrong with me. I feel fine."

"Missis Flinders" by Tess Slesinger (1932)

Introduction

In this short story, Tess Slesinger narrates a married couple's journey home from the maternity hospital where the titular woman has had a dilation and curettage procedure (D&C) to terminate her pregnancy. She switches between the present taxi ride with her husband and flashbacks of talking with the other women in the hospital while beginning to question the decision to have an abortion. This was first published in *Story*, a popular literary magazine founded the previous year.

"Missis Flinders" (*Story*, December 1932)

"Home you go!" Miss Kate, nodding in her white nurse's dress, stood for a moment—she would catch a breath of air—in the hospital door; "and thank you again for the stockings, you needn't have bothered"—drew a sharp breath and turning, dismissed Missis Flinders from the hospital, smiling, dismissed her forever from her mind.

So Margaret Flinders stood next to her basket of fruit on the hospital steps; both of them waiting, a little shame-faced in the sudden sun- shine, and in no hurry to leave the hospital—no hurry at al. It would be nicer to be alone, Margaret thought, glancing at the basket of fruit which stood respectable and a little silly on the stone step (the candy- bright apples were blushing caricatures of Miles: Miles' comfort, not hers). Flowers she could have left behind (for the nurses, in the room across the hall where they made tea at night); books she could have slipped into her suit-case; but fruit—Miles' gift, Miles' guilt, man's tribute to the Missis in the hospital—must be eaten; a half-eaten basket of fruit (she had tried to leave it: Missis Butter won't you… Missis Wiggam wouldn't you like… But Missis Butter had aplenty of her own thank you, and Missis Wiggam said she couldn't hold acids after a baby)—a half-eaten basket of fruit, in times like these, cannot be left to rot.

Down the street Miles was running, running, after a taxi. He was going after the taxi for her; it was for her sake he ran; yet this minute that his back was turned he stole for his relief and spent in running away, his shoulders crying guilt. And don't hurry, don't hurry, she said to them; I too am better off alone.

The street stretched in a long white line very finally away from the hospital, the hospital where Margaret Flinders (called there so solemnly Missis) had been lucky enough to spend only three nights. It would be four days before Missis Wiggam would be going home to Mister Wiggam with a baby; and ten possibly—the doctors were uncertain, Miss Kane prevaricated—before Missis Butter would be going home to Mister Butter without one. Zigzagging the street went the children; their cries and the sudden grinding of their skates she had listened to upstairs beside Missis Butter for three days. Some such child had she been—for the styles in children had not changed—a lean child gliding solemnly on skates and grinding them viciously at the nervous feet of grown-ups. Smile at these children she would not or could not; yet she felt on her face that smile, fixed, painful and frozen, that she had put there, on waking from ether three days back, to greet Miles. The smile spoke to the retreating shoulders of Miles: I don't need you; the smile spoke formally to life: thanks, I'm not having any. Not so the child putting the heels of his skates together Charlie Chaplin-wise and describing a scornful circle on the widest part of the sidewalk. Not so a certain little girl (twenty years back) skating past the wheels of autos, pursuing life in the form of a ball so red! so gay! better death than to turn one's back and smile over one's shoulder at life!

Upstairs Missis Butter must still be writhing with her poor caked breasts. The bed that had been hers beside Missis Butter's was empty now; Miss Kane would be stripping it and Joe would come in bringing fresh sheets. Whom would they put in beside Missis Butter, to whom would she moan and boast all night about the milk in her breasts that was turning, she said, into cheese?

Now Miles was coming back, jogging sheepishly on the running-board of a taxi, he had run away to the end of his rope and now was returning penitent, his eyes dog-like searching her out where she stood on the hospital steps (did they rest with complacence on the basket of fruit, his gift?), pleading with her, Didn't I get the taxi fast? like an anxious little boy. She stood with that smile on her face that hurt like too much ice-cream. Smile and smile; for she felt like a fool, she had walked open-eyed smiling into the trap (*Don't wriggle, Missis, I might injure you for life, Miss Kane had said cheerfully*) and felt the spring only when it was too late, when she waked from ether and knew like the thrust of a knife what she had ignored before. *Whatever did you do it for, Missis Flinders, Missis Butter was always saying; if there's nothing the matter with your insides—doesn't your husband …and Won't you have some fruit, Missis Butter, her calm reply: meaning, My husband gave me this fruit so what right have you to doubt that my husband.…* Her husband who now stumbled up the steps to meet her; his eyes he had sent ahead, but something in him wanted not to come, tripped his foot as he hurried up the steps.

"Take my arm, Margaret," he said. "Walk slowly," he said. The bitter pill of taking help, of feeling weakly grateful, stuck in her throat. Miles' face behind his glasses was tense like the face of an amateur actor in the rôle of a strike-leader. That he was inadequate for the part he seemed to know. And if he felt shame, shame in his own eyes, she could forgive him; but if it was only guilt felt man-like in her presence, a guilt which he could drop off like a damp shirt, if he was putting it all off on her for being a woman! "The fruit, Miles!" she said; "you've forgotten the fruit." "The fruit can wait," he said bitterly.

He handed her into the taxi as though she were a package marked glass—something, she thought, not merely troublesomely womanly, but ladylike. "Put your legs up on the seat," he said. "I don't want to, Miles." *Goodbye Missis Butter* Put your legs up on the seat. I don't want to—*Better luck next time Missis Butter* Put your legs *I can't make out our window, Missis Butter* Put your "All right, it will be nice and uncomfortable." (She put her legs up on the seat.) *Goodbye Missis But....* "Nothing I say is right," he said. "It's good with the legs up," she said brightly.

Then he was up the steps agile and sure after the fruit. And down again, the basket swinging with affected carelessness, arming him, till he relinquished it modestly to her outstretched hands. Then he seated himself on the little seat, the better to watch his woman and his woman's fruit; and screwing his head round on his neck said irritably to the man who had been all his life on the wrong side of the glass pane: "Charles street!"

"Hadn't you better ask him to please drive slowly?" Margaret said.

"I was just going to," he said bitterly.

"And drive slowly," he shouted over his shoulder.

The driver's name was Carl C. Strite. She could see Carl Strite glance cannily back at the hospital: Greenway Maternity Home; pull his lever with extreme delicacy as though he were stroking the neck of a horse. There was a small roar—and the hospital glided backward: its windows ran together like the windows of a moving train; a spurt—watch out for those children on skates!—and the car was fairly started down the street.

Goodbye Missis Butter I hope you get a nice roommate in my place, I hope you won't find that Mister B let the ice-pan flow over again—and give my love to the babies when Miss Kane stops them in the door for you to wave at—goodbye Missis Butter, really goodbye.

Carl Strite (was he thinking maybe of his mother; an immigrant German woman she would have been, come over with a shawl on her head and worked herself to skin and bone so the kids could go to school and turn out good Americans—and what had it come to, here he was a taxi-driver, and what taxi-drivers didn't know! what in the course of their lackeys' lives they didn't put up with, fall in with! well, there was one decent thing left in Carl Strite, he knew how to carry a woman home from a maternity hospital) drove softly along the curb....and the eyes of his honest puzzled gangster's snout photographed as "Your Driver" looked dimmed as though the glory of woman were too much for them, in a moment the weak cruel baby's mouth might blubber. Awful to lean forward and tell Mr Strite he was laboring under a mistake. Missis Wiggam's freckled face when she heard that Missis Butter's roommate ...maybe Missis Butter's baby had been born dead but anyway she had had a baby...whatever did you do it for Missis Flind....

"Well, patient," Miles began, tentative, nervous (bored? perturbed? behind his glasses?).

"How does it feel, Maggie?" he said in a new, small voice.

Hurt and hurt this man, a feeling told her. He is a man, he could have made you a woman. "What's a D and C between friends?" she said. "Nobody at the hospital gave a damn about my little illegality."

"Well, but I do," he protested like a short man trying to be tall.

She turned on her smile; the bright silly smile that was eating up her face.

Missis Butter would be alone now with no one to boast to about her pains except Joe who cleaned the corridors and emptied bed-pans—and thought Missis Butter was better than an angel because although she had incredible golden hair she could wise-crack like any brunette. Later in the day the eight-day mothers wobbling down the corridors for their pre-nursing constitutional would look in and talk to her; for wasn't Missis Butter their symbol and their pride, the one who had given up her baby that they might have theirs (for a little superstition is inevitable in new mothers, and it was generally felt that there must be one dead baby in a week's batch at any decent hospital) for whom they demanded homage from their visiting husbands? for whose health they asked the nurses each morning second only to asking for their own babies? That roommate of yours was a funny one, Missis Wiggam would say. Missis Wiggam was the woman who said big breasts weren't any good: here she was with a seven-pound baby and not a drop for it (here she would open the negligée Mister Wiggam had given her not to shame them before the nurses, and poke contemptuously at the floppy parts of herself within) while there was Missis Butter with no baby but a dead baby and her small breasts caking because there was so much milk in them for nothing but a....Yes, that Missis Flinders was sure a funny one, Missis Butter would agree.

"Funny ones", she and Miles, riding home with numb faces and a basket of fruit between them—past a park, past a museum, past elevated pillars—intellectuals they were, bastards, changelings....giving up a baby for economic freedom which meant that two of them would work in offices instead of one of them only, giving up a baby for intellectual freedom which meant that they smoked their cigarettes bitterly and looked out of the windows of a taxi onto streets and people and stores and hated them all. "We'd go soft," Miles had finally said, "we'd go bourgeois." Yes, with diapers drying on the radiators, bottles wrapped in flannel, the grocer getting to know one too well—yes, they would go soft, they might slump and start liking people, they might weaken and forgive stupidity, they might yawn and forget to hate. "Funny ones," class-straddlers, intellectuals, tight-rope-walking somewhere in the middle (how long could they hang on without falling to one side or the other? one more war? one more depression?); intellectuals, with habits generated from the right and tastes inclined to the left. Afraid to perpetuate themselves, were they? Afraid of anything that might loom so large in their personal lives as to outweigh other considerations? Afraid, maybe, of a personal life?

"Oh give me another cigarette," she said.

And still the taxi, with its burden of intellectuals and their inarticulate fruit-basket, its motherly, gangsterly, inarticulate driver, its license plates and its photographs all so very official, jogged on; past Harlem now; past fire-escapes loaded with flowerpots and flapping clothes; dingy windows opening to the soot-laden air blown in by the elevated roaring down its tracks. Past Harlem and through 125th street: stores and wise-cracks, Painless Dentists, cheap florists; Eighth Avenue, boarded and plastered, concealing the subway that was reaching its laborious birth beneath. But Eighth Avenue was too jouncy for Mr Strite's precious burden of womanhood (who was reaching passionately for a cigarette); he cut through the park, and they drove past quiet walks on which the sun had brought out babies as the Fall rains give birth to worms.

"But ought you to smoke so much, so soon after—so soon?" Miles said, not liking to say so soon after what. His hand held the cigarettes out to her, back from her.

"They do say smoking's bad for child-birth," she said calmly, and with her finger-tips drew a cigarette from his reluctant hand.

And tapping down the tobacco on the handle of the fruit-basket she said, "But we've got the joke on them there, we have." (Hurt and hurt this man, her feeling told her; he is a man and could have made you a woman.)

"It was your own decision too," he said harshly, striking and striking at the box with his match.

"This damn taxi's shaking you too much," he said suddenly, bitter and contrite.

But Mr Strite was driving like an angel. He handled his car as though it were a baby-carriage. Did he think maybe it had turned out with her the way it had with Missis Butter? I could have stood it better, Missis Butter said, if they hadn't told me it was a boy. And me with my fourth little girl, Missis Wiggam had groaned (but proudly, proudly); why I didn't even want to see it when they told me. But Missis Butter stood it very well, and so did Missis Wiggam. They were a couple of good bitches; and what if Missis Butter had produced nothing but a dead baby this year, and what if Missis Wiggam would bring nothing to Mister Wiggam but a fourth little girl this year—why there was next year and the year after, there was the certain little world from grocery-store to kitchen, there were still Mister Butter and Mister Wiggam who were both (Missis Wiggam and Missis Butter vied with each other) just crazy about babies. Well, Mister Flinders is different, she had lain there thinking (he cares as much for his unborn gods as I for my unborn babies); and wished she could have the firm assurance they had in "husbands," coming as they did year after year away from them for a couple of weeks, just long enough to bear them babies either dead-ones or girl-ones....good bitches they were: there was something lustful besides smug in their pride in being "Missis." Let Missis Flinders so much as let out a groan because a sudden pain grew too big for her groins, let her so much as murmur because the sheets were hot beneath her—and Missis Butter and Missis Wiggam in the security of their maternity-fraternity exchanged glances of amusement: SHE don't know what pain is, look at what's talking about PAIN....

"Mr Strite flatters us," she whispered, her eyes smiling straight and hard at Miles. (Hurt and hurt....)

"And why does that give you so much pleasure?" He dragged the words as though he were pounding them out with two fingers on the typewriter.

The name without the pain—she thought to say; and did not say. All at once she lost her desire to punish him; she no more wanted to "hurt this man" for he was no more man than she was woman. She would not do him the honor of hurting him. She must reduce him as she felt herself reduced. She must cut out from him what made him a man, as she had let be cut out from her what would have made her a woman. He was no man: he was a dried-up intellectual husk; he was sterile; empty and hollow as she was.

Missis Butter lying up on her pillow would count over to Missis Wiggam the fine points of her tragedy: how she had waited two days to be delivered of a dead baby; how it wouldn't have been so bad if the doctor hadn't said it was a beautiful baby with platinum-blond hair exactly like hers (and hers bleached unbelievably, but never mind, Missis Wiggam had come to believe in it like Joe and Mister Butter, another day and Missis Flinders herself, intellectual sceptic though she was, might have been convinced); and how they would pay the last instalment on—what a baby-carriage, Missis Wiggam, you'd never believe me!—and sell it second-hand for half its worth. I know when I was caught with my first, Missis Wiggam would take up the story her mouth had been open for. And that Missis Flinders was sure a funny one....

But I am not such a funny one, Margaret wanted, beneath her bright and silly smile, behind her cloud of cigarette smoke (for Miles had given in; the whole package sat gloomily on Margaret's lap) to say to them; even though in my "crowd" the girls keep the names they were born with, even though some of us sleep for a little variety with one another's husbands, even though I forget as often as Miles—Mister Flinders to you—to empty the pan under the ice-box. Still I too have known my breasts to swell and harden, I too have been unable to sleep on them for their tenderness to weight and touch, I too have known what it is to undress slowly and imagine myself growing night to night....I knew this for two months, my dear Missis Wiggam; I had this strange joy for two months, my dear Missis Butter. But there was a night last week, my good ladies, on coming home from a party, which Mister Flinders and I spent in talk—and damn fine talk, if you want to know, talk of which I am proud, and talk not one word of which you, with your grocery-and-baby minds, could have understood; in a régime like this, Miles said, it is a terrible thing to have a baby—it means the end of independent thought and the turning of everything into a scheme for making money; and there must be institutions such as there are in Russia, I said, for taking care of the babies and their mothers; why in a time like this, we both said, to have a baby would be suicide—goodbye to our plans, goodbye to our working out schemes for each other and the world—our courage would die, our hopes concentrate on the sordid business of keeping three people alive, one of whom would be a burden and an expense for twenty years.... And then we grew drunk for a minute making up the silliest names that we could call it if we had it, we would call it Daniel if it were a boy, call it for my mother if it were a girl—and what a tough little thing it is, I said, look, look, how it hangs on in spite of its loving mother jumping off tables and broiling herself in hot water....until Miles, frightened at himself, washed his hands of it: we mustn't waste any more time, the sooner these things are done the better. And I as though the ether cap had already been clapped to my nose, agreed off-handedly. That night I did not pass my hands contentedly over my hard breasts; that night I gave no thought to the nipples grown suddenly brown and competent; I packed, instead, my suit-case: I filled it with all the white clothes I own. Why are you taking white clothes to the hospital? Miles said to me. I laughed. Why did I? White, for a bride; white, for a corpse; white, for a woman who refuses to be a woman....

"Are you all right, Margaret?" (They were out now, safely out on Fifth Avenue, driving placidly past the Plaza where ancient coachmen dozed on the high seats of the last hansoms left in New York.)

"Yes, dear," she said mechanically, and forgot to turn on her smile. Pity for him sitting there in stolid New England inadequacy filled her. He was a man, and he could have made her a woman. She was a woman, and could have made him a man. He was not a man; she was not a woman. In each of them the life-stream flowed to a dead-end.

And all this time that the blood, which Missis Wiggam and Missis Butter stored up preciously in themselves every year to make a baby for their husbands, was flowing freely and wastefully out of Missis Flinders—toward what? would it pile up some day and bear a book? would it congeal within her and make a crazy woman?—all this time Mr Strite, remembering, with his pudgy face, his mother, drove his taxi softly along the curb; no weaving in and out of traffic for Mr Strite, no spurting at the corners and cheating the side-street traffic, no fine heedless rounding of rival cars for Mr Strite; he kept his car going at a slow and steady roll, its nose poked blunt ahead, following the straight and narrow—Mr Strite knew what it was to carry a woman home from the hospital.

But what in their past had warranted this? She could remember a small girl going from dolls to books, from books with colored pictures to books with frequent conversations; from such books to the books at last that one borrowed from libraries, books built up of solemn text from which you took notes; books which were gray to begin with, but which opened out to your eyes subtle layers of gently shaded colors. (And where in these texts did it say that one should turn one's back on life? Had the coolness of the stone library at college made one afraid? Had the ivy nodding in at the open dormitory windows taught one too much to curl and squat looking out?) And Miles? What book, what professor, what strange idea, had taught him to hunch his shoulders and stay indoors, had taught him to hide behind his glasses? Whence the fear that made him put, in cold block letters, implacably above his desk, the sign announcing him "Not at Home" to life?

Missis Flinders, my husband scaled the hospital wall at four o'clock in the morning, frantic I tell you.... But I just don't understand you, Missis Flinders (if there's really nothing the matter with your insides), do you understand her, Missis Wiggam, would your husband?...Why goodness, no, Mister Wiggam would sooner...! And there he was, and they asked him, Shall we try an operation, Mister Butter? scaled the wall...shall we try an operation? (Well, you see, we are making some sort of protest, my husband Miles and I; sometimes I forget just what.) If there's any risk to Shirley, he said, there mustn't be any risk to Shirley... Missis Wiggam's petulant, childish face, with its sly contentment veiled by what she must have thought a grown-up expression: Mister Wiggam bought me this negligée new, surprised me with it, you know—and generally a saving man, Mister Wiggam, not tight, but with three children—four now! Hetty, he says, I'm not going to have you disgracing us at the hospital this year, he says. Why the nurses will all remember that flannel thing you had Mabel and Suzy and Antoinette in, they'll talk about us behind our backs. (It wasn't that I couldn't make the flannel do again, Missis Butter, it wasn't that at all.) But he says, Hetty, you'll just have a new one this year, he says, and maybe it'll bring us luck, he says—you know, he was thinking maybe this time we'd have a boy... Well, I just have to laugh at you, Missis Flinders, not wanting one, why my sister went to doctors for five years and spent her good money just trying to have one....Well, poor Mister Wiggam, so the negligée didn't work, I brought him another little girl—but he didn't say boo to me, though I could see he was disappointed. Hetty, he says, we'll just have another try! oh I thought I'd die, with Miss Kane standing right there you know (though they do say these nurses....);but that's Mister Wiggam all over, he wouldn't stop a joke for a policeman....No, I just can't get over you, Missis Flinders, if Gawd was willing to let you have a baby—and there really isn't anything wrong with your insides?

Miles' basket of fruit standing on the bed-table, trying its level inadequate best, poor pathetic inarticulate intellectual basket of fruit, to comfort, to bloom, to take the place of Miles himself who would come in later with Sam Butter for visiting hour. Miles' too-big basket of fruit standing there, embarrassed. Won't you have a peach, Missis Wiggam (I'm sure they have less acid)? Just try an apple, Missis Butter? Weigh Miles' basket of fruit against Mister Wiggam's negligée for luck, against Mister Butter scaling the wall at four in the morning for the mother of his dead baby. Please have a pear, Miss Kane; a banana, Joe? How they spat the seeds from Miles' fruit! How it hurt her when, unknowing, Missis Butter cut away the brown bruised cheek of Miles' bright-eyed, weeping apple! Miles! they scorn me, these ladies. They laugh at me, dear, almost as though I had no "husband," as though I were a "fallen woman". Miles, would you buy me a new negligée if I bore you three daughters? Miles, would you scale the wall if I bore you a dead baby?....Miles, I have an inferiority complex because I am an intellectual.... But a peach, Missis Wiggam! can't I possibly tempt you?

To be driving like this at mid-day through New York; with Miles bobbing like an empty ghost (for she could see he was unhappy, as miserable as she, he too had had an abortion) on the side-seat; with a taxi-driver, solicitous, respectful to an ideal, in front; was this the logical end of that little girl she remembered, of that girl swinging hatless across a campus as though that campus were the top of the earth? And was this all they could give birth to, she and Miles, who had closed up their books one day and kissed each other on the lips and decided to marry?

And now Mr Strite, with his hand out, was making a gentle right-hand turn. Back to Fifth Avenue they would go, gently rolling, in Mr Strite's considerate charge. Down Fourteenth Street they would go, past the stores unlike any stores in the world: packed to the windows with imitation gold and imitation embroidery, with imitation men and women coming to stand in the doorways and beckon with imitation smiles; while on the sidewalks streamed the people unlike any other people in the world, drawn from every country, from every stratum, carrying babies (the real thing, with pinched anaemic faces) and parcels (imitation finery priced low in the glittering stores). There goes a woman, with a flat fat face, will produce five others just like herself, to dine off one-fifth the inadequate quantity her Mister earns today. These are the people not afraid to perpetuate themselves (forbidden to stop, indeed) and they will go on and on until the bottom of the world is filled with them; and suddenly there will be enough of them to combine their wild-eyed notions and take over the world to suit themselves. While I, while I and my Miles, with out good clear heads will one day go spinning out of the world and leave nothing behind…only diplomas crumbling in the museums…

The mad street ended with Fifth Avenue; was left behind.

They were nearing home. Mr Strite, who had never seen them before (who would never again, in all likelihood, for his territory was far uptown) was seeing them politely to the door. As they came near home all of Margaret's fear and pain gathered in a knot in her stomach. There would be nothing new in their house; there was nothing to expect; yet she wanted to find something there that she knew she could not find, and surely the house (once so gay, with copies of old paintings, with books which lined the walls from floor to ceiling, with papers and cushions and typewriters) would be suddenly empty and dead, suddenly, for the first time, a group of rooms unalive as rooms with "For Rent" still pasted on the windows. And Miles? did he know he was coming home to a place which had suffered no change, but which would be different forever afterward? Miles had taken off his glasses; passed his hand tiredly across his eyes; was sucking now as though he expected relief, some answer, on the tortoise-shell curve which wound around his ear.

Mr Strite would not allow his cab to cease motion with a jerk. Mr Strite allowed his cab to slow down even at the corner (where was the delicatessen that sold the only loose ripe olives in the Village), so they tolled softly past No. 14; on past the tenement which would eventually be razed to give place to modern three-room apartments with In-a-Dor beds; and then slowly, so slowly that Mr Strite must surely be an artist as well as a man who had had a mother, drew up and slid to a full stop before No. 60, where two people named Mister and Missis Flinders rented themselves a place to hide from life (both life of the Fifth Avenue variety, and life of the common, or Fourteenth Street, variety: in short, life).

So Miles, with his glasses on his nose once more, descended; held out his hand; Mr Strite held the door open and his face most modestly averted; and

Margaret Flinders painfully and carefully swung her legs down again from the seat and alighted, step by step, with care and confusion. The house was before them; it must be entered. Into the house they must go, say farewell to the streets, to Mr Strite who had guided them through a tour of the city, to life itself; into the house they must go and hide. It was a fact that Mister Flinders (was he reluctant to come home?) had forgotten his key; that Missis Flinders must delve under the white clothes in her suit-case and find hers; that Mr Strite, not yet satisfied that his charges were safe, sat watchful and waiting in the front seat of his cab. Then the door gave. Then Miles, bracing it with his foot, held out his hand to Margaret. Then Mr Strite came rushing up the steps (something had told him his help would be needed again!), rushing up the steps with the basket of fruit hanging on his arm, held out from his body as though what was the likes of him doing holding a woman's basket just home from the hospital.

"You've forgotten your fruit, Missis!"

Weakly they glared at the fruit come to pursue them; come to follow them up the stairs to their empty rooms; but that was not fair: come, after all, to comfort them. "You must have a peach," Margaret said.

No, Mr Strite had never cared for peaches; the skin got in his teeth. "You must have an apple," Margaret said.

Well, no, he must be getting on uptown. A cigarette (he waved it, deprecated the smoke it blew in the lady's face) was good enough for him.

"But a pear, just a pear," said Margaret passionately.

Mr Strite wavered, standing on one foot. "Maybe he doesn't want any fruit," said Miles harshly.

"Not want any fruit!" cried Margaret gayly, indignantly. Not want any fruit?—ridiculous! Not want the fruit my poor Miles bought for his wife in the hospital? Three days I spent in the hospital, in a Maternity Home, and I produced, with the help of my husband, one basket of fruit (tied with ribbon, pink—for boys). Not want any of our fruit? I couldn't bear it, I couldn't bear it…

Mr Strite leaned over; put out a hand and gingerly selected a pear— "For luck," he said, managing an excellent American smile. They watched him trot down the steps to his cab, all the time holding his pear as though it were something he would put in a memory book. And still they stayed, because Margaret said foolishly, "Let's see him off"; because she was ashamed, suddenly, before Miles; as though she had cut her hair unbecomingly, as though she had wounded herself in some unsightly way—as though (summing up her thoughts as precisely, as decisively as though it had been done on an adding machine) she had stripped and revealed herself not as a woman at all, but as a creature who would not be a woman and could not be a man. And then they turned (for there was nothing else to stay for, and on the street and in the sun before Missis Salvemini's fluttering window-curtains they were ashamed as though they had been naked or dead)—and went in the door and heard it swing to, pause on its rubbery hinge, and finally click behind them.

References

Adashi, Eli Y., et al. 2022. The next two decades of mifepristone at FDA: History as destiny. *Contraception* 109: 1–7, https://doi.org/10.1016/j.contraception.2022.01.016.

Brodie, Janet Farrell. 1994. Contraception and Abortion in Nineteenth-Century America. Ithaca: Cornell University Press.

Brodie, Janet Farrell. 2002. Mifepristone in the Context of American Abortion History, *Women & Politics*, 24: 101–119. https://doi.org/10.1300/J014v24n03_06

Brookes, Barbara. 1988. *Abortion in England, 1900–1967*. London: Croom Helm.

Eig, Jonathan. 2014. *The Birth of the Pill: How Four Crusaders Reinvented Sex and Launched a Revolution*. New York: W. W. Norton & Company.

Ellertson, Charlotte. 1996. History and Efficacy of Emergency Contraception: Beyond Coca-Cola. *International Family Planning Perspectives* 22:52–56 https://doi.org/10.2307/2950731

Engelman, Peter C. 2011. *A History of the Birth Control Movement in America*. Santa Barbara: Praeger.

Gordon, Linda. 2002. *The Moral Property of Women: A History of Birth Control Politics in America*. Urbana: University of Illinois Press.

McLaren, Angus. 1990. *A History of Contraception: From Antiquity to the Present Day*. Oxford: Basil Blackwell.

Mohr, James C. 1978. Abortion in America: The Origins and Evolution of National Policy. New York: Oxford University Press.

Reilly, Philip. 1991. The Surgical Solution: A History of Involuntary Sterilization in the United States. Baltimore: Johns Hopkins University Press.

Roberts, Dorothy. 2016. Killing the Black Body: Race, Reproduction, and the Meaning of Liberty. New York: Vintage Books.

4

Breast & Gynecological Cancers

Introduction

Through much of history from ancient times into the early twentieth century, cancer was considered a woman's disease primarily because breast cancer was more easily diagnosed than other cancers. Even with twenty-first-century diagnostic tools, the World Health Organization's International Agency for Research on Cancer lists breast cancer as the most common cancer worldwide, representing 12.5% of all cases in 2020. Gynecological cancers—including cervical, uterine, ovarian, vulvar, and vaginal—combined to account for 7.7% of cases. When those numbers are limited to women patients, breast cancer represents the most common form of cancer (25.8%), and the combined gynecological cancers are second (16%) (Ferlay et al. 2020). Historically, cancers of the breast and the reproductive organs were referred to more broadly as "women's cancers," which is evident in popular literature about cancer through at least the 1950s (Gardner 2006, p. 17). These cancers have also been commonly associated with women's behaviors around reproduction, including whether and when they had children and whether or how long they nursed any children.[1]

---

[1] Certainly, people of all gender identities can have breast cancer. This form of cancer was not on the World Cancer Research Fund's chart of global cancer incidence in men, which lists the 27 most common. The American Cancer Society (2022) describes the incidence in men as "rare, accounting for less than 1% of breast cancer cases in the US."

History of Breast and Gynecological Cancer Diagnosis and Treatment

The history of cancer, particularly breast cancer, can be traced back to ancient Greece and Persia, as theories arose about what caused cancer and shaped the suggested treatments for it (Lerner 2001; Olson 2002). Through much of that time, cancer has been seen as a woman's disease, particularly because the position of breast cancer meant patients and doctors could see and feel a growth unlike tumors in the brain, stomach, uterus, or any other part of the human body. Cervical cancer was similarly considered more "external" in a way that made it easier to diagnose than internal cancers that were only confirmed postmortem (Moscucci 2016). This more external position also led to differences in treatment, with surgical removal of the tumor or the whole breast or cervix when possible, even if a patient was unlikely to survive such a procedure before antiseptic surgical practices and the availability of anesthesia. Approaches to treatment resulted from the varying theories about whether cancer was a local issue or a systemic one. Over the centuries, these views about the nature of cancer followed larger medical beliefs including Hippocrates's and Galen's humoral theory that suggested cancer came from an excess of black bile, which was the prevailing belief from the fifth century BCE through the seventeenth century.[2]

In the eighteenth and nineteenth centuries, medical debates reconsidered whether cancer was a local issue or a systematic one that impacted the entire body, which shaped the types of treatment available to and preferred by both doctors and their patients. In addition to humoral beliefs, some physicians associated breast cancer with a traumatic injury to the breast or the restrictive clothing worn by women or cervical cancer with scars from tears during childbirth. With the simultaneous rise of medical research in the mid-nineteenth century, "women with breast cancer became scientific objects as well as patients, subject to the whims of male physicians afflicted with gender biases and scientific detachment" (Olson 2002, p. 64). Such research led to the development of the radical mastectomy near the turn of the twentieth century, which was the primary treatment for decades. In the 1930s and 1940s, Geoffrey Keynes and Robert McWhirter discovered that a modified mastectomy followed by radiation had the same survival rates as the radical mastectomy with less physical impact on the bodies of women patients (pp. 89–92). For cervical cancer too, radiation "produced results comparable to those of surgery in

---

[2] Olson (2002) explains the slow demise of humoral theory and its impact on treatments for breast cancer, noting "By the 1760s, no physician with any self-respect offered black bile diagnoses" (29).

operable cases" while providing "an alternative to 'mutilating' gynecological surgery" (Moscucci 2016, p. 5). Around the same time, the development of chemotherapy expanded the possible treatment options, but the radical mastectomy was a frequent treatment through much of the twentieth century. And even with the scientific progress, "physicians were not much better in 1950 at curing breast cancer than they had been in 1900" (Olson 2002, p. 99). Even as breast cancer has become less of a death sentence, the treatment options have continued to bring together a combination of surgical and nonsurgical approaches to reach remission for many patients and extend survival rates for decades rather than months.

Regardless of the treatment approach or type of cancer, doctors have agreed on the importance of early diagnosis for centuries. Where early detection was recommended by individual doctors in their publications or in their direct interactions with patients, the twentieth century saw a concerted effort through national awareness campaigns and the development of diagnostic measures like George N. Papanicolaou's vaginal smear (now called a Pap smear) and breast self-examination and mammography. Early detection efforts have led to preventative approaches in the twenty-first century with testing for the genetic predisposition to cancer and the choice for some women to have prophylactic surgery.

The Rise of Radical Surgical Treatments

For centuries, many treatments relied on alternative nonsurgical approaches that included plasters and poultices with ingredients based on the provider's views about cancer. For those that believed in Galen's humoral theory, the compounds addressed the black bile associated with cancer, while others trained in chemistry often used otherwise poisonous combinations in measured doses in their attempt to find a universal cure for cancer. These nonsurgical treatments relied on a combination of traditional remedies and medical advances as they experimented with mercury, lead, blood transfusions, hemlock, electricity, and carbonic acid among other purported cures (Kaartinen 2016, pp. 27–35). Compression therapy in both the nineteenth and early twentieth century combined plasters and linen compresses with pressure from metal plates and rollers (Aronowitz 2007, p. 41). Other doctors experimented with injections of a serum like William Coley's attempts to "provok[e] immune reactions against cancer...with heat-killed bacteria" (p. 140). These treatments could reduce the size of tumors, but most patients still died from their cancer (p. 41).

Surgical techniques evolved in the early modern period, as German surgeons recommended mastectomies from the early seventeenth century and French surgeons did so by the turn of the eighteenth century. This time also saw many medical professionals including a grand tour of continental Europe as part of their training, which ensured that these practices spread to Britain and America as well (Olson 2002).[3] As humoral beliefs were fully replaced by other scientific theories, doctors considered cancer as a local disease that, if removed fully enough and early enough, could be cured. For breast cancer, doctors emphasized the importance of early diagnosis and treatment, though women's fears about the painful treatments led some to hide their symptoms for as long as possible. With gynecological cancers, their placement in the body meant that early diagnosis was rare, so doctors sought to treat any abnormal symptoms in the hopes of preventing cervical or uterine cancer from developing. For both forms of cancer, these treatments included not only surgery with a knife or scalpel but also cautery with hot irons or with caustic medicines.

From the eighteenth century, doctors across Europe recommended removal of more than the cancerous breast during a mastectomy, and by the middle of the nineteenth century, some were attempting an *en bloc* approach which removed the breast and surrounding muscle and lymph nodes without cutting the tumor. For many surgeons, though, such an extreme surgery was still too risky. Several key medical advances in the nineteenth century made possible the development of the radical mastectomy. First, doctors needed anesthesia to resolve the issue of performing a painful surgery on wide-awake patients or those sedated only with alcohol, which produced unstable results. The medical use of ether began in 1846 in an operation on a facial tumor and became connected with women's bodies because of its use during childbirth. Though anesthesia like ether or chloroform was not used widely until late in the nineteenth century, its availability helped to facilitate a move toward surgical treatments for many serious maladies. Another key advancement in this period followed the early nineteenth-century development of the microscope, which German doctor Rudolf Virchow used to initiate our modern understanding of pathology and cellular theory with a series of published papers in the 1840s. By noting differences in the cells of some tumors, Virchow offered surgeons the ability to distinguish between benign and malignant tumors and to make more informed decisions about treating cancer (Olson 2002). Finally,

---

[3] Based on these and other factors, Kaartinen (2016) confidently suggests "that surgical operations for breast cancers became more common" starting in the late seventeenth and early eighteenth centuries (p. 39).

the infections following an operation could be as risky as the surgery itself until advancements toward germ theory and antiseptic medical practices spread. Among other doctors across Europe, Louis Pasteur's analysis of microbes under a microscope and work on treating postpartum infections and Joseph Lister's 1867 *Antiseptic Principle of the Practice of Surgery* led to the eventual changes to surgical practices that would reduce deadly infections.

These advances paved the way for William Stewart Halsted to develop and encourage the widespread use of the radical mastectomy, an operation used in the treatment of breast cancer that removed "the cancerous breast, nearby lymph nodes, and the two chest wall muscles on the affected side" in a single piece (Lerner 2001, p. 4). Halsted's medical theories clearly depended on German predecessors, among other continental influences, as he visited and learned from doctors treating breast cancer throughout Europe. After Halsted presented the procedure in the final decades of the nineteenth century, the procedure came to be known as the Halsted radical mastectomy and was the preferred treatment by many doctors through much of the twentieth century.

Similarly, to treat gynecological cancers in the second half of the nineteenth century, doctors explored surgical treatment options though long-term survival after the operation was still rare. Surgeons split between those that preferred a vaginal hysterectomy, which removed the cervix and the lower part of uterus, and those that followed Halsted's approach and developed a radical abdominal hysterectomy, which removed "the uterus, part of the vagina, ovaries, fallopian tubes, and abdominal lymph nodes" (Löwy 2011, p. 41).

By the 1940s and 1950s, some surgeons expanded the radical operations into superradical ones that removed even more of the flesh or organs near the cancerous parts. For breast cancer, this could be "interscapulothoracic ('forequarter') amputations, which entailed separation of the clavicle (collarbone), scapula (shoulder blade), and an arm." When "cervical, uterine, or ovarian cancers involved multiple pelvic organs or were otherwise untreatable," superradical operations removed "not only the woman's gynecological organs, but also the bladder and rectum" resulting in the patient "permanently pass[ing] both their stool and urine" into a colostomy bag (Lerner 2001, pp. 72–73). Overall, forms of radical surgical treatments for cancer continued to be popular in the medical profession and expected by patients well into the 1960s and 1970s.

The Fall of Radical Surgical Treatments

Though many patients had feared a radical operation to treat their cancer for decades, the mid-twentieth century brought support from surgeons who "argue[d] that smaller operations could often achieve as much as larger procedures, while causing many fewer physical and psychological effects" (Lerner 2001, p. 64). These doctors suggested a modified radical mastectomy that removed a much smaller portion of the pectoral muscle, a simple mastectomy that removed the breast but not the lymph nodes, or a lumpectomy that removed the cancerous tumor along with a small amount of surrounding tissue. Similarly, for gynecological cancers, options included a modified radical hysterectomy that removed less of the vagina and tissues around the uterus, a simple hysterectomy that removed the uterus and cervix typically leaving the ovaries and fallopian tubes, or a trachelectomy that removed the cervix and the upper part of the vagina but allowed patients to retain their ability to carry a pregnancy. After research in the 1930s and 1940s developed tools and procedures for chemical treatments, some doctors followed these less-invasive operations with radiotherapy or chemotherapy. Beginning in the 1950s, the wide range of treatment options were studied with randomized controlled trials, which prevented surgeons from exaggerating claims about the efficacy of their preferred treatment. Many doctors turned away from the more radical operations as the longer-term results like ten-year survival rates were reported and medicine and society changed in other ways.

Surgical treatments also fell out of favor as the women's rights movement and second-wave feminism changed medicine by empowering women to pursue careers in medicine and to speak out about their bodies and their healthcare. Though "in the United States the ratio of women doctors stagnated at around 5 percent until the 1960s" and was just double that in Great Britain, numbers in both countries slowly but steadily increased from there; by 1985, 14 percent of physicians in the United States were women (Morantz-Sanchez 2000, p. xxi, ix). The lived experiences of many women doctors gave them the empathy needed to rethink the disfiguring and disabling radical treatments. Around the same time, feminist activists worked together to claim agency over their bodies and their medical treatment. As publications like *Our Bodies, Ourselves* (1971) from the Boston Women's Health Book Collective connected the feminist movement with women's health, an increasing number of famous women publicly shared their own experiences with cancer and resisting the still-standard radical operations. As cancer and women's health became less taboo, coverage of the topic in periodicals brought awareness to the general public with more articles on women's cancers published per year and more focus on patient rights.[4] Ellen Leopold (1999) directly connects women's "growing awareness of the overuse of hysterectomies" for minor concerns with a larger issue of mistrusting doctors who could extend a woman's consent mid-surgery to remove more of a woman's breast or reproductive organs than she expected (205–206). Also, a patient's power over her own body extended to the option for reconstructive surgery following a mastectomy. A radical mastectomy created a body unable to support breast reconstruction, and thus took choice away from the patient a central concern for women of this period. All of these factors combined to give women patients more of a voice in their treatments and the opportunity to question the necessity of radical and super-radical operations.

Psychological Effects of Breast and Gynecological Cancer and Treatments

Throughout this history of approaches to breast and gynecological cancers and the evolutions in treatment options, cancer has consistently caused negative psychological effects for patients. For any life-threatening or terminal illness, diagnosis alone is a significant source of trauma, but in many cases, the treatment options only compound their distress. Until the late nineteenth century, women endured surgery without anesthesia and suffered intense pain from post-surgical infections, and they rarely received reliable pain medication for the suffering caused by alternative treatments that relied on compresses and caustics to reduce the size of tumors. All treatment options, surgical or not, were (and generally still are) accompanied by side effects that could be uncomfortable at best and debilitating at worst. Even the promise of a "cure" was far from permanent, as many doctors used the word to describe a patient living for several years after treatment. Halsted used three years as his benchmark, a span which had expanded to five years by the 1920s (Lerner 2001).

Fear around this experience of diagnosis and treatment as well as the expectation of eventual death from cancer led many women to conceal their symptoms for as long as possible. Additionally, consulting with a doctor represented the end of a patient's autonomy as she submitted to the expertise of medical

---

[4] According to Montini and Ruzek (1989), the average number of magazine articles on breast cancer published per year increased and from 4 in the late 1960s to 20 from 1974 through 1984. In the 1970s, the focus on patient rights appeared in one in four articles on breast cancer (13).

professionals for treatment. Through the nineteenth century, patients feared being advised to undergo surgery at all, but even after surgery was less medically risky in the mid-twentieth century, the absence of informed consent meant a woman could go under anesthesia uncertain of what the full procedure would include. Surgeons would begin with a biopsy and decide whether to continue with a radical mastectomy while the patient was on the operating table. Activists in the 1970s fought for informed consent with language that echoed that of the pro-choice movement, working toward a two-step procedure that separated the biopsy from the treatment and allowed a patient to understand her diagnosis before considering treatment options. Once a woman underwent surgical treatment for either breast or gynecological cancers, further psychological effects resulted from damage to or complete loss of the body parts most closely associated with femininity. Removal of the breast (or more with a radical surgery) could leave a woman visibly disfigured with further challenges in using prosthetic materials or having breast reconstruction. Treatments for gynecological cancers could cause fertility loss or the inability to carry a pregnancy in addition to hormonal side effects. The psychological effects of these cancers from the moment a patient felt concern about a symptom through the aftermath of her treatment cannot be understated.

Cultural Shifts and the Rise of the Cancer Narrative

Until the mid-twentieth century, most stories about women's experiences with cancer are included only in their letters and diaries, in the memoirs written by their family and friends, or in fictional representations. Since then, however, several factors have led to the publication of more cancer narratives, including widespread marketing around cancer awareness and prevention along with the destigmatization of facing cancer and talking about bodies and illnesses. In addition to advice books and articles offering women information about cancer symptoms and treatments, magazines like *Good Housekeeping*, *Ladies Home Journal*, *Ebony*, and *Essence* printed stories from average people who faced cancer and included "an undercurrent that suggested the urgent need to break the silence about discussing breast cancer in public places" (Knopf-Newman 2004, p. 19). Though many of these narratives show women following dominant medical advice about treatment, another central message is how the process of narrating one's experience is also therapeutic in dealing with the trauma.

In the early 1970s, famous and well-connected women publicly shared their experiences with breast cancer, raising awareness about the disease and the options for treatment. For example, when former child actor Shirley Temple Black announced her cancer in 1973, she wrote in *McCall's* magazine that she believed women should be able to consent to the extent of surgical treatment done to their bodies, famously saying after her own research into her treatment options, "The doctor can make the incision; I'll make the decision." The next year, First Lady Betty Ford's modified radical mastectomy was shared in a press conference and followed by intimate photos of the President and First Lady in her hospital suite. Just three weeks later, Nelson Rockefeller announced in a press conference that his wife Happy was undergoing a radical mastectomy. In 1976, singer and young mother Minnie Riperton shared her breast cancer diagnosis on *The Tonight Show* after undergoing a radical mastectomy.

The decades since have seen such an explosion of narratives that scholars have defined their qualities as a genre and analyzed the work of counternarratives. Thomas Couser (1997) suggests that, though breast cancer narratives are "conditioned by the physical manifestations of the disease and the medical protocols of treatment," they are ultimately "women's responses to the disease, individually and collectively" (p. 37). Because he focuses on the women patients facing breast cancer, Couser describes the breast cancer narrative as "an autobiographical… subgenre" that emerged in the 1970s and 1980s (p. 39). Similarly, Mary K. DeShazer (2013) uses the term *mammographies* to signify not only the technological and diagnostic tool but also "the documentary imperative that drives [women patients'] written and visual mappings of the breast cancer experience" (p. 2). Emilia Nielsen (2019) introduces counternarratives that "resist standardized cancer stories of hope and courage…because, for many women, a breast cancer diagnosis is fraught with the conflicting emotions of anxiety, anger, and sadness" (p. 3). Though these analyses focus on breast cancer, their observations also apply to narratives about gynecological cancers, even if those books may receive less attention.

Themes and Topics in Selections

Across the texts presented in this chapter, several key ideas recur and offer the opportunity for comparison.

Hiding Cancer and Fear of Surgical Treatment

The psychological effects described above led many women to conceal from their doctors and their family and friends the discovery of cancer symptoms. Additionally, through much of history, the surgeons who could treat cancers were not only men but often unfamiliar ones. A local doctor who treated other illnesses in the family and might have delivered their babies rarely had the experience or training to treat cancer, so if a woman's doctor suspected cancer, he would likely refer her to another doctor. This resulted in many women not consulting a doctor at all until the cancer was more advanced and thus more difficult to treat.

Nearly every selection in this chapter acknowledges this reality of cancer before the 1950s, as both real and fictional women delay consultation about concerning symptoms and seek alternative treatments or otherwise try to avoid surgery. Conversely, most doctors writing the medical advice texts selected here remind women of the importance of seeing a doctor as quickly as possible in order to begin treatment.

Risks of Some Alternative Treatments

Women sought out the alternative treatments described above for two primary reasons. First, the fear of an operation—particularly one before anesthesia or antiseptic surgical practices—made nonsurgical options appealing. Also, for women afraid of the stigma associated with a cancer diagnosis, avoiding a mastectomy offered the ability to keep their condition secret from others.

Alternative medicine as a form of manipulation appears in Tynan's *The House on the Bogs*, where the treatment promoted is by a maid and not someone in the established medical field. Gosse's narrative of his wife's experiences with alternative treatments is, in part, meant to warn others of the dangers associated with this kind of treatment. Additionally, Dufferin's journal mentions ignoring a friend's advice about consulting such a practitioner, while several of the mainstream doctors warn women readers against being manipulated, including Kellogg and the physician contributing to the *Englishwoman's Review*.

Class in Treatment Options

For many women patients, their treatment options and decisions were driven by their social class. Through the nineteenth century, doctors treated wealthier patients in their homes, reducing the risk of infection and ensuring some level of privacy. In that time, hospitals were primarily used by the poor, as many patients relied on charity medical care from these institutions or the generosity of doctors.

The experience of poverty on the patient's treatment options appears in Brown's "Rab and His Friends" and Tynan's "Willie." More privileged patients are included in Smith's and, Burney's accounts of their mastectomies, and Tynan's *The House on the Bogs*. Gosse's account of his wife's treatment offers a middle-class experience, as the family had access to the best doctors but felt financial strain while pursuing treatment.

"Some Account of a Pamphlet Lately Published" (1761)

Introduction

This essay reviews a pamphlet by Dr. John Andree, in which he questions the claims of Viennese doctor Anton von Störck's treatise about using hemlock to cure cancer. The anonymous reviewer quotes heavily from Andree's account of the negative effects of using hemlock, including a specific case of a woman with breast cancer. *The London Magazine*, which published this review, which published this review, was a monthly periodical that presented essays on a variety of topics meant to appeal to a broad but educated audience. This review of a specialized pamphlet represents an early attempt to enlighten patients and their families of the risks associated with some purported cures for cancer.

"Some Account of a Pamphlet Lately Published, Intitled Observations upon a Treatise on the Virtues of Hemlock, in the Cure of Cancers, Written by Dr. Storck, &c." (*The London Magazine, or Gentleman's Monthly Intelligencer*, July 1761)

The Doctor,[5] whose abilities, and whose veracity are too well known to be disputed, says, in his preface, "When Dr. Storck's treatise first appeared, recommending hemlock for the cure of cancers, seemingly with the sanction of the celebrated baron Van Swieten, M.D. physician to the empress of Germany; I was induced, among many others, to try the success of this important dis-

---

[5] Dr. John Andree, writer of the pamphlet being reviewed,

covery. But finding, upon repeated trials, my expectations frustrated, and hearing that others had met with no better success than myself; that some curable scirrhuses were, during the use of the extract of hemlock, instead of mending, brought to the state of deplorable cancers; I then examined Dr. Storck's cases again, with more attention, and thought them exceptionable in many material circumstances: Whereupon I determined not to remain silent in a matter so interesting to the publick, but to communicate my sentiments upon the several cases, produced by the doctor, with some observations of my own, as a caution to others, not to continue this remedy, when the tumour goes on increasing and assuming a cancerous aspect; as, I am sorry to say, has been too much the case, for fear of its coming to that degree of inveteracy, as to elude all physical and chirurgical assistance afterwards." In p. 3, the doctor says, after mentioning the affair of the *solanum lethale*,[6] "The physical alarm is lately raised again, by a tract imported from the imperial city of Vienna, published by the learned Dr. Storck, recommending the *cicuta*, or hemlock, for the cure of cancers, scirrhous and edematous tumours, malignant and fistulous ulcers and cataracts, The learned writer sets out with a description of the plant, and then names it *cicuta vulgaris*. Accordingly the common hemlock has been under trial here some time, but finding it did not answer the character given of it, I am informed, that application has been made to Dr. Storeck, who says it is the cicuta latifolia; which, it is rather wished than hoped, may prove more effectual than the other, it being much more of the same nature and quality."

...

"…A lady of consideration, who has been long of a bad habit of body, was afflicted with a cancer in her breast, which had ulcerated, but was extracted by Mr. Guy, an eminent surgeon of this city, (whose practice in that way has met with extraordinary success) about a year and a half before: And being subject to be frequently ailing from her childhood, on account of a bad humour she had about her, was advised to a kind of diet-drink, by an ignorant person; which was said to have done great cures in those disorders. This, at first, she thought, did her service; but soon after heated her to such a degree, that the issue in her arm discharged a great quantity of blood, and the breast that had been cured before, was very much inflamed.----She sent for an eminent physician in that state, who ordered her two *cicuta* pills every day. After the second dose, she was taken with a dizziness in the head, and sickness. On taking the fourth dose, she became paralytic all over, lost her speech, and for several days

---

[6] Solanum lethale is a poisonous plant also known as belladonna or deadly nightshade, which was used medically as an anesthetic or to relieve pain.

seemed to be dying. By the assistance of cardiac, &c. medicines, she recovered from this dangerous situation; but the menses she had upon her, when she began taking the pills, studently stopped, and she has but once since had an appearance of them, and that so little as scarce to be discerned. Several new complaints also arose, as a fever, pains in the back and loins, and abdomen; irregular stools, attended with griping, loss of appetite and of strength. In this fate I found her, and ordered her to be blooded, which had been objected to before, as thinking that to be the time when she used to have her menses. This gave her great relief, and by means of small doses of rhubarb, nervous and absorbent medicines, and a restorative diet, she became pretty well, expect a great nervous weakness, which I fear she will hardly get the better of. We observe in this case, that the *cicuta* is not *a very innocent remedy*, as the learned doctor seems to pronounce it to be; and that his second corollary, where he says, *that it does not hinder any of the natural functions of the body, the secretions and excretions,* stands upon no better a foundation. It, however, behoves my impartiality and candour, in the examination of this matter, to mention that this lady was of the age, when the menses commonly go off; but as she had had them hitherto regularly, their sudden obstruction may not be improperly imputed to the effect of the *cicuta*.——Emmenagogues she could not bear, because they heated her too much. Repeated small bleedings were indicated; but could not be administered, on account of her nervous weakness and impaired strength….Some advocates for this practice may pretend we have not had a fair trial of it, as the *cicuta* was gathered in autumn, when its virtue is greatly decayed; and, therefore, have still great expectations from it when gathered in its full vigour. We make no objection to it being tried fairly, provided it is not done to the prejudice of mankind; but as its power in the weak state seemed rather to be injurious to the human body, we should apprehend it may still be more dangerous when it is more vigorous. Although this must be left to time and experience to determine, we would have the publick reflect upon a passage in the *Memoires de Madame de Motteville*, where mention is made, that the *cicuta* was applied in France above a hundred years ago, to the breast of the queen of Lewis the thirteenth, for a cancer; of which at last she died. This was done for a fortnight together; but disordered her so much, that they were obliged to leave it off. Now if this plant had not been in some kind of reputation, in that disorder, it would, in all probability, not have been applied to so great a personage; and its disuse since, proves plainly, that no good was done with it at that time….And, to contribute my mite to this great work, I have, at this time, under trial, a medicine of no noxious quality, which seems to promise well for the cure of scirrhuses and, perhaps, may do service in cancers; but I forbear mentioning anything of its efficacy, till I have found it serviceable by sufficient experiments, and then intend to make it publickly known, for the service of the community.——We mention this chiefly to encourage others to fall into the same kind of pursuits of investigating the virtues of plants experimentally, not only for this, but various other diseases; especially, as some chymists vend many counterfeit medicines for the sake of greater lucre, by which the physician's expectations are frequently disappointed; and for which reason we shall be necessarily compelled to go to that shop, where no adulteration is practised, viz. the vegetable creation, which never varies; wherein, we apprehend, the sovereign remedy for the cancer may be found; chymical preparations, and ponderous medicines, being experienced hitherto to be inefficacious."…The following hint, in regard to uterine fluxes, &c. may be of the utmost service, and eminently displays the skill and humanity of the worthy author. "It cannot be thought a wide digression, if we throw in here a practical observation, of great consequence to the fair sex; which is, that as they are liable to immoderate fluxes, upon this[7] and many other occasions, they should not be treated with restringent or styptic medicines, because these are apt to occasion scirrhuses in the womb, ovary, or dropsy of the uterus, ovary, &c. but with alternatives agglutinating and corroborating remedies; which effect a safe cure, not followed by any bad consequences; and hope this intimation will save the lives of many valuable women. The same observation and treatment hold good with regard to the piles in both sexes…."

The Woman of Letters, or The History of Miss Fanny Belton by Maria Smyth (1783)

Introduction

In this epistolary novel, Fanny Belton is a clergyman's daughter seeking work in London when her misery is balanced with an encounter with Mrs. Perry, a young mother dying from breast cancer. Mrs. Perry represents a common trope in such narratives: a pious woman who becomes increasingly selfless and devout in the face of the compounding difficulty of her illness and suffering. In this case, the characters believe Mrs. Perry's cancer was caused by an injury to her breast, an idea that appears in other texts from this period, including Edgeworth's *Belinda*.

---

[7] Original Note: *the menses.*

Excerpts from Letter XVI

I was much affected to day by the following scene of wretchedness.

...

My heart, you know, my Lucy, is ever open to a tale of woe.—I heard the above sad story with great attention and pity.

"Pray, madam," said, I, "what is her disorder?"

"A cancer in her breast," she replied, "confirm'd cancer,—which must inevitably be her end in a very few months.—But her fortitude, her resignation is beyond imagination; and were it not for the support of the religion, she never, I am convinced, could endure what she does.—I call'd into her room yesterday morning, and for the first time, saw her weeping."—"I am ashamed of these tears, Madam," (said she, forcing a sweet languid smile) "but my little Billy, here, has been telling me I shall not die."—"No, my poor mama shall not die—shall she, Mrs. Williams," (said the pretty fellow) "for what she's such a little baby, as sister Sally do, and I do, without her?"

The wretched mother cast her eyes to heaven! and with a silent, earnest address, seem'd, to implore its aid for her precious children.———"When I am gone," said she, "my dear, you will have a *friend* that will never forsake you."—"But shall I indeed?"—said the sweet innocent.

"Heavens!" said I, "good madam, who, or what is this poor woman?—Is she young?"

"By what I can find," she replied, "she has been genteely bred, and well-educated; but unfortunately has highly disoblig'd her friends by marriage.—Her husband, I understand, is the most vile wretch, and has left her absolutely to starve with these poor children—the youngest not a year old.—The brutality of her husband has been the cause of this dreadful malady in her breast; a cruel blow occasioned it."

Good Mrs. Barlow has had a surgeon sense for her to look at the cancer, whose opinion is, it is absolutely incurable. He says, she may languish on a few months longer, and that's the utmost that can be expected.

Poor young creature! She is, it seems, about twenty-two years of age.

"Think, Miss Belton." continued Mrs. Williams, "what must be the amazing industry of this unhappy woman, who, in the midst of the most excruciating pains of this shocking disease, yet endeavours to support her little ones by the labor of her hands! her ingenious employment is making artificial flowers, which she sells to the shops.—On her first coming to my house, now two months since, she used to crawl out herself to dispose of them, but now, as her disease is daily getting ground, she is not able.

...

What a scene I have just been witness to!—I can say with Shakespear's Miranda, "that the *very virtue* of compassion, is awaken'd in my breast."

My good landlady and I have been to see the above-mention'd poor industrious wretch. On our entering her little garret, Mrs. Williams said, "I have brought you, Mrs. Perry, a young lady to look at your ingenious manufactory. "I turn'd my head and saw, sitting up in her bed, supported by bolsters, an amiable young woman—pale—and emaciated.—"Want, *staring* in her haggard eye;"—busily employ'd in making a very beautiful carnation.—On one side, on a small pillow, lay, in a sweet sleep, a little infant,—and on the other, a bible,—and before her stood, a large band-box, with a great variety of curious artificial flowers. "How do you to day," (ask'd Mrs. Williams) "are you a little easier than you were yesterday?"

"I thank, heaven," answer'd the patient sufferer, "I have had a tolerable night for *me*, madam"—looking up with a sweet smile.

Letters Relating to Abigail Adams Smith's Breast Cancer (1811)

Introduction

In 1811, Abigail Adams Smith, adult daughter of the second President of the United States John Adams, was diagnosed with breast cancer and endured a mastectomy. In the collection of letters printed here, Abigail Smith Adams informs her daughter's husband William Stephens Smith of the prognosis from several doctors in Boston. Abigail Adams Smith writes to Benjamin Rush, her father's trusted confidant, for a second opinion. Rather than replying directly to Smith, Rush responds to her father, strongly recommending a mastectomy and suggesting that John and Abigail Adams should gently inform their daughter. Finally, John Adams reports to Rush the details of the operation and his hope for his daughter's recovery. Smith lived nearly two years after the mastectomy, though she suffered pain as the cancer had metastasized.

From Abigail Smith Adams to William Stephens Smith

Quincy August 28th 1811
    My Dear Sir

your Letter of August 12th I received in the absence of Mrs Smith, who was upon a visit to mrs Guild, and therefore I could not communicate it to her; she past Several days, in Boston at Dr welch's, and as I had requested Dr warren was consulted in conjunction with Dr Welch upon her complaint, and their opinion was Similar to Dr Holbrook's who is a Skilfull physician, and practises in our Family. Dr Tufts alone varies in some measure from them, he is at a loss as to its natures; but the result is by no means to do any thing to worry or irritate the part, by no means to [...] it. would it not be best having advised with Surgeons and Physicians, to follow their advice? She is not taking even the hemlock pills—a Lady of my acquaintance labourd under a similar Tumour and was advised to have it removed, but upon a consultation with a Gentleman of the profession, he prevaild upon her to defer it for a time. She did so and lived to the Age of 82 without any further trouble from it—I know it will be a Source of anxiety to herself, and Friends. I pray that it may never be more So—

...

I am dear Sir with Sentiments / of Love and affection, / your Mother
A Adams

From Abigail Adams Smith to Benjamin Rush

Quincy [*12*] Septr 1811

you will I hope pardon the Liberty I have taken to address myself to you Sir upon a Subject which has become very interesting to myself. since I have been on a visit to my Parents, I have met with a volume of your Medical inquiries, in which are containd some observations upon the use of Arsenic in the cure of Cancers and schirrous complaints—about May 1810 I first perceived a hardness in my right Breast just above the nipple which occasioned me an uneasy sensation, like a burning sometimes an itching & at time a deep darting pain through the Breast, but without any discolouration at all. it has continued to Contract and the Breast has become much smaller than it was. the tumor appears now about the size of a Cap and does not appear to adhere but to be loose—I applied to a Physician and he recommended me to apply a Plaister of the cicuta which I did and kept it on several weeks but did not find any good affect from it it appeard to me to increase the uneasiness I therefore took it off. I have also taken a considerable of cicuta in Pills, but I thought they produced a heaviness in my head & have for some time discontinued them I came to since I have been here I have consulted several Physicians upon the Subject they have all advised me not to make any outward application to it—and as it has not affected the State of my health they do not recommend me to use any medicine—Still I am uneasy upon the Subject—for I think I observe it becoming harder and a little redness at times on the skin Dr Warren who has seen it told me that in its present state he would not advise me to do anything for it but if it should enflame I had better apply for surgical aid—this is a remedy that I dont know in any Event I could consent to submit to—certainly I should wish to try every other possible expedient first. and if in the course of your researches you should have discovered any thing that you find of use in this state of it, you would confer a great obligation upon me by communicating it

I am Sir with great respect your obedient Servant
A Smith

From Benjamin Rush to John Adams

Philadelphia Septr 20th: 1811

My dear Sir

I shall begin my letter by replying to your daughters. I prefer giving my Opinion & Advice in you her Case in this way. You and Mrs Adams may communicate it gradually and in such a manner as will be least apt to distress and alarm her.

After the experience of more than 50 years in cases similar to hers, I must protest agst: all local applications, and internal medicines for her relief. They now and then cure, but in 19 Cases Out of 20 in tumors in the *breast*, they do harm, or suspend the disease Until it passes beyond that time in which the only radical remedy is ineffectual. This remedy is the knife. From her account of the *Moving* state of the tumor it is now in a proper Situation for the Operation. Should She wait 'till it suppurates, or even inflames much, it may be too late. The pain of the Operation is much less than her fears represent it to be. I write this from experience having about two Years ago had a tumor of perhaps a larger Size cut out by Dr Physick from my Neck. I was surprized when the Doctor's assistant told me the operation was finished, and could not help saying After Cæsar when he had finished his conquests—"and is this All."—I repeat again—let there be no delay in flying to the knife. Her time of life—calls for expedition in this business, for tumors such as hers tend much more rapidly to cancers after 45, than in more early life. I sincerely sympathize with her, and with you and your dear Mrs Adams in this family Affliction, but it will be but for a few minutes if She submits to have it extirpated, & if not, it will probably be a Source of distress and pain to you all for years to come.

It shocks shocks me to think of the Consequences of procrastination in her case.

And now for your letter. …

Adieu—Ever yours

Benjn: Rush

From Abigail Smith Adams to William Stephens Smith

Quincy Septr 27th 1811

dear Sir

I yesterday received your Letter, and at the Same time, the President received the one inclosed from dr Rush which I think it my duty, altho a distressing and painfull one, to me, to communicate the contents to you by the earliest opportnty

you will See by the Letter, that Mrs Smith wrote her case to dr Rush, which her Father inclosed with a request that he would give his candid opinion. Mrs Smith was induced to write to the doctor from having Read in his Medical works a treatise upon this Subject. If the opperation is necessary as the dr States it to be, and as I fear it is, the Sooner it is done the better provided Mrs Smith can bring her mind, as I hope She will to consent to it. dr Warren of Boston is considerd the first Surgeon there; and has performed the greatest opperations. in this case he will no doubt call in Skillfull assistants. I hope mrs Smith will write her mind to you, and if She consents that you will be with her. every assistance and accommodation in the power of all her Friends here, will most Cheerfully and readily be given her, and I pray heaven to Support her, and her Friends through the painfull tryal. I am dear Sir / affectionatly yours

A Adams

PS we think Mr Charles Adams better—Mrs Smith will write by the next post. She must take time to weigh well what her duty is

From John Adams to Benjamin Rush

Quincy October 13. 1811

Dear Rush

Sobrius esto! Recollect your own Non Nobis!

Your Letter of the 20th. of September I communicated to Mrs Adams as you advised. Mrs Adams to her Daughter, After a reasonable Time for

Deliberation and Reflections the Heroine determined. The Mother and the Daughter went to Boston and consulted Dr Warren Junior, Dr Welsh, Dr Warren Junior having previously consulted Dr Tufts and Dr Holbrook. The Physicians and Surgeons all unanimously pronounced Dr Rush's opinion and Advice, to be exactly and perfectly in all Points agreable to their own, and the Plan was laid and the Catastrophy resolved.

On Tuesday the Eighth of October, a day memorable in my little Annals, the operation was performed in Presence of the two Dr Warrens, Dr Welsh and Dr Holbrook, by Dr Warren Senior. The operation was twenty five Minutes in performing, and the dressing an hour longer.

The Surgeons all agree that in no Instance did they ever witness a Patient of more Intrepidity than she exhibited through the whole Transaction.

They all affirm that the morbid substance is totally eradicated and nothing left but Flesh perfectly sound

They all Agree that the Probability of compleatt and ultimate success is as great as in any Instance that has fallen under their Experience.

Yesterday October 12 The Surgeons met again and dressed the Wound and unanimously declare it in as good a State as they could expect.

Had not your Letter overcome all her Scruples and Timidity, I believe she would have returned before now to Smiths Valley, which would have been to her The Valley of Jehoshaphat.

Oh! that a vaccine Inoculation could be discovered [...] for this opprobrium of Philosophy and Midicine, The Cancer, This Physical disgrace of human Nature!

Neither you nor I have much Superstition in our Natures or our Creeds. But neither of Us can refuse to acknowledge a Providence in this Instance. She accidentally as the world says read your Book wrote you a Letter, received your answer altered her Plan, postponed her Journey home, and as I sincerely hope and devoutly pray saved her Life.

I rejoice however still with trembling. I know the Uncertainty that still remains: and that our only ultimate Resource is Resignation.

We are all very sensible of our obligation to you, and pray you to accept our cordial Thanks

John Adams

From Benjamin Rush to John Adams

Philadelphia Octobr 18th: 1811
My dear old friend,

All my family rejoice with yours in the happy issue of the operation performed upon Mrs Smiths breast. The enclosed letter[8] is intended as an answer to her's to me, and to serve the further purpose of exciting in her a belief that her Cure will be radical & durable. I consider her as rescued from a premature grave.

…

Adieu my dear Sir. With love & congratulations to all your family I am ever yrs
Benjn: Rush

Account from Paris of a Terrible Operation by Frances Burney D'Arblay (1812)

Introduction

This account from British novelist Frances "Fanny" Burney D'Arblay about her mastectomy has become one of the most common breast cancer narratives written before the 1950s and is often used to represent more broadly the experience of breast cancer in the nineteenth century. In the letter from Paris to her family in London, Burney recounts months of events with detail on her full journey from discovering a lump through the gruesome details of her mastectomy to her eventual recovery. Burney's experience is unique in several ways. As the wife of an officer in Napoleon's army, Burney had access to French military surgeons who performed her mastectomy in her home. Because of Napoleonic Wars and her husband's military status, Burney was unable to leave France, and thus needed to write a letter to update and inform her concerned family who remained in England. Also, Burney lived a remarkable 29 years after her mastectomy in a time when such an operation often failed to prevent recurrence or extend the patient's life beyond a few years at the longest. This text directly reflects what is written in the manuscript version of the letter, so archaic spelling and minor errors have been preserved.

Account from Paris of a Terrible Operation—1812

P.S. I have promised my dearest Esther a Volume – & here it is: I am at this moment quite well – so are my Alexanders. Read, therefore, this narrative at

---

[8] In his edition to Rush's letters, Butterfield suggests the letter to Abigail Adams Smith could not be found.

your leisure, & without emotion – for all has ended happily. I will send the rest by the very first opportunity: I seize this present with eagerness – oh let none – none pass by that may being me a return! – I have no more yet written.

March 22.

1812

Separated as I have now so long—long been from my dearest Father—Brothers—Sisters—Nieces, and Native Friends, I would spare, at least, their kind hearts any grief for me but what they must inevitably feel in reflecting upon the sorrow of such absence to one so tenderly attached to all her first and for-ever so dear and regretted ties—nevertheless, if they should hear that I have been dangerously ill from any hand but my own, they might have doubts of my perfect recovery which my own alone can obviate. And how can I hope they will escape hearing what has reached Seville to the South, and Constantinople to the East? from both I have had messages—yet nothing could urge me to this communication till I heard that M. Boinville had written it to his Wife, without any precaution, because in ignorance of my plan of silence. Still I must hope it may never travel to my dearest Father—But to You, my beloved Esther, who, living more in the World, will surely hear it ere long, to you I will write the whole history, certain that, from the moment you know any evil has befallen me your kind kind heart will be constantly anxious to learn its extent and its circumstances, as well as its termination.

About August, in the year 1810, I began to by annoyed by a small pain in my breast, which went on augmenting from week to week, yet, being rather heavy than acute, without causing me any uneasiness with respect to consequences: Alas, "what was ignorance?" The most sympathising of Partners, however, was more disturbed: not a start, not a wry face, not a movement that indicated pain was unobserved, and he early conceived apprehensions to which I was a stranger. He pressed me to see some Surgeon; I revolted from the idea, and hoped, by care and warmth, to make all succour unnecessary. Thus passed some months, during which Madame de Maisonneuve, my particularly intimate friend, joined with M. d'Arblay to press me to consent to an examination. I thought their fears groundless, and could not make so great a conquest over my repugnance. I relate this false confidence, now, as a warning to my dear Esther—my Sisters and Nieces, should any similar sensations excite similar alarm.

M. d'Arblay now revealed his uneasiness to another of our kind friends, Mme de Tracy, who wrote to me a long and eloquent Letter upon the subject, that began to awaken very unpleasant surmizes: and a conference with her ensued, in which her urgency and representations, aided by her long experience of disease, and most miserable existence by art, subdued me, and, most painfully and reluctantly, I ceased to object, and M. d'Arblay summoned a physician—M. Bourdois? Maria will cry;—No, my dear Maria, I would not give your beau frere that trouble; not him, but Dr Jouart, the physician of Miss. Potts. Thinking but slightly of my statement, he gave me some directions that produced no fruit—on the contrary, I grew worse, and M. d'Arblay now would take no denial to my consulting M. Dubois, who had already attended and cured me in an abscess of which Maria, my dearest Esther, can give you the history.

M. Dubois, the most celebrated surgeon of France, was then appointed accoucheur to the Empress, and already lodged in the Tuilleries, and in constant attendance: but nothing could slacken the ardour of M. d'Arblay to obtain the first advice. Fortunately for his kind wishes, M. Dubois had retained a partial regard for me from the time of his former attendance, and, when applied to through a third person, he took the first moment of liberty, granted by a *promenade* taken by the Empress, to come to me. It was now I began to perceive my real danger, M. Dubois gave me a prescription to be pursued for a month, during which time he could not undertake to see me again, an pronounced nothing—but uttered so many charges to me to be tranquil, and to suffer no uneasiness, that I could not but suspect there was room for terrible inquietude.

My alarm was encreased by the non-appearance of M. d'Arblay after his departure. They had remained together some time in the Book room, and M. d'Arblay did not return—till, unable to bear the suspence, I begged him to come back. He, also, sought then to tranquilize me—but in words only; his looks were shocking! his features, his whole face displayed the bitterest woe. I had not, therefore, much difficulty in telling myself what he endeavoured not to tell me—that a small operation would be necessary to avert evil consequences!—Ah, my dearest Esther, for this I felt no courage—my dread and repugnance, from a thousand reasons *besides* the pain, almost shook my faculties, and, for some time, I was rather confounded and stupefied than affrighted.—Direful, however was the effect of this interview; the pains became quicker and more violent, and the hardness of the spot affected encreased. I took, but vainly, my proscription, and every symtom grew more serious.

At that time, M. de Narbonne spoke to M. d'Arblay of a Surgeon of great eminence, M. Larrey, who had cured a polonoise lady of his acquaintance of a similar malady; and, as my horror of an operation was insuperable, M. de Narbonne strongly recommended that I should have recourse to M. Larrey. I thankfully caught at any hope; and another friend of M. d'Arblay gave the same counsel instant, which other, M. Barbier Neuville, has an influence irresistible over this M. Larrey, to whom he wrote the most earnest injunction that he would use every exertion to rescue me from what I so much dreaded. M. Larrey came, though very unwillingly, and full of scruples concerning M. Dubois; nor would he give me his services till I wrote myself to state my affright at the delay of attendance occasioned by the present high office and royal confinement of M. Dubois, and requesting that I might be made over to M. Larrey. An answer such as might be expected arrived, and I was now put upon a new *regime*, and animated by fairest hopes.—

M. Larrey has proved one of the worthiest, most disinterested, and singularly excellent of men, endowed with real Genius in his profession, though with an ignorance of the World and its usages that induces a *naiveté* that leads those who do not see him thoroughly to think him not alone simple, but weak. They are mistaken; but his attention and thoughts having exclusively turned one way, he is hardly awake any other. His directions seemed all to succeed, for though I had still cruel seizures of terrible pain, the fits were shorter and more rare, and my spirits revived, and I went out almost daily, and quite daily received to my Apartment some friend or intimate acquaintance, contrarily to my usual mode of *sauvagerie*—and what friends I have found! what kind, consoling, zealous friends during all this painful period! In fine, I was much better, and every symptom of alarm abated. My good M. Larrey was enchanted, yet so anxious, that he forced me to see le Docteur Ribe, the first anatomist, he said, in France, from his own fear lest he was under any delusion, from the excess of his desire to save me. I was as rebellious to the first visit of this famous anatomist as Maria will tell you I had been to that of M. Dubois, so odious to me was this sort of process: however, I was obliged to submit: and M. Ribe confirmed our best hopes—

Here, my dearest Esther, I must grow brief, for my theme becomes less pleasant—Sundry circumstances, too long to detail, combined to counter-act all my flattering expectations, and all the skill, and all the cares of my assiduous and excellent Surgeon. The principal of these evils were—the death, broke to me by a newspaper! of the lovely and loved Princess Amelia—the illness of her venerated father[9]—and the sudden loss of my nearly adored—my Susan's nearly worshipped Mr Lock—which terrible calamity reached me in *a few lines* from Fanny Waddington, when I knew not of any illness or fear!—Oh my Esther, I must indeed be brief, for I am not yet strong enough for sorrow.—The good M. Larrey, when he came to me next after the last of these trials, was quite thrown into a consternation, so changed he found all for the

---

[9] King George III

worse—"Et qu'est il donc arrive?"[10] he cried, and presently, sadly, announced his hope of dissolving the hardness were nearly extinguished. M. Ribe was now again called in—but he only corroborated the terrible judgement; yet they allowed me to my pleadings some further essays, and the more easily as the weather was not propitious to any operation. My Exercise, at this time, though always useful and chearing, occasioned me great suffering in its conclusion, from mounting up three pair of stairs: my tenderest Partner, therefore, removed me to La Rue Mirmenil, where I began my Paris residence nearly 10 Years ago!—*quite* 10 next Month! Here we are *au premier*[11] —but alas—to no effect! once only have I yet descended the short flight of steps from which I had entertained new hopes.

A Physician was now called in, Dr Moreau, to hear if he could suggest any new means: but Dr Larrey had left him no resources untried. A formal consultation now was held, of Larrey, Ribe, and Moreau—and, in ftine, I was formally condemned to an operation by all Three. I was as much astonished as disappointed—for the poor breast was no where discoloured, and not much larger than its healthy neighbour. Yet I felt the evil to be deep, so deep, that I often thought if it could not be dissolved, it could only with life be extirpated. I called up, however, all the reason I possessed, or could assume, and told them that—if they saw no other alternative, I would not resist their opinion and experience—the good Dr Larrey, who, during his long attendance had conceived for me the warmest friendship, had now tears in his Eyes; from my dread he had expected resistance. He proposed again calling in M. Dubois. No, I told him, if I could not by himself be saved, I had no sort of hope elsewhere, and, if it must be, what I wanted in courage should be supplied by Confidence. The good man was now dissatisfied with himself, and declared that I ought to have the First and most eminent advice his Country could afford; "Vous êtes si considerée, Madame, said he, ici, que le public même sera mecontent si vous n'avez pas tout le secour que nous avons à vous offrir.—"[12] () Yet this modest man is premier chirurgien de la Garde Imperiale,[13] and had been lately created a Baron for his eminent services!—M. Dubois, he added, from his super-skill and experience, might yet, perhaps, suggest some cure. This conquered me quickly, ah—Send for him! Send for him! I cried—and Dr Moreau received the commission to consult with him.—

---

[10] "And so, what is going on?"
[11] On the first floor.
[12] "You are so esteemed here, Madam, that the public itself would be unhappy if you did not receive all the help that we have to offer.—"
[13] First Surgeon of the Imperial Guard of Napoleon I.

What an interval was this! Yet my poor M. d'Arblay was more to be pitied than myself, though he knew not the terrible idea I had internally annexed to the trial—but Oh what he suffered!—and with what exquisite tenderness he solaced all that I had to bear! My poor Alex I kept as much as possible, and as long, ignorant of my situation.—M. Dubois behaved extremely well, no pique intervened with the interest he had professed in my well-doing, and his conduct was manly and generous. It was difficult still to see him, but he appointed the earliest day in his power for a general and final consultation. I was informed of it only on the Same day, to avoid any useless agitation. He met here Drs Larrey, Ribe, and Moreau. The case, I saw, offered uncommon difficulties, or presented eminent danger, but the examination over, they desired to consult together. I left them—what an half hour I passed alone!—M. d'Arblay was at his office. Dr Larrey then came to summon me. He did not speak, but looked very like my dear Brother James, to whom he has a personal resemblance that has struck M. d'Arblay as well as myself. I came back, and took my seat, with what calmness I was able. All were silent, and Dr Larrey, I saw, hid himself nearly behind my Sofa. My heart beat fast: I saw all hope was over. I called upon them to speak. M. Dubois then, after a long and unintelligible harangue, from his own disturbance, pronounced my doom. I now saw it was inevitable, and abstained from any further effort. They received my formal consent, and retired to fix a day.

All hope of escaping this evil now at an end, I could only console or employ my Mind in considering how to render it less dreadful to M. d'Arblay. M. Dubois had pronounced "il faut s'attendre à souffrir, Je ne veux pas vous tromper—Vous Souffrirez—vous souffrirez *beaucoup!*—"[14] M. Ribe had *charged* me to cry! to withhold or restrain myself might have seriously bad consequences, he said. M. Moreau, in echoing this injunction, enquired whether I had cried or screamed at the birth of Alexander—Alas, I told him, it had not been possible to do otherwise; Oh then, he answered, there is no fear!—What terrible inferences were here to be drawn! I desired, therefore, that M. d'Arblay might be kept in ignorance of the day might be kept in ignorance of the day till the operation should be over. To this they agreed, except M. Larrey, with high approbation: M. Larrey looked dissentient, but was silent. M. Dubois protested he would not undertake to act, after what he had seen of the agitated spirits of M. d'Arblay if he were present: nor would he suffer me to know the time myself over night; I obtained with difficulty a promise of 4 hours warning, which were essential to me for sundry regulations.

---

[14] "You must expect to suffer, I do not want to deceive you—you will suffer—you will suffer *very much!*"

From this time, I assumed the best spirits in my power, *to meet the coming blow*;—and support my too sympathising Partner. They would let me make no preparations, refusing to inform me what would be necessary; I have known, since, that Mme de Tessé, an admirable old friend of M. d'Arblay, now mine, equally, and one of the first of her sex, in any country, for uncommon abilities, and nearly universal knowledge, had insisted upon sending me all that might be necessary, and of keeping me in ignorance. M. d'Arblay filled a Closet with Charpie, compresses, and bandages—All that to *me* was owned, as wanting, was an arm Chair and some Towels.—Many things, however, joined to the depth of my pains, assured me the business was not without danger. I therefore made my Will—unknown, to this moment, to M. d'Arblay, and entrusted it privately to M. La Tour Maubourg, without even letting my friend his Sister, Mme de Maisonneuve, share the secret. M. de Maubourg conveyed it for me to Maria's excellent M. Gillet, from whom M. de Maubourg brought me directions. As soon as I am able to go out I shall reveal this clandestine affair to M. d'Arblay—till then, if might still affect him. Mme de Maisonneuve desired to be present at the operation;—but I would not inflict such pain. Mme de Chastel belle soeur de Mme de Boinville, would also have sustained the shock; but I secured two Guards, one of whom is known to my two dear Charlottes, Mme Soubiren, portiere de l'Hotel Marengo: a very good Creature, who often amuses me by repeating "*ver. vell, Mawm;*" which she tells me she learnt of Charlotte the younger, whom she never names but with rapture, The other is a workman whom I have often employed. The kindnesses I received at this period would have made me for-ever love France, had I hitherto been hard enough of heart to hate it—but Mme d'Henin—the tenderness she shewed me surpasses all description. Twice she came to Paris from the Country, to see, watch and sit with me; there is nothing that can be suggested of use or comfort that she omitted. She loves me not only from her kind heart, but also from her love of Mrs. Lock, often, often, exclaiming "Ah! si votre Angelique amie étoit ici!—"[15] But I must force myself from these episodes, though my dearest Esther will not think them *de trop*.[16]

After sentence thus passed, I was in hourly expectation of a summons to execution; judge, then to my surprise to be suffered to on full 3 Weeks in the same state! M. Larrey from time to time visited me, but pronounced nothing, and was always melancholy. At length, M d'Arblay was told that he waited himself for a Summons! and that, a formal one, and in writing! *I* could not give one. A *consent* was my utmost effort. But poor M. d'Arblay wrote a desire

---

[15] "Ah! if your angelic friend were here!—"
[16] Too much.

that the operation, if necessary, might take place without further delay. In my own mind, I had all this time been persuaded there were hopes of a cure: why else, I thought, let me know my doom thus long? But here I must account for this apparently useless, and therefore cruel measure, though I only learnt it myself 2 months afterwards. M. Dubois had given his opinion that the evil was too far advanced for any remedy; that the cancer was already internally declared; that I was inevitably destined to that most frightful of deaths, and that an operation would but accelerate my dissolution. Poor M. Larrey was so deeply affected by this sentence, that—as he has lately told me, he regretted to his Soul ever having known me, and was upon the point of demanding a commission to the furthest end of France in order to force me into other hands. I had said, however, he remembered, once, that I would far rather suffer a quick end without, than a lingering life with this dreadfullest of maladies: he finally, therefore, considered it might be possible to save me by the trial, but that without it my case was desperate, and resolved to make the attempt. Nevertheless, the responsibility was too great to rest upon his own head entirely; and therefore he waited the formal summons.—

In fine, One morning—the last of September, 1811, while I was in Bed, and M. d'Arblay was arranging some papers for his office, I received a Letter written by M. de Lally to a Journalist, in vindication of the honoured memory of his Father against the assertions of Mme du Deffand. I read it aloud to My Alexanders, with tears of admiration and sympathy, and then sent it by Alex. to its excellent Author, as I had promised the preceding evening.

I then then dressed, aided, as usual for many months, by my maid, my right arm being condemned to total inaction; but not yet was the grand business over, when another Letter was delivered to me—another, indeed!—'twas from M. Larrey, to acquaint me that at 10 o'clock he should be with me, properly accompanied, and to exhort me to rely as much upon his sensibility & his prudence, as upon his dexterity and his experience; he charged to secure the absence of M. d'Arblay—and told me that the young Physician who would deliver me this *announce* would prepare for the operation, in which he must lend his aid: and also that it had been the decision of the consultation to allow me but two hours' notice.—judge, my Esther, if I read this unmoved!—yet I had to disguise my sensations and intentions from M. d'Arblay!

Dr Aumont, the Messenger and terrible Herald, was in waiting; M. d'Arblay stood by my bedside; I affected to be long reading the Note, to gain time for forming some plan, and such was my terror of involving M. d'Arblay in the unavailing wretchedness of witnessing what I must go through, that it conquered every other, and gave me the force to act as if I were directing some third person. The detail would be too *Wordy*, as James says, but the *wholesale* is—I called Alex to my Bedside, and sent him to inform M. Barbier Neuville, chef du division du Bureau de M. d'Arblay that *the moment was come*, and I entreated him to write a summons upon urgent business for M. d'Arblay and to detain him till all should be over. Speechless and appalled, off went Alex, and, as I have since heard, was forced to sit down and sob in executing his commission.

I then, by the maid, sent word to the young Dr Aumont that I could not be ready till one o'clock: and I finished my breakfast, and—not with much appetite, you will believe! forced down a crust of bread, and hurried off, under various pretences, M. d'Arblay. He was scarcely gone, when M Du Bois arrived: I renewed my request for one o'clock: the rest came; all were fain to consent to the delay, for I had an apartment to prepare for my banished Mate. This arrangement, and those for myself, occupied me completely. Two engaged nurses were out of the way—I had a bed, Curtains, and heaven knows what to prepare—but business was good for my nerves. I was obliged to quit my room to have it put in order—Dr Aumont would not leave the house; he remained in the Salon, folding linen!—He had demanded 4 or 5 old and fine left off under Garments—I glided to our Book Cabinet: sundry necessary works and orders filled up my time entirely till One O'clock, When all was ready—but Dr Moreau then arrived, with news that M. Dubois could not attend till three. Dr Aumont went away—and the Coast was clear. This, indeed, was a dreadful interval. I had no longer anything to do—I had only to think—Two Hours thus spent seemed never-ending.

I would fain have written to my dearest Father—to You, my Esther—to Charlotte James—Charles—Amelia Lock—but my arm prohibited me: I strolled to the Sallon—I saw it fitted with preparations, and I recoiled—But I soon returned; to what effect disguise from myself what I must so soon know?—yet the sight of the immense quantity of bandages, compresses, sponges, Lint—made me a little sick:—I walked backwards and forwards till I quieted all emotion, and became, by degrees, nearly stupid - torpid, without sentiment or consciousness;—and thus I remained till the Clock struck three.

A sudden spirit of exertion then returned,—I defied my poor arm, no longer worth sparing, and took my long banished pen to write a few words to M. d'Arblay— and a few more for Alex, in case of a fatal result. These short billets I could only deposit safely, when the Cabriolets—one—two—three—four—succeeded rapidly to each other in stopping at the door. Dr Moreau instantly entered my room, to see if I were alive. He gave me a wine cordial, and went to the Sallon. I rang for my Maid and Nurses,—but before I could speak to them, my room, without previous message, was entered by 7 Men in black, Dr Larry, M. Dubois, Dr Moreau, Dr Aumont, Dr Ribe, and a pupil of Dr Larry, and another of M. Dubois. I was now awakened from my stupor—and by a sort of indignation—Why so many? and without leave?—But I could not utter a syllable.

M. Dubois acted as Commander in Chief. Dr Larry kept out of sight; M. Dubois ordered a Bed stead into the middle of the room. Astonished, I turned to Dr Larry, who had promised that an Arm Chair would suffice; but he hung his head, & would not look at me. Two *old mattrasses* M. Dubois then demanded, and an old Sheet. I now began to tremble violently, more with distaste and horror of the preparations even than of the pain. These arranged to his liking, he desired me to mount the Bed stead. I stood suspended, for a moment, whether I should not abruptly escape—I looked at the door, the windows—I felt desperate—but it was only for a moment, my reason then took the command, and my fears and feelings struggled vainly against it. I called to my maid—she was crying, and the two Nurses stood, transfixed, at the door. "Let those women all go!" cried M. Dubois. This order recovered me my Voice—"No," I cried, "let them stay! *qu'elles restent*!"[17]

This occasioned a little dispute, that re-animated me—The Maid, however, and one of the nurses ran off—I charged the other to approach, and she obeyed. M. Dubois now tried to issue his commands *en militaire*, but I resisted all that were resistable—I was compelled, however, to submit to taking off my long robe de Chambre, which I had meant to retain—Ah, then, how did I think of My Sisters!—not one, at so dreadful an instant, at hand, to protect—adjust—guard me—I regretted that I had refused Mme de Maisonneuve—Mme Chastel—no one upon whom I could rely—my departed Angel!—how did I think of her!—how did I long—long for my Esther—my Charlotte!—

My distress distress was, I suppose, apparent, though not my Wishes, for M. Dubois himself now softened, and spoke soothingly. "Can *You*," I cried, "feel for an operation that, to *You*, must seem so trivial?"—"Trivial?" he repeated—taking up a bit of paper, which he tore, unconsciously, into a million of pieces, "*oui—c'est peu de chose—mais*"[18] — he stammered, and could not go on. No one else attempted to speak, but I was softened myself, when I saw even M. Dubois grow agitated, while Dr Larry kept always aloof, yet a glance shewed me he was pale as ashes. I knew not, positively, then, the immediate danger, but every thing convinced me danger was hovering about me,

---

[17] "*Let them stay!*"
[18] "*Yes—it's a small thing—but*"—

and that this experiment could alone save me from its laws. I mounted, therefore, unbidden, the Bed stead—and M. Dubois placed me upon the mattrass, and spread a cambric handkerchief upon my face.

It was transparent, however, and I saw, through it, that the Bedstead was instantly surrounded by the 7 men and my nurse. I refused to be held; but when, Bright through the cambric, I saw the glitter of polished Steel—I closed my Eyes. I would not trust to convulsive fear the sight of the terrible incision. A silence the most profound ensued, which lasted for some minutes, during which, I imagine, they took their orders by signs, and made their examination—Oh what a horrible suspension!—I did not breathe—and M. Dubois tried vainly to find any pulse. This pause, at length, was broken by Dr Larry, who, in a voice of solemn melancholy, said "Qui me tiendra ce sein?[19]—"

No one answered; at least not verbally; but this aroused me from my passively submissive state, for I feared they imagined the whole breast infected—feared it too justly,—for, again through the Cambric, I saw the hand of M. Dubois held up, while his forefinger first described a straight line from top to bottom of the breast, secondly a Cross, and thirdly a circle; intimating that the Whole was to be taken off. Excited by this idea, I started up, threw off my veil, and, in answer to the demand "Qui me tiendra ce sein?" cried "C'est moi, Monsieur!"[20] and I held My hand under it, and explained the nature of my sufferings, which all sprang from one point, though they darted into every part. I was heard attentively, but in utter silence, and M. Dubois then replaced me as before, and, as before, spread my veil over my face. How vain, alas, my representation! immediately again I saw the fatal finger describe the Cross—and the circle—Hopeless, then, desperate, and self-given up, I closed once more my Eyes, relinquishing all watching, all resistance, all interference, and sadly resolute to be wholly resigned.

My dearest Esther,—and all my dears to whom she communicates this doleful ditty, will rejoice to hear that this resolution once taken, was firmly adhered to, in defiance of a terror that surpasses all description, and the most torturing pain. Yet—when the dreadful steel was plunged into the breast—cutting through veins—arteries—flesh—nerves—I needed no injunctions not to restrain my cries. I began a scream that lasted unintermittingly during the whole time of the incision—and I almost marvel that it rings not in my Ears still! so excruciating was the agony. When the wound was made, and the instrument was withdrawn, the pain seemed undiminished, for the air that

---

[19] Who will hold this breast for me?—
[20] "I will, Sir!"

suddenly rushed into those delicate parts felt like a mass of minute but sharp and forked poniards, that were tearing the edges of the wound—but when again I felt the instrument—describing a curve—cutting against the grain, if I may so say, while the flesh resisted in a manner so forcible as to oppose and tire the hand of the operator, who was forced to change from the right to the left—then, indeed, I thought I must have expired.

I attempted no more to open my Eyes,—they felt as if hermetically shut, and so firmly closed, that the Eyelids seemed indented into the Cheeks. The instrument this second time withdrawn, I concluded the operation over—Oh no! presently the terrible cutting was renewed—and worse than ever, to separate the bottom, the foundation of this dreadful gland from the parts to which it adhered—Again all description would be baffled—yet again all was not over,—Dr Larry rested but his own hand, and—Oh Heaven!—I then felt the Knife rackling against the breast bone—scraping it!—This performed, while I yet remained in utterly speechless torture, I heard the Voice of Mr Larry,—(all others guarded a dead silence) in a tone nearly tragic, desire everyone present to pronounce if anything more remained to be done; The general voice was Yes,—but the finger of Mr Dubois—which I literally *felt* elevated over the wound, though I saw nothing, and though he touched nothing, so indescribably sensitive was the spot—pointed to some further requisition—and again began the scraping!—and, after this, Dr Moreau thought he discerned a peccant attom (fragments of diseased [peccant] breast tissue)—and still, and still, M. Dubois demanded attom after attom.—

My dearest Esther, not for days, not for Weeks, but for Months I could not speak of this terrible business without nearly again going through it! I could not *think* of it with impunity! I was sick, I was disordered by a single question—even now, 9 months after it is over, I have a headache from going on with the account! and this miserable account, which I began 3 Months ago, at least, I dare not revise, nor read, the recollection is still so painful.

To conclude, the evil was so profound, the case so delicate, and the precautions necessary for preventing a return so numerous, that the operation, including the treatment and the dressing, lasted 20 minutes! a time, for sufferings so acute, that was hardly supportable—However, I bore it with all the courage I could exert, and never moved, nor stopt them, nor resisted, nor remonstrated, nor spoke - except once or twice, during the dressings, to say "Ah Messieurs! que je vous plains!—" ("Ah Sirs! how I pity you!—") for indeed I was sensible to the feeling concern with which they all saw what I endured, though my speech was principally—*very* principally meant for Dr Larry. Except this, I uttered not a syllable, save, when so often they re-commenced, calling out "Avertissez moi, Messieurs! Avertissez moi!—" ("Warn me, Sirs!

warn me!") Twice, I believe, I fainted; at least, I have two total chasms in my memory of this transaction, that impede my tying together what passed.

When all was done, and they lifted me up that I might be put to bed, my strength was so totally annihilated, that I was obliged to be carried, and could not even sustain my hands and arms, which hung as if I had been lifeless; while my face, as the Nurse has told me, was utterly colourless. This removal made me open my Eyes—and I then saw my good Dr Larry, pale nearly as myself, his face streaked with blood, its expression depicting grief, apprehension, and almost horrour.

When I was in bed,—my poor M. d'Arblay—who ought to write you himself his own history of this Morning—was called to me—and afterwards our Alex.— No! No my dearest & ever more dear friends, I shall not make a fruitfull attempt. No language could convey what I felt in the deadly course of these seven hours. Nevertheless, every one *of you my dearest dearest friends*, can guess, must even know it. Alexander had no less feeling, but showed more fortitude. He, perhaps will be more able to describe to you, nearly at least, the torturing state of my poor heart & soul. Besides, I must own, to you, that these details which were, till just now quite unknown to me, have almost killed me, & I am only able to thank God that this more than half Angel has had the sublime courage to deny herself the comfort I might have afforded her, to spare me, not the sharing of her excruciating pain, that was impossible, but the witnessing so terrific a scene, & perhaps the remorse to have rendured it more tragic! For I don't flatter myself that I could have got through it – I must confess it. Thank Heaven! She is now surprisingly well, & in good spirits, & we hope to have many many still happy days. May that of piece soon arrive, and enable me to embrace better thus with my pen my beloved & ever ever more dear friends of the town & country. Amen. Amen! [In Frances Burney D'Arblay's Handwriting]:

God bless my dearest Esther – I fear this is all written confusedly, but I cannot read it & I can write it no more, therefor I entrust you to let all my dear brethren male & female take a perusal and that you will lend it also to my father & most beloved Mrs. Angerstein, who will pardon, I will know, my opening myself – which is sparing her, a separate letter upon such a theme. My dearest Esther & my dearest Mrs. Locke live so little in the world, that I flatter myself they will never hear of this adventure. I earnestly desire it may never reach them. My kind Miss Cambridge & Miss Baker, also, may easily escape it. I leave all others, & all else, to your own decision.

I ought to have mentioned Sarah when I regretted & sighed for my sisters, for I am sure she would gladly & affectionately have nursed me had she been at hand: but at that critical moment I only thought of those who had already – &

so often – had opportunity as well as soul to demonstrate their tenderness. And she who is gone is ever, & on all occasions, still present to me. Adieu, adieu, my beloved Esther –

Letter to Kitty Barry Blackwell by Elizabeth Blackwell (1887)

Introduction

Elizabeth Blackwell was the first woman to attend medical school in the United States and first female student to publish a medical article in the United States. With her sister Emily, she founded the New York Infirmary for Women and Children as well as a medical college for women. Additionally, Blackwell worked with Florence Nightingale, Sophia Jex-Blake, and Elizabeth Garrett Anderson to establish the first medical school for women in England. In this letter to Katherine "Kitty" Barry, the Irish orphan she adopted in 1856, Blackwell begins a memoir in which she describes her resistance to pursuing medicine until a family friend faced what was probably uterine cancer and had delayed seeking treatment because of discomfort with male doctors. She concludes with her views on abortionist Madame Restell, a reminder of Blackwell's socially conservative views and Christian beliefs. This letter is placed chronologically with the period it describes (the mid-1840s) rather than the date of its composition.

Letter to Begin Memoir

Rock House. Hastings.
  Jan. 2nd. 1887.
  My dear child,
    …
  First of all I will try and tell you why I tried to become a doctor; for I had become a member of the medical profession, several years before I saw you. You know that my father emigrated from Bristol where I was born, to New York, in 1832 – the cholera year. I remember that we buried seven steerage passengers during our voyage of more than seven weeks; and we found New York comparatively deserted from fear of cholera, when we reached there in October.
    *****

1844–1845. When I returned to Cincinnati, I found my family established in the pleasant suburb of Walnut Hills. This was the site of a rather famous theological seminary of which Dr Lyman Beecher was the President. Prof. Stowe who had married Harriet Beecher was settled here; and with other teachers in the college, and the older the students of theology, formed a very intelligent society of a rather liberal presbyterian cast. In this healthy and rapidly growing settlement on the table land of the beautiful Ohio hills, our family remained for several years.

It was during the Autumn and Winter that I now passed with my family on Walnut Hills, that the possibility of studying for the medical profession, and becoming a regular physician, was first suggested me – an idea which was destined to mould so completely my whole future life. The idea was first forced upon my attention by a valued lady friend of the family (Mrs Donaldson) who was a sufferer from a most painful disease requiring surgical intervention. She was a woman of must refined delicacy as well as intelligence. She represented to me, that the character of the treatment she was compelled to undergo, was far more painful when than the disease itself, and she implored me to reflect, how all that additional suffering could be avoided, if her surgeon were a woman; and she asked me whether I had health, leisure, and cultivated intelligence, it was not a positive duty to devote them to the service of suffering women.

The thought of studying medicine was to me so utterly repugnant, that I instantly put it aside, and tried to forget it. I had always despised the body, has the greatest hinderance to all that I most valued. I disliked everything that related to our physical organization, even studies in natural history were antipathetic to me. I cannot at all trace the source where I derived this contempt for the body; but I well remember trying as a child again and again to subdue my body. When going to school in New York I had tried to go without food for days, and I had tried to sleep on the bare floor. I was ashamed of physical ailments, and when exposed to intermittent fever in an unhealthy country house, I used to shut myself up in a dark closet when I felt the deadly chill creeping on (in spite of my desperate efforts to walk it off) so that no one should know of the attacks.

This spirit of asceticism and deep rooted opposition to the conditions of human existence was rudely shocked by Mrs Donaldson's prayer that I should become a physician; and doubtless had the proposition continued to present itself in relation to the special studies requisite for such a course, I should never have taken the matter up. But as the idea would occur to me again and again, other and quite different aspects of the question presented themselves.

Much was said in the public press of that date, respecting a notorious abortionist living in New York – a certain Madame Restell, who had a luxurious establishment, a fine carriage, a pew in a fashionable church, and was really a very clever woman. She was always spoken of as "a female physician"; and the term, then, meant an abortionist. This seemed to me a really wicked perversion of what should be a very honourable position and title. I keenly felt the degradation involved in the unnatural and wicked career of this fashionable woman whom the one-sided law vainly tried to stop.

Swedenborg's phrase "redeem the halls" often occurred to me; and the question, whether it would not be a glorious moral battle to redeem the title "female physician" to a really true and noble signification, continually forced itself upon me.

The Ladies' Medical Friend by W. Hamilton Kittoe (1845)

Introduction

Dr. William Hamilton Kittoe's *The Ladies' Medical Friend* includes information on treating diseases specific to women, information on infant care for mothers, and an appendix of prescriptions. The opening of the book lists his qualifications with M.D. after his name, his role as surgeon and accoucheur, and the location of his home in London as well as the hours he is available to consult patients. In the preface, Kittoe suggests that women readers will find the guide particularly useful in an emergency, noting that "in all serious cases, the information given is only to be adopted till professional aid can be procured, and that in others, a medical man may be consulted effectually, with a due regard to that delicacy so indispensable with the female character." The guide includes a brief discussion of cancer of the womb and a much more detailed section on cancer in the breast. In both sections, the emphasis is on nonsurgical treatments. Before discussing diseases of the breast, Kittoe discusses representations of the female breast in art and literature and in cultural beliefs throughout Europe, an approach wholly unlike other such guides of the period.

Cancer of the Womb

The womb which only weighs between two and three ounces, or perhaps a little more in the virgin, and adult state of women who have never borne children may be increased by disease so as to fill the entire cavity of the belly, causing not only derangement of the bladder and intestines, but of every organ of the body. Instances are on record where the disorganized mass has weighed one hundred pounds avoirdupois. There is however great consolation in knowing that vast and inestimable relief may be afforded to the sufferer in every derangement of this organ and its appendages, although their true nature cannot in all cases be discovered during life, and even were this possible, they might not be curable. In this complaint the system is to be improved by tonics and chalybeates, combined with mild laxatives; where the digestive powers are disordered some slight alterative may be necessary; pain must be relieved by anodynes administered in liberal doses. In cancerous and other malignant disorders of the womb, injections of the different preparations of iodine and chlorine are to be employed, but never without the sanction of a medical practitioner; opium in all its forms may be given by night to relieve pain and procure sleep, which is of great importance, in as much as it assists materially in supporting the powers of the constitution. Hemlock and belladonna are medicines which should always have a trial; plasters composed of these remedies will be advantageously applied over the loins, in most instances very signal relief being afforded by their use. The bowels must be induced to act daily by enemas or very mild aperients, as castor oil or lenitive electuary, all violent purgatives will be certain to do mischief. The mind is to be soothed and tranquillized by every possible means; the sufferer should never be permitted to despond, on the contrary, is to be cheered and led to hope for improvement; rest with a recumbent position is indispensable; the diet must be light, plain, but nourishing; where there is great languor, with depression of mind, a little light wine will be of service. Such are the general indications in this very melancholy disorder, but the treatment will require to be modified according to the constitution of the individual and the nature of the case.

Excerpts from "On the Breast and its Diseases"

A beautiful female bosom has at all periods been an object of admiration with the other sex. The poet has eulogized it, the painter has delineated, and the statuary modelled it. In fact, it is the received opinion in most countries that a woman cannot be perfect, however beautiful she may be, without a finely formed breast. There are, however, some strange exceptions to this rule. The most singular and unnatural custom prevails in Spain of destroying it, similar to the absurd usage in China of cramping and deforming the feet. It is esteemed a mark of beauty in the Spanish female to have no bosom; as soon as it begins to be developed, it is compressed with pieces of lead, and tight bandages, in this manner it is rendered nearly flat, and in some instances totally obliterated. The ancients, however, formed a very different estimate of feminine beauty and symmetry, as may be discovered from the Greek poets, who ever neglect in their description of female loveliness to introduce the epithet of full-bosomed…

The eminent artists of antiquity however never represented the breast with much protuberance or elevation; in the statue of Venus we invariably find the natural proportions strictly carried out. The Grecian ladies used a powder in order to prevent their breasts from in becoming too large, they also employed bandages for the same purpose; some authors recommend powdered mint to be applied in order to check their growth. It may be important to remark that the breasts are the first parts of the frame which are subject to be affected with fat or emaciation; in the latter instance, frictions with the hand or a soft flesh brush for an hour or two every day will increase their growth; nothing prevents this in so great a degree as the artificial padding so much employed to supply natural deficiency, with the exception perhaps of the artificial breast made of India rubber. Should there on the other hand be great luxuriance, bandaging must be employed, and if this does not succeed, the lead as used by the Spanish ladies very probably will. The most certain method of reducing their size with which I am acquainted, is by means of an internal remedy of extraordinary power, that was discovered while it was employed to destroy wens and other tumours. As so powerful a remedy may not be safe to employ in every instance internally, I have given in my Appendix a form for its preparation as an ointment for external use.

A very erroneous opinion prevails among the higher orders that suckling tends to injure the beauty of the bosom, such an idea cannot be too strongly discountenanced and exploded, the very opposite being the fact; for the milk which is prepared in the breast, as the natural food of the infant, not finding an outlet, distends and disorganises the form of the part; instead of which, if it were regularly drawn off by suckling, such would never occur. I am, however, happy in being enabled to state that this unnatural and absurd notion is fast fading away; indeed nothing would so effectually tend to alienate the love of the mother for her offspring as a practice of this nature, an affection which (ought not) in fact never can decay…

The female breast, from its very delicate structure, is liable to many affections, some of which are of a very serious nature. Tumours are frequently met with of various kinds, yet they are rarely dangerous, though some attain a most astounding size; those of an irritable nature are found in girls from fifteen to twenty-five years of age; if they are not examined very gently and tenderly the patient will suffer severely for hours, or even days afterwards, so very great is their sensibility; they are usually accompanied with pain, always aggravated prior to the monthly evacuations; this indeed is a certain criterion of their being connected with an unhealthy state of the menstrual functions, the breast invariably being in close sympathy with the womb. The treatment must be directed to restoring these functions to a healthy tone, and will be found laid down under the head of menstruation. Simple tumours of the breast are commonly found in women of good constitution and healthy appearance; this tumour is a moveable swelling, has an irregular, or what is professionally termed, lobulated feel, that is, being divided into various parts by bands or threads; in size it varies from that of a filbert or wall-nut to a goose-egg or orange; its cause is not well known, in general it may be traced to the pressure of stays or ill-constructed corsets, the evil consequences of which have been already noticed. In the treatment we must employ tonics, alteratives, blisters, disculent ointments or plasters: a nourishing diet, with regular exercise, and change of air. Encysted tumours, that is, such as are enclosed in bags, are of two species, they in general contain a fluid, sometimes a thin gelatinous substance, the former is however the most frequent; when they have acquired any considerable magnitude a slight inflammatory action takes place and they ulcerate, this frequently occurs; the contents are then discharged, and what is termed adhesive inflammation takes place; the cyst or cavity being by such action destroyed, another forms, which undergoes the same process and is again obliterated in a similar manner; this is commonly a disease of advanced life.

Cancer

Women are, unfortunately, frequently the victims of this dreadful disease, and the breast and womb appear to be the organs most predisposed to its attacks; celibacy, as well as the final cessation of the menses, conduce to its production and development; hence unmarried females, past the meridian of life, are too frequently its prey; next to these are mothers who have never suckled their children (for it may be laid down as a decided maxim, that a milk-abscess never degenerates into a cancer); next follow women who are past child-bearing; and lastly, such as have borne children and suckled them with their own milk.

Symptoms

In the commencement, a small, hard tumour, possessing excessive hardness, is discovered; it is indolent, free from pain, and usually circumscribed; after a time, a sense of uneasiness and itching are occasionally felt, succeeded by pricking, shooting, acute darting, and hot lancinating pains; the surface of the tumour becomes irregular, wrinkled, or puckered, and feels knotty: sometimes the nipple is drawn in, and at length wholly disappears, the surrounding veins are swollen, and have a tortuous appearance.

The glands in the arm-pit and above the collar bone now begin to enlarge, but are free from pain; in this stage the malady is termed a schirrous, and when ulceration takes place, cancer. Previous to the formation of a sore, the skin assumes a dull red, or livid appearance, when it gives way, a thin unhealthy matter is discharged, the ulcer soon enlarges, its edges become hard, ragged, and either turned inwards, upwards, or backwards; its entire surface is unequal; in some parts are deep excavations, whilst in others there are considerable elevations. In many instances there will be an attempt to form granulations, or an approach to healing on some parts of the surface, but the effort generally proves deceitful and abortive; spongy fungous flesh speedily following which disappears, returning again either on the same or different parts of the wound; from these surfaces blood is discharged, which, with the increase of pain and irritation, undermines the strength and produces hectic fever; other symptoms attend this malady in its progress, as pain in different parts resembling rheumatism, cough, swelling of the arms and hands on the affected side; sometimes small hard tumours form at at (*sic*) a little distance round the edge of the ulcerations; such are the prominent features of this horrible disorder in the female breast, but there is very considerable diversity in its appearances in different instances; for example, there is what is vulgarly called stone cancer, on account of its extreme hardness and size, another kind, termed indolent cancer, and a third variety entitled soft cancer; the stony cancer is undoubtedly the most unfavourable species, inasmuch as it exceeds all the others in the severity of its symptoms, running its course very rapidly. The indolent, from its name, is slow in its march, and its symptoms comparatively mild, rarely creating much alarm; the last description, or soft cancer, is frequently the one which is apt to be mistaken for other tumours; its progress is slow, and its symptoms mild, seldom causing any uneasiness, till it is too late to apply a remedy. The causes which induce cancer, are long continued derangement of the digestive functions, anxiety of mind, blows, and that peculiar change the female constitution undergoes at the cessation of the monthly evacuations; the more remote are age, cold, variable climate, sedentary habits, celibacy and scrofula. It is worthy of remark, that this malady, is never one of early life, it chiefly commences between the ages of forty and fifty, though it is now and then met with about thirty-five; there is not unfrequently a scrofulous swelling of the breasts occurring in women of that habit, but this is commonly before the the (sic) time of life at which cancer develops (sic) itself. Notwithstanding what has been stated of the distinguishing features of this disorder, it undoubtedly requires very nice discrimination to decide upon the true nature of tumours and ulcerations, in order to decide which are cancerous and which are not.

Treatment

In this most untractable of all human maladies a cure is of rare occurrence, and for this reason, it occurs at a period of life, when the energies of the body begin to decline, or in constitutions enfeebled by previous anxiety, excessive fatigue, or internal disease; the sufferers in every case should make use of such diet as is capable of improving the general health and strength; eating moderately, and at regular hours, of such animal and vegetable food as is most easy of digestion, and contains the largest proportion of nourishment in the smallest possible bulk; the secretion of the bowels must, when defective, be rendered healthy; the remedies chiefly to be depended on are, hemlock, arsenic, iron, iodine, and opium, the two first and the fourth appear to have been by far the most successful. Where there is much pain, from a quarter to half a grain of muriate of morphia must be adminstered (sic) at bed-time, and a sixth of a grain every four or six hours during the day, if urgent necessity demands it. Operations for the removal of cancerous breast are never or rarely performed by men of judgment, in fact they are very seldom advised, even in scirrhous or unbroken cancer, except the tumour is very small, and prior to the occurrence of pain. Indeed, I am well convinced that after the commencement of severe pain, the use of the knife is not only useless, but will aggravate the patient's sufferings and accelerate the fatal termination of the case.

Those who reside at a distance from London, should reflect seriously before they put a friend or relative to the pain, inconvenience and expense of a journey; as it is by no means an uncommon circumstance for the metropolitan surgeon to give an opinion diametrically opposite to that of the country practitioner; and in no instance should an operation be performed, without some previous course of alterative remedies, of which small doses of blue pill, hemlock and a free use of sarsaparilla, in a concentrated from, should form a part.

"Cancer Said To Be Cured By Mesmerism" (1848)

Introduction

Though German doctor Franz Anton Mesmer developed his clinical technique in the eighteenth century, mesmerism was popular across Europe in the nineteenth century. In Britain, its most famous practitioner was Dr. John Elliotson, Professor of Medicine at University College London and physician at University College Hospital. Elliotson's demonstrations of mesmerism attracted large crowds (including a young Charles Dickens) as he performed the technique on young women. Eventually, Elliotson's work was discredited and his popularity diminished. In the coverage of breast cancer in this period, mesmerism was used for sedation during operations and touted as a miracle cure, as seen in this excerpt. The anonymous reporter presents to the broad audience of *Chambers's Edinburgh Journal* a summary of an article from *The Zoist*, Elliotson's periodical about mesmerism and phrenology, demonstrating a curiosity about the healing power of the practice.

"Cancer Said to Be Cured By Mesmerism" (*Chambers's Edinburgh Journal*, 9 December 1848)

The October number of a periodical work called the *Zoist* contains an account by Dr Elliotson of a case of cancer alleged to be cured by mesmerism. The patient, Miss Barber, presented herself to Dr. E. in March 1843, with an intensely hard tumour in the breast, of about a year and a-half's standing. The doctor commenced subjecting her to mesmeric treatment, with a view to her being rendered and sensible to the pain of the operation which he then thought inevitable. After daily 'passes'[21] for a month, she attained a slight degree of 'susceptibility;' her pains during this time and for some months after lessened, and she improved in complexion; but the disease still went on; and many surgeons who saw the breast declared it a case of decided cancer, for which nothing could be done for excision of the part. Dr. Elliotson continued to throw her into the mesmeric sleep every day during the ensuing winter, and she at length became liable to fall into a state of perfect rigidity, during which her arms, unconsciously on her part, would follow those with the operator, from whose fingers on those occasions she beheld a stream of colourless fluid, passing towards her. The summer of 1844 saw her pain diminished, her

---

[21] In passes, the mesmerist moved their hands along the patient's body to and from the diseased parts.

strength increased, the cancerous sallowness gone, and a warty-looking substance had dropped from the breast, leaving a sound smooth surface.

In autumn, Dr. Elliotson being abroad on a tour, the operations were performed by another person, but less regularly. The bad symptoms then returned with great virulence, and the diseased mass was found to have adhered to the ribs. Regular operations being resumed, an improvement recommenced; and in the summer of 1846 the pain had entirely ceased. During 1847 that disease steadily gave way. The mass had not only become much less, but detached from the ribs. At length, during the present year, under the constant daily practice of the mesmeric passes, the cancer has been pronounced to be '*entirely dissipated*; the breast is perfectly flat; the skin rather thicker and firmer than before the disease existed. Not the smallest lump is now to be found; nor is there the slightest tenderness of the bosom person or armpit.' The quondam patient lives at Mrs Gower's, No. 12 New St., Dorset Square, open to any examination or interrogation on the subject.

Assuming that the account of the case is correct, it is certainly a remarkable one. Here, fortunately, for the mesmerists, there ought to be no dubiety about the means of the cure; for cancer is universally regarded by the profession as incurable by anything but the knife, and the knife, as we see, has not been employed. The doctors will scoff; but is scoffing in such a case strictly rational? Would it not be better to investigate, and ascertain if there be not, in certain operations inferring a nervous intercommunication, a sanatory influence capable of affecting great good for suffering humanity? It is surely but the simplest dictate of common sense, as well as benevolent feeling, which would prompt an unprofessional person to point out this course as preferable to the eternal gabble of a barren scepticism.

Memoirs about Emily Gosse's Breast Cancer by Philip Henry Gosse (1857) and Edmund Gosse (1907)

Introduction

Emily Gosse married naturalist Philip Henry Gosse in 1848 and was herself a prolific writer of religious texts, including religious poems, articles in religious periodicals, and more than sixty tracts. Shortly after her death, Emily's husband Philip composed a narrative of her final illness to circulate privately among friends who would want to remember her final days. Because Emily was a writer of religious tracts, Philip saw his wife's faith though her final, and very painful, illness as a testament, explaining in the preface: "the Lord may possibly make use of this simple record of one of his servants, for the stirring up of the faith and love of those who knew her not, and thus to the extension of his own glory" (iv). Throughout the narrative of Emily's nine-month-long journey, Philip describes Emily sharing her faith with those she met during her treatment. Because of his hope that Emily's story would inspire others, Philip shows little reticence and includes specific medical terms to describe Emily's condition and the severity of her suffering throughout the process. Emily Gosse's son Edmund, painter and critic, included a narrative of his mother's illness from his perspective as a seven-year-old child in his memoir. Unlike his father, Edmund is extremely reticent in his description of his mother's illness, going so far as to censor the word *cancer* from the dialogue that represents the first time he realized his mother was ill. Edmund's observation of the illness as a child is unique and reflects the trauma of caring for his mother during her final illness and death.

Excerpts from *A Memorial of the Last Days on Earth of Emily Gosse* by Philip Henry Gosse

About the end of April, 1856, my beloved Emily became conscious of a hard lump in her left breast, the first intimation of that dreadful disease, which was commissioned to dissolve her earthly house of this tabernacle in nine short months.

...

Slightly alarmed at the lump in her breast, my dearest Emily took the first opportunity of showing it to her tried friend, Miss Stacey, of Tottenham, who immediately accompanied her to Dr. Laseron. She returned to me in the afternoon, met me with her usual quiet smile, and with unbroken calmness told me that he pronounced it cancer! The next day we consulted a relative of my own, an eminent physician, by whose recommendation we saw the first authority on cancer in London, Mr. Paget:[22] by both the case was declared to be indubitable cancer, and the instant excision was recommended.

But my relative had heard of an American, who professed to cure cancer by a new process, without the need of an operation; and as he was said to invite

---

[22] Sir James Paget (1814–1899) was a surgeon at St. Bartholomew's and started treating Queen Victoria and the royal family in 1858. He published widely, but his 1874 report "On disease of the mammary areola producing cancer of the mammary gland" led to the disease being called Paget's disease of the mammary nipple and areola. *ODNB*.

the notice of the faculty, Dr. S—— kindly offered to attend on one of his public days, and let us know the result. He accordingly went, and, from his report, we determined to consult the American physician, residing at Pimlico.

On our visit, he professed to be in possession of a secret medicament, by the external application of which to a cancer the diseased portion gradually became dead, spontaneously separated from the healthy flesh, and soughed away, leaving a cavity, which soon healed, and the patient was well. He showed us photographs of many patients in different stages of cure, many large tumours preserved in spirit, which had been sloughed away under his treatment, and, what was still more to the point, we saw one of his patients dressed. This was a middle-aged woman, suffering under cancer of one breast, who told us she had been three weeks under Dr. F——.[23] We saw the large tumour, dark, hard, and apparently dead, deeply scored across, and divided by a distinct line of demarcation from the white living flesh around. We saw that when the doctor applied his fingers, there was a separation, all round, of the dead tumour from the healthy flesh, so that we could see to the depth of an inch or more, in which there was no union of part with part, except that of a few mucous threads, which he divided with scissors. The woman declared that the pain of the process was not worth speaking of.[24]

These things we saw, but for others we were dependent on testimony only; as, for instance, the painlessness of the treatment, in which, to judge from what my beloved Emily subsequently underwent, as well as others who were treated coetaneously with her, I believe we were greatly deceived. We asked concerning the probabilities of the cure being a complete one. Dr. F—— assured us that he, and the few co-possessors of the secret in the United States, had found that, out of every 100 cases treated, not more than twenty instances occurred of a return or reappearance of the disease; whereas, in ordinary surgical practice, as many as 80 per cent. is about the average of recurrence.

…

After much prayer, then, we were perfectly agreed that the American's mode of treatment seemed to promise best. According to the sources of information open to us, it appeared to present comparative freedom from pain in the process, and a far greater probability in the ultimate cure. With the knowledge we afterwards attained, we should no doubt have decided far otherwise; but it was not the Lord's will that we *should* decide differently, and therefore He saw

---

[23] Dr. Jesse Weldon Fell was a fellow of the New York Academy of Medicine and published a book titled *A Treatise on Cancer, and Its Treatment* in 1857. See Croft for more about his work.

[24] Note in Original Text: We left her under the doctor's hands; but my wife soon afterwards saw her again, and learned that the tumour actually came away at that same dressing, after we had left the house.

fit to withhold form us that knowledge. He surely guided us, however, with the infinite wisdom, to fulfil his purpose, which was infinitely good.

On the 12th of May, my dearest wife was placed under the care of Dr. F——. He conceived hopes that the tumour might be dispersed or absorbed without extraction; and at all events recommended that this alternative should be tried for some time. He distinctively assured us, over and over, that even should this hope be disappointed, the tumour would not be in a condition appreciably less favourable for the extractive treatment, after the lapse of a few months, than at that time; and he entertained confidence that the case was one which he should be able to bring to a happy issue.

He commenced by applying two or three kinds of ointment to the breast; using them alternatively on successive days; and this mode of treatment was continued until the end of August. It involved the necessity of my beloved wife's going from Islington to Pimlico three times a-week—a wearisome task, but which greatly opened up to her, what she greatly loved and valued, opportunities of serving her Lord in testimony, both by distribution of Gospel Tracts, and by conversation with strangers.

…

One of the unguents employed was attended with pain, presently causing a gnawing or aching in the breast, which at times was scarcely supportable. No marked changed occurred in the appearance of feeling of the tumour throughout the summer. It certainly had not extended, and we fancied its volume was slightly diminished. It was not the seat of any pain, except what was produced by the application.

Professional engagement called me to Tenby, on the coast of South Wales, during the month of September; and it had been a subject of some solicitude with us, whether that sweet companionship, which had never been interrupted more than a few days at a time since our union, would be vouchsafed to us there Dr. F——, however, had from time to time encouraged us to expect it; and when the time arrived, he gave his full and hearty consent, furnishing my dear Emily with a supply of his medicaments, and giving her instructions for their application. His confidence had by this time communicated itself to us, so that our minds scarcely contemplated a fatal issue, except as a very improbable, or at least very remote, contingency.

Our sojourn at Tenby continued from the 29th of August to the 2d of October. During the first three weeks my Emily was ill with general weakness and headache; and afterwards, the use of the ointments furnished by Dr. F—— produced such intense aching and "drawing" pain in the tumour, that altogether it was a time of much suffering. There were few days, however, in which she was not to be seen according to her custom, on the sand, offering her tracts to visitors, conversing with a bathing-woman, or sitting on the rocks by the side of some nursery governess or mother, sowing, in her own effective way, the good seed of the kingdom.

…

We returned home on the 2d of October, and immediately saw Dr. F———, who advised the removal of the tumour. The lack of any apparent result from the five months' attempt to disperse it, had led us to look to such a course as the most hopeful. On the 10th, therefore, my beloved, accompanied by our little boy,[25] her faithful companion and assiduous nurse throughout her trial, removed to a lodging in Pimlico, uncomfortable in many respects, but presenting the advantage of being next door to Dr. F———'s own residence. The next morning, October 11th, the process of extraction commenced.

The whole surface of the left breast, an area of four inches in diameter, was wetted with nitric acid, applied by means of a small bit of sponge tied to the end of a stick. The object of this application was to remove the skin. The smart was very trying, and continued for several hours augmenting; the effect being to blister and destroy the whole skin, exactly as if a severe burn had taken place.

On the succeeding day, the doctor proceeded to incise the tumour, in order that it might be penetrated by the peculiar medicament which he used for its separation. With the scalpel he drew, on the surface of the new exposed flesh, a series of parallel scratches, about half an inch apart, reaching from the top to the bottom. When these were made, a plaister of a purple mucilaginous substance was spread over the whole. The next day, on renewing this plaister, the scalpel was passed again along the scratches, deepening them a very little; and a fresh plaister was applied. By the daily repetition of this operation, the scratches were in a few days deepened into long parallel cuts or scores, into which narrow strips of linen rag, covered with the purple mucilage, were pressed, instead of the common plaister. Every day these strips of rag were renewed, and the scores were made deeper and deeper.

The effect of this application was very distressing. In about an hour after its renewal every morning, the breast began to be the seat of an aching, piercing pain, under which my beloved sufferer was fain to wander up and down her narrow room, leaning now and then her head upon the mantel-piece or against the wall, unable from the agony to lie, sit, or stand. For several hours this continued, after which the intensity of the anguish commonly abated. Abatement of suffering, however, was the most she could look for; suffering never *ceased* from the beginning of the operation, till her spirit was freed from the worn-out body.

---

[25] Their seven-year-old son Edmund Gosse details his memory of the experience in *Father and Son*.

Her sleep was greatly disturbed by the pain. In health she had been accustomed to sleep well, and had been generally able to forget herself in a few moments after lying down, whether by day or night. But from the commencement of the extraction to her departure, it was a rare thing with her to be unconscious more than half an hour at a time, and a large portion of every night was passed in the wakefulness of pain. From the first she was unable to lie down, so that the repose she took was in a semi-recumbent position, propped up by pillows. The progress of the operation was attended by considerable aching, and loss of muscular power, in the left arm, which prevented her from reclining at all on that side; hence she was reduced to use the half-sitting posture, varied occasionally by a very slight leaning over to the right side.

The only sleep she obtained, for the most part of the time she was at Pimlico, was induced by opiates. We were very reluctant to use them, but Dr. F—— urged them upon my beloved as absolutely necessary, and the experience, that sleep was out of the question naturally, induced her to yield. She took the preparation known as Battley's Sedative, commencing with twelve drops, but at length taking twenty to twenty-five drops nightly.

The scoring of the tumour was not attended with any pain. The purple mucilaginous substance had evidently a caustic power, killing the flesh so far as it penetrated. It has, too, an antiseptic property; for the part so destroyed had no tendency to decomposition; it was brought to a woody hardness, and a deep black colour, without the least odour. It was one merciful mitigation of her sufferings, that, all the time she was under Dr. F——, not the slightest offensive odour was perceptible from the disease.

When the incisions had reached the depth of about an inch and a quarter, the operator announced that he had reached the bottom of the cancer. He now scored no more, but applied a "girdle," or annular plaister, around the line where the killed tumour adjoined the living flesh; a line which was marked with perfect definiteness. The object was now to promote a suppuration, whereby the tumour should be gradually detached from the flesh, and sloughed off, like a stone dropped out of a basin. It was nearly four weeks after the removal of the skin that the "girdle" was first put on, and two weeks more before the tumour came away. A furrow, gradually deepening, formed between the living flesh and the hard and black tumour, and this was filled with pus. The sensation now became that of a heavy weight dragging at the breast, and this feeling increased as the connexion between the parts daily diminished. At length, on Sunday, the 23d of November, to our delight, the great insensible tumour fell out of its cavity, hanging only by a slender fleshly thread, which presently yielded, and the breast was relieved of its load—the dead body that it had so long carried about.

There it lay on the table, a hard and solid block of black substance, resembling in size and shape a penny bun, deeply scored on one surface, and on the other nearly smooth. And on the breast of my beloved sufferer was the corresponding cavity, raw and partly lined with pus, but presenting an apparently healthy appearance.

This was the point to which our hopes had been directed for six weeks past; hopes not unmingled with fears, however; for we had ascertained that, not unfrequently, after the main tumour had come away, as in this instance, a piece of the diseased flesh was left—a sort of offshoot of the tumour, in the bottom of the cavity, imbedded in the flesh. In such case, there was no alternative but to treat this piece with the purple mucilage, like the original tumour.

With anxious hearts we awaited Dr. F———'s verdict. It was two days before he would venture to decide, and those days were precious to my beloved. The sense of ease produced by the removal of the dead weight, and the intermission of the gnawing medicament, were delightful, notwithstanding the soreness of the open wound; while the hopefulness arising from the consciousness that one important stage was passed, added mental to the bodily relief.

The cup was soon dashed from our lips; for the doctor presently announced that there was a large piece on the outer edge of the cavity, which, though he could not say it was actually cancerous, he deemed it prudent to take away. The whole painful process had now to be gone over again, with the exception of the application of the nitric acid. It was with heavy hearts we heard these tidings; my beloved's nervous system was one peculiarly sensitive to pain; but she resigned herself to the new torture with calm submission to her Father's will. Indeed, amidst all the sighs and moans wrung from her in the course of this sore affliction, I never heard her utter a single murmuring word; not an expression, not a look, that intimated a doubt of the loving-kindness of the Lord. She delighted to dwell on his goodness; and it was often, when others, less instructed in God's school, might have failed to trace it, peculiarly manifested it to her, because of her quick understanding in the fear of the Lord. "How merciful it is of the Lord that—" was so frequent a commencement of her sentences, as to be recognized as quite characteristic by those who were intimate with her.

Nearly four weeks more of the grinding, wearing agony were now to be borne; by which time the continued pain, the sleepless nights, and the violence done to the whole system by the destruction of so large a portion of the tissues, had accomplished a work but too perceptible. Her strength was greatly reduced; to the last she crawled in every morning from her lodgings to Dr.

F——'s (now removed to Warwick Square) and back, a distance of about a quarter of a mile, but it was a slow process, not performed without assistance, and it left her much exhausted; yet she always enjoyed the fresh air, and the effort.

…

On the 17th of December, the second portion of the tumour which had been treated since the 23d of November, a mass about as large as a hen's egg, from the outer side of the breast, detached itself; and again hope was raised. This hope was not, however, unmixed; for both on the inner and on the outer side of the wound, on the surface that had hitherto appeared sound, indications had begun to manifest themselves that gave us anxiety. Pimples were forming, especially under the arm; and though Dr. F—— had hitherto treated them lightly, we did not feel able to rely on his opinion with the same buoyant confidence as at first. As before, he waited a few days before he would give any information as to the course he would follow, now that this epoch was reached.

At length, on Monday the 22d, he said, after examining the wound, "Mrs. Gosse, I'm very sorry for this. I shall have to take out another piece under the arm." Her heart sank at this announcement, but she replied, "And what then, Doctor?" "Then I must treat this other part on the inner side of the breast." "But how do you account for this spreading of the disease beyond the part you have all along been dealing with?" "Oh, 'tis in your blood."

She said no more, but calmly took her leave; and in the afternoon, when I returned to her from my daily work, she told me of the result. Worn down as she was, she felt that she could not undergo the pain of a third, and then a fourth process, the unintermitted agony of which she had sufficiently proved; especially as there seemed no reasonable hope that the merely local mode of treatment hitherto pursued would, if continued, overtake a disease which had already spread so far beyond the area originally attacked. We had, moreover, been all along assured that cancer was a local, and not a constitutional disease; and therefore the announcement that it was seated in the blood, while indeed we had good reason to believe it true, took us by surprise, as contrary to the statements we had all along relied on. The question, too, was obvious, "What is the use of a merely local treatment of a disease which is seated in the blood?"[26]

…

---

[26] Note in Original Text: Of Dr. F——'s personal kindness and attention to my beloved sufferer, I would speak most gratefully; he did all he could for her; and I do not hesitate to affirm that he is in possession of a very important discovery; but its value in cases of real cancer, I feel assured, has been much overrated. I do not think I am offending against the golden law of love, in giving my opinion on a mode of treatment whose claim is before the public, and on the efficacy of which health and life depend.

It is a solemn position to be placed in when one is called to choose between rival systems of medicine, with the feeling that life and death are in the balance. My Emily had no confidence in allopathy, the old drug system; and I had no more than herself. She had long been a firm advocate of homœopathy; and though my mind was not made up, my predilections rather inclined that way. We decided on a homœopathic course.

Without an hour's needless delay, I removed her from Pimlico to her own home in Islington. The increase to her comfort from being thus at home was a matter of much thankfulness; and it was most providential that it happened when it did, as she sank so rapidly, that if it had been delayed a few days later, I doubt if she could have been removed at all. She bore the journey well, very much enjoying the fresh air as she passed through the streets.

Indeed the luxury of air was enjoyed too freely, for she preferred to have the glass of the carriage down all the way; and as her cough was much aggravated afterwards, I fear she caught cold. During the greater portion of her residence at Pimlico, her sufferings had been much augmented by a harassing cough, the paroxysms of which shook her debilitated frame terribly, and still further weakened it.

During the three weeks that followed her return home, she suffered very much from sleeplessness. The regular administration of opium, to which she had been so long accustomed, was *suddenly* given up, perhaps not quite wisely; and the usual phenomena resulted—fits of exceeding depression at the usual hour of the opiate, the most painful restlessness, and inability to remain for more than a moment in one place or position; and dreary sleepless nights. About the time just named, the middle of January, the cancer began rapidly to assume a very virulent appearance; the cavity produced by the extraction of the tumours was somewhat diminished in the area, and skinned over, except in the centre, where there was a mass of raw fungoid flesh, on which a fetid pus copiously formed. The pimples around increased in number, and some of them were attended with a smarting, stinging pain. A large area on all sides of the wound became swollen, livid, and quite hard to the touch. There was no shooting or lancinating pain in any part, but a burning heat in the rough pimply surface beneath the armpit, with aching in the shoulder and arm reaching down to the hand. This arm, the left, was now become useless. These local sufferings were accompanied by shifting rheumatoid pains in the body, alternations of burning feverishness and sudden chills, paroxysms of coughing, and great debility. She was scarcely able now to rise from a chair.

I now called in another homœopathic physician.[27] He gave no hope of recovery, but thought there was no probability of speedy decease. He examined the chest by auscultation, and declared that two diseases were present, either of which might be the immediate cause of death. Besides the cancerous taint which was pervading the whole blood, there was a diseased condition of the lungs, of old standing, which would probably have given no trouble but for the weakening of the whole system, during the long process of agony to which the patient had been subjected; the lungs were now in an emphysematous condition. He despaired of being able to remove, or even seriously to arrest, either of these developments, but hoped to alleviate the sufferings of the patient.

Accordingly, no sooner had my beloved wife begun to take his prescriptions, than she found marked relief. Throughout the first week there was a very manifest improvement; the pains were greatly mitigated; the restlessness and depression nearly disappeared; and the progress of the cancer, so far as we were cognizant of it, was arrested. In the succeeding week, these favourable indications were scarcely diminished; but the cough had all along been most distressing. From this time until her death this was the most trying symptom. The cancer gave little pain in the part affected; but bodily vigour sank rapidly, and appetite was nearly gone. The cough, however, occurred in terrific paroxysms, especially during the night, tearing and shaking the frame, and almost depriving her of sleep. Whenever she lay quiet and unconscious for half an hour, we considered it quite a matter for congratulation.

…

Another proof of the mercifulness of God in hearing prayer, was the mitigation of actual pain as the closing scene drew on. Her nervous system, though in general, through life, she had enjoyed even robust health, was peculiarly sensitive to pain; so that what to many could have been only a slight inconvenience, often quite unfitted her for every duty. Knowing, as we did, in what terrible agony cancer often ends, we looked forward with somewhat of foreboding anxiety to the future; and our eyes were lifted up unto the Lord, that He would spare his trembling child the depth of the affliction. And He graciously did. The worst pain was endured at Pimlico; after her return home, there was comparatively little from this source; the increase of the tumour being in no wise a measure of her bodily suffering.

---

[27] In *The Life of Philip Henry Gosse*, Edmund Gosse provides John Epps's name as the homœopathic doctor whose treatment gave his mother relief from her suffering (270). Edmund later married one of Epps's nieces.

There was enough, however, remaining. She could not be raised in the bed without strong pains in the loins; her nights, from the terrible paroxysms of coughing, were frequently wretched; the power of using the lower limb as well as the upper, on the left side, was almost wholly lost; bed-sores appeared; breathing was performed with increased difficulty.

From *Father and Son: A Study of Two Temperaments* by Edmund Gosse

It was not, however, until the course of my seventh year that the tragedy occurred, which altered the whole course of our family existence. My Mother had hitherto seemed strong and in good health; she had even made the remark to my Father, that 'sorrow and pain, the badges of Christian discipleship', appeared to be withheld from her.

…

But a symptom began to alarm her, and in the beginning of May, having consulted a local physician without being satisfied, she went to see a specialist in a northern suburb in whose judgement she had great confidence. This occasion I recollect with extreme vividness. I had been put to bed by my Father, in itself a noteworthy event. My crib stood near a window overlooking the street; my parents' ancient four-poster, a relic of the eighteenth century, hid me from the door, but I could see the rest of the room. After falling asleep on this particular evening, I awoke silently, surprised to see two lighted candles on the table, and my Father seated writing by them. I also saw a little meal arranged.

While I was wondering at all this, the door opened, and my Mother entered the room; she emerged from behind the bed-curtains, with her bonnet on, having returned from her expedition. My Father rose hurriedly, pushing back his chair. There was a pause, while my Mother seemed to be steadying her voice, and then she replied, loudly and distinctly, 'He says it is—' and she mentioned one of the most cruel maladies by which our poor mortal nature can be tormented. Then I saw them hold one another in a silent long embrace, and presently sink together out of sight on their knees, at the farther side of the bed, whereupon my Father lifted up his voice in prayer. Neither of them had noticed me, and now I lay back on my pillow and fell asleep.

Next morning, when we three sat at breakfast, my mind reverted to the scene of the previous night. With my eyes on my plate, as I was cutting up my food, I asked, casually, 'What is—?' mentioning the disease whose unfamiliar name I had heard from my bed. Receiving no reply, I looked up to discover why my question was not answered, and I saw my parents gazing at each other with lamentable eyes. In some way, I know not how, I was conscious of the presence of an incommunicable mystery, and I kept silence, though tortured with curiosity, nor did I ever repeat my inquiry.

About a fortnight later, my Mother began to go three times a week all the long way from Islington to Pimlico, in order to visit a certain practitioner, who undertook to apply a special treatment to her case.[28] This involved great fatigue and distress to her, but so far as I was personally concerned it did me a great deal of good. I invariably accompanied her, and when she was very tired and weak, I enjoyed the pride of believing that I protected her. The movement, the exercise, the occupation, lifted my morbid fears and superstitions like a cloud. The medical treatment to which my poor Mother was subjected was very painful, and she had a peculiar sensitiveness to pain.

…

Fortunately my Father was able to take us away in the autumn for six weeks by the sea in Wales, the expenses of this tour being paid for by a professional engagement, so that my seventh birthday was spent in an ecstasy of happiness, on golden sands, under a brilliant sky, and in sight of the glorious azure ocean beating in from an infinitude of melting horizons. Here, too, my Mother, perched in a nook of the high rocks, surveyed the west, and forgot for a little while her weakness and the gnawing, grinding pain.

But in October, our sorrows seemed to close in upon us. We went back to London, and for the first time in their married life, my parents were divided. My Mother was now so seriously weaker that the omnibus journeys to Pimlico became impossible. My Father could not leave his work and so my Mother and I had to take a gloomy lodging close to the doctor's house. The experiences upon which I presently entered were of a nature in which childhood rarely takes a part. I was now my Mother's sole and ceaseless companion; the silent witness of her suffering, of her patience, of her vain and delusive attempts to obtain alleviation of her anguish. For nearly three months I breathed the atmosphere of pain, saw no other light, heard no other sounds, thought no other thoughts than those which accompany physical suffering and weariness. To my memory these weeks seem years; I have no measure of their monotony. The lodgings were bare and yet tawdry; out of dingy windows we looked from a second storey upon a dull small street, drowned in autumnal fog. My Father came to see us when he could, but otherwise, save when we made our morning expedition to the doctor, or when a slatternly girl

---

[28] This partitioner was Dr. Jesse Weldon Fell, a fellow of the New York Academy of Medicine who published a book titled *A Treatise on Cancer, and Its Treatment* in 1857. See Croft for more about his work.

waited upon us with our distasteful meals, we were alone, without any other occupation than to look forward to that occasional abatement of suffering which was what we hoped for most.

It is difficult for me to recollect how these interminable hours were spent. But I read aloud in a great part of them. I have now in my mind's cabinet a picture of my chair turned towards the window, partly that I might see the book more distinctly, partly not to see quite so distinctly that dear patient figure rocking on her sofa, or leaning, like a funeral statue, like a muse upon a monument, with her head on her arms against the mantelpiece. I read the Bible every day, and at much length; also,—with I cannot but think some praiseworthy patience,—a book of incommunicable dreariness, called Newton's 'Thoughts on the Apocalypse'.

…

As my Mother's illness progressed, she could neither sleep, save by the use of opiates, nor rest, except in a sloping posture, propped up by many pillows. It was my great joy, and a pleasant diversion, to be allowed to shift, beat up, and rearrange these pillows, a task which I learned to accomplish not too awkwardly. Her sufferings, I believe, were principally caused by the violence of the medicaments to which her doctor, who was trying a new and fantastic 'cure', thought it proper to subject her. Let those who take a pessimistic view of our social progress ask themselves whether such tortures could today be inflicted on a delicate patient, or whether that patient would be allowed to exist, in the greatest misery in a lodging with no professional nurse to wait upon her, and with no companion but a little helpless boy of seven years of age. Time passes smoothly and swiftly, and we do not perceive the mitigations which he brings in his hands. Everywhere, in the whole system of human life, improvements, alleviations, ingenious appliances and humane inventions are being introduced to lessen the great burden of suffering.

If we were suddenly transplanted into the world of only fifty years ago, we should be startled and even horror-stricken by the wretchedness to which the step backwards would reintroduce us. It was in the very year of which I am speaking, a year of which my personal memories are still vivid, that Sir James Simpson received the Monthyon prize as a recognition of his discovery of the use of anaesthetics.[29] Can our thoughts embrace the mitigation of human torment which the application of chloroform alone has caused? My early experiences, I confess, made me singularly conscious, at an age when one should

---

[29] See Chap. 2 on popular and medical considerations of chloroform in the mid-nineteenth century. Sir James Simpson began using ether as anesthesia for childbirth in 1847, which was met with great opposition for decades. He received the Monthyon prize by the French Academy of Sciences, for "most important benefits done to humanity" in 1856.

know nothing about these things, of that torrent of sorrow and anguish and terror which flows under all footsteps of man.

....

In my Mother's case, the savage treatment did no good; it had to be abandoned, and a day or two before Christmas, while the fruits were piled in the shop-fronts and the butchers were shouting outside their forests of carcases, my Father brought us back in a cab through the streets to Islington, a feeble and languishing company. Our invalid bore the journey fairly well, enjoying the air, and pointing out to me the glittering evidences of the season, but we paid heavily for her little entertainment, since, at her earnest wish the window of the cab having been kept open, she caught a cold, which became, indeed, the technical cause of a death that no applications could now have long delayed.

Yet she lingered with us six weeks more, and during this time I again relapsed, very naturally, into solitude. She now had the care of a practised woman, one of the 'saints' from the Chapel, and I was only permitted to pay brief visits to her bedside. That I might not be kept indoors all day and everyday, a man, also connected with the meeting-house, was paid a trifle to take me out for a walk each morning. This person, who was by turns familiar and truculent, was the object of my intense dislike.

...

After our return to Islington, there was a complete change in my relation to my Mother. At Pimlico, I had been all-important, her only companion, her friend, her confidant. But now that she was at home again, people and things combined to separate me from her. Now, and for the first time in my life, I no longer slept in her room, no longer sank to sleep under her kiss, no longer saw her mild eyes smile on me with the earliest sunshine. Twice a day, after breakfast and before I went to rest, I was brought to her bedside; but we were never alone; other people, sometimes strange people, were there. We had no cosy talk; often she was too weak to do more than pat my hand; her loud and almost constant cough terrified and harassed me. I felt, as I stood, awkwardly and shyly, by her high bed, that I had shrunken into a very small and insignificant figure, that she was floating out of my reach, that all things, but I knew not what nor how, were coming to an end. She herself was not herself; her head, that used to be held so erect, now rolled or sank upon the pillow; the sparkle was all extinguished from those bright, dear eyes. I could not understand it; I meditated long, long upon it all in my infantile darkness, in the garret, or in the little slip of a cold room where my bed was now placed; and a great, blind anger against I knew not what awakened in my soul.

"Rab and His Friends" by John Brown (1858)

Introduction

John Brown's experiences while apprenticing under surgeon James Syme led him to opt for the life of a physician and inspired the story "Rab and His Friends," originally published in his 1858 *Horæ Subsecivæ*. In the Preface to a later illustrated edition of the short story, Brown describes a sense of urgency in the need to retell the story of breast cancer patient Ailie Noble, her husband James, and their dog Rab. He explains how the story "came on me at intervals almost painfully, as if demanding to be told, as if I heard Rab whining at the door to get in or out…or as if James was entreating me on his deathbed to tell all the world what his Ailie was" (117). Not only is the story a fictionalized account of Ailie's illness, but it is also Brown's own narrative about treating a breast cancer patient. "Rab and His Friends" opens with two violent dogfights, the second of which begins with a small dog attacking Rab, a mastiff, and ends with Rab quickly killing it. This opening episode explains Brown's connection to Rab and his owners and demonstrates Rab's strength and his avoidance of violence until it is necessary. The story quickly moves on to a time six years later where the text printed here begins.

Excerpt from "Rab and His Friends"

Six years have passed,—a long time for a boy and a dog: Bob Ainslie is off to the wars; I am a medical student, and clerk at Minto House Hospital. Rab I saw almost every week, on the Wednesday; and we had much pleasant intimacy. I found the way to his heart by frequent scratching of his huge head, and an occasional bone. When I did not notice him he would plant himself straight before me, and stand wagging that bud of a tail, and looking up, with his head a little to the one side. His master I occasionally saw; he used to call me "Maister John," but was laconic as any Spartan.

One fine October afternoon, I was leaving the hospital, when I saw the large gate open, and in walked Rab, with that great and easy saunter of his. He looked as if taking general possession of the place; like the Duke of Wellington entering a subdued city, satiated with victory and peace. After him came Jess, now white from age, with her cart, and in it a woman carefully wrapped up,— the carrier leading the horse anxiously, and looking back. When he saw me, James (for his name was James Noble) made a curt and grotesque "boo," and said, "Maister John, this is the mistress; she's got a trouble in her breest,—some kind o' an income, we're thinkin'."

By this time I saw the woman's face; she was sitting on a sack filled with straw, her husband's plaid round her, and his big-coat, with its large white metal buttons, over her feet.

I never saw a more unforgettable face,—pale, serious, *lonely*,[30] delicate, sweet, without being at all what we call fine. She looked sixty, and had on a mutch, white as snow, with its black ribbon; her silvery, smooth hair setting off her dark-gray eyes,—eyes such as one sees only twice or thrice in a lifetime, full of suffering, full also of the overcoming of it; her eyebrows black and delicate, and her mouth firm, patient, and contented, which few mouths ever are.[31]

As I have said, I never saw a more beautiful countenance, or one more subdued to settled quiet. "Ailie," said James, "this is Maister John, the young doctor; Rab's freend, ye ken. We often speak aboot you, doctor." She smiled, and made a movement, but said nothing, and prepared to come down, putting her plaid aside and rising. Had Solomon, in all his glory, been handing down the Queen of Sheba at his palace gate, he could not have done it more daintily, more tenderly, more like a gentleman, than did James the Howgate carrier, when he lifted down Ailie his wife. The contrast of his small, swarthy, weather-beaten, keen, worldly face to hers—pale, subdued, and beautiful—was something wonderful. Rab looked on concerned and puzzled, but ready for anything that might turn up,—were it to strangle the nurse, the porter, or even me. Ailie and he seemed great friends.

"As I was sayin', she's got a kind o' trouble in her breest, doctor: wull ye tak' a look at it?" We walked into the consulting-room, all four, Rab grim and comic, willing to be happy and confidential if cause could be shown, willing also to be the reverse on the same terms. Ailie sat down, undid her open gown and her lawn handkerchief round her neck, and, without a word, showed me her right breast. I looked at and examined it carefully,—she and James

---

[30] Note in Original Text: It is not easy giving this look by one word: it was expressive of her being so much of her life alone.

[31] Note in Original Text:

Black brows, they say,

Become some women best; so that there be not
Too much hair there, BUT IN A SEMICIRCLE
OR A HALF-MOON MADE WITH A PEN.
—A WINTER' TALE.

watching me, and Rab eying all three. What could I say? There it was, that had once been so soft, so shapely, so white, so gracious and bountiful, so "full of all blessed conditions,"—hard as a stone, a centre of horrid pain, making that pale face, with its gray, lucid, reasonable eyes, and its sweet resolved mouth, express the full measure of suffering overcome. Why was that gentle, modest, sweet woman, clean and lovable, condemned by God to bear such a burden?

I got her away to bed. "May Rab and me bide?" said James. "YOU may; and Rab, if he will behave himself." "I'se warrant he's do that, doctor;" and in slunk the faithful beast. I wish you could have seen him. There are no such dogs now. He belonged to a lost tribe. As I have said, he was brindled, and gray like Rubislaw granite; his hair short, hard, and close, like a lion's; his body thick-set, like a little bull,—a sort of compressed Hercules of a dog. He must have been ninety pounds' weight, at the least; he had a large blunt head; his muzzle black as night, his mouth blacker than any night, a tooth or two—being all he had—gleaming out of his jaws of darkness. His head was scarred with the records of old wounds, a sort of series of fields of battle all over it; one eye out, one ear cropped as close as was Archbishop Leighton's father's; the remaining eye had the power of two; and above it, and in constant communication with it, was a tattered rag of an ear, which was forever unfurling itself, like an old flag; and then that bud of a tail, about one inch long, if it could in any sense be said to be long, being as broad as long,—the mobility, the instantaneousness of that bud were very funny and surprising, and its expressive twinklings and winkings, the intercommunications between the eye, the ear, and it, were of the oddest and swiftest.

Rab had the dignity and simplicity of great size; and, having fought his way all along the road to absolute supremacy, he was as mighty in his own line as Julius Caesar or the Duke of Wellington, and had the gravity[32] of all great fighters.

You must have often observed the likeness of certain men to certain animals, and of certain dogs to men. Now, I never looked at Rab without thinking of the great Baptist preacher, Andrew Fuller.[33] The same large, heavy,

---

[32] Note in Original Text: A Highland game-keeper, when asked why a certain terrier, of singular pluck, was so much more solemn than the other dogs, said, "Oh, sir, life's full o' sairiousness to him: he just never can get eneuch o' fechtin'."

[33] Note in Original Text: Fuller was in early life, when a farmer lad at Soham, famous as a boxer; not quarrelsome, but not without "the stern delight" a man of strength and courage feels in their exercise. Dr. Charles Stewart, of Dunearn, whose rare gifts and graces as a physician, a divine, a scholar, and a gentleman live only in the memory of those few who knew and survive him, liked to tell how Mr. Fuller used to say that when he was in the pulpit, and saw a buirdly man come along the passage, he would instinctively draw himself up, measure his imaginary antagonist, and forecast how he would deal with him, his hands meanwhile condensing into fists and tending to "square." He must have been a hard hitter if he boxed as he preached,—what "The Fancy" would call an "ugly customer."

menacing, combative, sombre, honest countenance, the same deep inevitable eye, the same look,—as of thunder asleep, but ready,—neither a dog nor a man to be trifled with.

Next day, my master, the surgeon, examined Ailie. There was no doubt it must kill her, and soon. It could be removed; it might never return; it would give her speedy relief: she should have it done. She curtsied looked at James, and said, "When?" "To-morrow," said the kind surgeon,—a man of few words. She and James and Rab and I retired. I noticed that he and she spoke little, but seemed to anticipate everything in each other.

The following day, at noon, the students came in, hurrying up the great stair. At the first landing-place, on a small well-known black board, was a bit of paper fastened by wafers, and many remains of old wafers beside it. On the paper were the words, "An operation to-day.—J.B., *Clerk*"

Up ran the youths, eager to secure good places: in they crowded, full of interest and talk. "What's the case?" "Which side is it?"

Don't think them heartless; they are neither better nor worse than you or I; they get over their professional horrors, and into their proper work; and in them pity, as an *emotion* ending in itself or at best in tears and a long-drawn breath, lessens,—while pity, as a *motive* is quickened, and gains power and purpose. It is well for poor human nature that it is so.

The operating theatre is crowded; much talk and fun, and all the cordiality and stir of youth. The surgeon with his staff of assistants is there. In comes Ailie: one look at her quiets and abates the eager students. That beautiful old woman is too much for them; they sit down, and are dumb, and gaze at her. These rough boys feel the power of her presence. She walks in quickly, but without haste; dressed in her mutch, her neckerchief, her white dimity short-gown, her black bombazine petticoat, showing her white worsted stockings and her carpet shoes. Behind her was James with Rab. James sat down in the distance, and took that huge and noble head between his knees. Rab looked perplexed and dangerous; forever cocking his ear and dropping it as fast.

Ailie stepped up on a seat, and laid herself on the table, as her friend the surgeon told her; arranged herself, gave a rapid look at James, shut her eyes, rested herself on me, and took my hand. The operation was at once begun; it was necessarily slow; and chloroform—one of God's best gifts to his suffering children—was then unknown. The surgeon did his work. The pale face showed its pain, but was still and silent. Rab's soul was working within him; he saw that something strange was going on,—blood flowing from his mistress, and she suffering; his ragged ear was up, and importunate; he growled and gave now and then a sharp impatient yelp; he would have liked to have done something to that man. But James had him firm, and gave him a *glower* from time to time, and an intimation of a possible kick;—all the better for James, it kept his eye and his mind off Ailie.

It is over: she is dressed, steps gently and decently down from the table, looks for James; then, turning to the surgeon and the students, she curtsies and in a low, clear voice begs their pardon if she has behaved ill. The students—all of us—wept like children; the surgeon happed her up carefully, and, resting on James and me, Ailie went to her room, Rab following. We put her to bed. James took off his heavy shoes, crammed with tackets, heel-capt and toe-capt, and put them carefully under the table, saying, "Maister John, I'm for nane o' yer strynge nurse bodies for Ailie. I'll be her nurse, and I'll gang aboot on my stockin' soles as canny as pussy." And so he did; and handy and clever and swift and tender as any woman was that horny-handed, snell, peremptory little man. Everything she got he gave her: he seldom slept; and often I saw his small shrewd eyes out of the darkness, fixed on her. As before, they spoke little.

Rab behaved well, never moving, showing us how meek and gentle he could be, and occasionally, in his sleep, letting us know that he was demolishing some adversary. He took a walk with me every day, generally to the Candlemaker Row; but he was sombre and mild, declined doing battle, though some fit cases offered, and indeed submitted to sundry indignities, and was always very ready to turn, and came faster back, and trotted up the stair with much lightness, and went straight to that door.

Jess, the mare, had been sent, with her weather-worn cart, to Howgate, and had doubtless her own dim and placid meditations and confusions on the absence of her master and Rab and her unnatural freedom from the road and her cart.

For some days Ailie did well. The wound healed "by the first intention;" for, as James said, "Oor Ailie's skin's ower clean to beil." The students came in quiet and anxious, and surrounded her bed. She said she liked to see their young, honest faces. The surgeon dressed her, and spoke to her in his own short kind way, pitying her through his eyes, Rab and James outside the circle,—Rab being now reconciled, and even cordial, and having made up his mind that as yet nobody required worrying, but, as you may suppose, semper paratus.

So far well; but four days after the operation my patient had a sudden and long shivering, a "groosin'," as she called it. I saw her soon after; her eyes were too bright, her cheek colored; she was restless, and ashamed of being so; the balance was lost; mischief had begun. On looking at the wound, a blush of red told the secret: her pulse was rapid, her breathing anxious and quick; she wasn't herself, as she said, and was vexed at her restlessness. We tried what we could. James did everything, was everywhere; never in the way, never out of it; Rab subsided under the table into a dark place, and was motionless, all but his eye, which followed every one. Ailie got worse; began to wander in her mind, gently; was more demonstrative in her ways to James, rapid in her questions, and sharp at times. He was vexed, and said, "She was never that way afore,— no, never." For a time she knew her head was wrong, and was always asking our pardon,—the dear, gentle old woman: then delirium set in strong, without pause. Her brain gave way, and then came that terrible spectacle,—

> The intellectual power, through words and things,
> Went sounding on its dim and perilous way;

she sang bits of old songs and Psalms, stopping suddenly, mingling the Psalms of David, and the diviner words of his Son and Lord, with homely odds and ends and scraps of ballads.

Nothing more touching, or in a sense more strangely beautiful, did I ever witness. Her tremulous, rapid, affectionate, eager, Scotch voice, the swift, aimless, bewildered mind, the baffled utterance, the bright and perilous eye, some wild words, some household cares, something for James, the names of the dead, Rab called rapidly and in a "fremyt" voice, and he starting up, surprised, and slinking off as if he were to blame somehow, or had been dreaming he heard. Many eager questions and beseechings which James and I could make nothing of, and on which she seemed to set her all and then sink back ununderstood. It was very sad, but better than many things that are not called sad. James hovered about, put out and miserable, but active and exact as ever; read to her, when there was a lull, short bits from the Psalms, prose and metre, chanting the latter in his own rude and serious way, showing great knowledge of the fit words, bearing up like a man, and doting over her as his "ain Ailie." "Ailie, ma woman!" "Ma ain bonnie wee dawtie!"

The end was drawing on: the golden bowl was breaking; the silver cord was fast being loosed; that *animula blandula, vagula, hospes, comesque*,[34] was about to flee. The body and the soul—companions for sixty years—were being sundered, and taking leave. She was walking, alone, through the valley of that shadow into which one day we must all enter; and yet she was not alone, for we know whose rod and staff were comforting her.

One night she had fallen quiet, and, as we hoped, asleep; her eyes were shut. We put down the gas, and sat watching her. Suddenly she sat up in bed, and, taking a bed-gown which was lying on it rolled up, she held it eagerly to

---

[34] Allusion to first lines of dying emperor Hadrian's poem in Latin in which he addresses his soul.

her breast,—to the right side. We could see her eyes bright with a surprising tenderness and joy, bending over this bundle of clothes. She held it as a woman holds her sucking child; opening out her night-gown impatiently, and holding it close, and brooding over it, and murmuring foolish little words, as over one whom his mother comforteth, and who sucks and is satisfied. It was pitiful and strange to see her wasted dying look, keen and yet vague,—her immense love.

"Preserve me!" groaned James, giving way. And then she rocked backward and forward, as if to make it sleep, hushing it, and wasting on it her infinite fondness. "Wae's me, doctor! I declare she's thinkin' it's that bairn." "What bairn?" "The only bairn we ever had; our wee Mysie, and she's in the Kingdom forty years and mair." It was plainly true: the pain in the breast, telling its urgent story to a bewildered, ruined brain, was misread and mistaken; it suggested to her the uneasiness of a breast full of milk, and then the child; and so again once more they were together, and she had her ain wee Mysie in her bosom.

This was the close. She sank rapidly: the delirium left her; but, as she whispered, she was "clean silly;" it was the lightening before the final darkness. After having for some time lain still, her eyes shut, she said, "James!" He came close to her, and, lifting up her calm, clear, beautiful eyes, she gave him a long look, turned to me kindly but shortly, looked for Rab but could not see him, then turned to her husband again, as if she would never leave off looking, shut her eyes and composed herself. She lay for some time breathing quick, and passed away so gently that, when we thought she was gone, James, in his old-fashioned way, held the mirror to her face. After a long pause, one small spot of dimness was breathed out; it vanished away, and never returned, leaving the blank clear darkness without a stain. "What is our life? it is even a vapor, which appeareth for a little time, and then vanisheth away."

Rab all this time had been fully awake and motionless: he came forward beside us: Ailie's hand, which James had held, was hanging down; it was soaked with his tears; Rab licked it all over carefully, looked at her, and returned to his place under the table.

James and I sat, I don't know how long, but for some time, saying nothing: he started up abruptly, and with some noise went to the table, and, putting his right fore and middle fingers each into a shoe, pulled them out, and put them on, breaking one of the leather latchets, and muttering in anger, "I never did the like o' that afore!"

I believe he never did; nor after either. "Rab!" he said, roughly, and pointing with his thumb to the bottom of the bed. Rab leaped up, and settled himself, his head and eye to the dead face. "Maister John, ye'll wait for me," said the carrier; and disappeared in the darkness, thundering downstairs in his heavy shoes. I ran to a front window; there he was, already round the house, and out at the gate, fleeing like a shadow.

I was afraid about him, and yet not afraid: so I sat down beside Rab, and, being wearied, fell asleep. I awoke from a sudden noise outside. It was November, and there had been a heavy fall of snow. Rab was *in status quo*; he heard the noise too, and plainly knew it, but never moved. I looked out; and there, at the gate, in the dim morning,—for the sun was not up,—was Jess and the cart, a cloud of steam rising from the old mare. I did not see James; he was already at the door, and came up the stairs and met me. It was less than three hours since he left, and he must have posted out—who knows how?—to Howgate, full nine miles off, yoked Jess, and driven her astonished into town. He had an armful of blankets, and was streaming with perspiration. He nodded to me, spread out on the floor two pairs of clean old blankets having at their corners "A. G., 1794," in large letters in red worsted. These were the initials of Alison Graeme, and James may have looked in at her from without—himself unseen but not unthought of—when he was "wat, wat, and weary," and, after having walked many a mile over the hills, may have seen her sitting, while "a' the lave were sleepin'," and by the firelight working her name on the blankets for her ain James's bed.

He motioned Rab down, and, taking his wife in his arms, laid her in the blankets, and happed her carefully and firmly up, leaving the face uncovered; and then, lifting her, he nodded again sharply to me, and, with a resolved but utterly miserable face, strode along the passage, and down-stairs, followed by Rab. I followed with a light; but he didn't need it. I went out, holding stupidly the candle in my hand in the calm frosty air; we were soon at the gate. I could have helped him, but I saw he was not to be meddled with, and he was strong and did not need it. He laid her down as tenderly, as safely, as he had lifted her out ten days before,—as tenderly as when he had her first in his arms when she was only "A. G.,"—sorted her, leaving that beautiful sealed face open to the heavens; and then, taking Jess by the head, he moved away. He did not notice me; neither did Rab, who presided behind the cart.

I stood till they passed through the long shadow of the College and turned up Nicolson Street. I heard the solitary cart sound through the streets and die away and come again; and I returned, thinking of that company going up Libberton Brae, then along Roslin Muir, the morning light touching the Pentlands and making them like on-looking ghosts, then down the hill through Auchindinny woods, past "haunted Woodhouselee;" and as daybreak came sweeping up the bleak Lammermuirs, and fell on his own door, the company would stop, and James would take the key, and lift Ailie up again, laying her on her own bed, and, having put Jess up, would return with Rab and shut the door.

James buried his wife, with his neighbors mourning, Rab watching the proceedings from a distance. It was snow, and that black ragged hole would look strange in the midst of the swelling spotless cushion of white. James looked after everything; then rather suddenly fell ill, and took to bed; was insensible when the doctor came, and soon died. A sort of low fever was prevailing in the village, and his want of sleep, his exhaustion, and his misery made him apt to take it. The grave was not difficult to reopen. A fresh fall of snow had again made all things white and smooth; Rab once more looked on, and slunk home to the stable.

And what of Rab? I asked for him next week at the new carrier who got the good-will of James's business and was now master of Jess and her cart. "How's Rab?" He put me off, and said, rather rudely, "What's YOUR business wi' the dowg?" I was not to be so put off. "Where's Rab?" He, getting confused and red, and intermeddling with his hair, said, "'Deed, sir, Rab's deid." "Dead! what did he die of?" "Weel, sir," said he, getting redder, "he didna exactly dee; he was killed. I had to brain him wi' a rackpin; there was nae doin' wi' him. He lay in the treviss wi' the mear, and wadna come oot. I tempit him wi' kail and meat, but he wad tak' naething, and keepit me fra feedin' the beast, and he was aye gur gurrin', and grup gruppin' me by the legs. I was laith to mak' awa wi' the auld dowg, his like wasna atween this and Thornhill,—but, 'deed, sir, I could do naething else." I believed him. Fit end for Rab, quick and complete. His teeth and his friends gone, why should he keep the peace and be civil?

He was buried in the braeface, near the burn, the children of the village, his companions, who used to make very free with him and sit on his ample stomach as he lay half asleep at the door in the sun, watching the solemnity.

"Extracts from My Case-Book. By an Old Physician" (1858)

Introduction

The Englishwoman's Review was a weekly newspaper that emphasized the roles of their women readers and wives and mothers. In this short piece, the anonymous doctor associates his work with mainstream medical practice through a condemnation of "ignorant quacks." For this audience of women readers, the doctor spends little time explaining the treatment and instead focuses on the issue of women hiding their maladies and delaying treatment.

Extracts from my Case-Book. By an Old Physician (*The Englishwoman's Review*, 23 October 1858)

ON CANCER.—In my long practice I have often found cases where the patients, particularly ladies advanced in years, have concealed cancer, even from their intimate friends, till it has been too late to get relief; in other cases I have known instances of their applying to ignorant quacks, thus losing the precious time in which, by judicious treatment, relief might have been obtained. I have found that if a cancerous breast is removed by an operation, if the cancerous diathesis is not got out of the system by proper medicines and *diet*, it generally forms in the other breast, or some other part, in two or three years; whereas I have found, after I had performed the operation, and put the patient under a proper régime, that it has not been the case. Therefore, I advise my fair country women to seek the best advice in an early stage, though many tumours are not cancerous, and may be dispersed by bringing the system into a healthy state.
W. J.

Diary of Helen Blackwood, Lady Dufferin and Claneboye, Countess of Gifford (1867)

Introduction

Writer Helen Selina Blackwood, Lady Dufferin and Claneboye, faced breast cancer in 1866 and 1867. Seven months after a mastectomy, her cancer returned, and in her final months, she recorded the progression of her illness in a diary addressed to her adult son. The journal entries from 1 January to 15 March 1867 demonstrate her worsening symptoms while she actively concealed her prognosis from her son and his family. She addresses the diary to her son with the expectation that he will read her entries after her death from breast cancer. Three months after the last entry in the journal, she died on 13 June 1867.

January 1st

My dearly loved and most loving son! I shall keep this little record of my thoughts and inmost feelings for you as something to speak to you when I am no longer with you, and because there are many things that come into my mind which I am forced to keep from you now (to spare your kind warm heart), but which would, I think, comfort you could I share them with you. They shall be posthumous confidences, and will lose nothing in your eyes by that condition. I believe that although you are ignorant of my real state, the Gracious God—who has shown us both so many mercies—is teaching you by secret instincts that I am soon to leave you. I felt that so strongly the day we left Clandeboye. Do you remember coming through the gallery where H[35] and I were sitting waiting to see you start, and opening your arms to me, embracing me so tenderly, as if we were parting for a long time, the *Home Farewell*, and I recognized it as such, and blessed you and yours, oh so fervently! before I left the house. May Peace and innocent Joy and lasting Happiness dwell with you there for ever. May your children grow up round you—and my dear good Harriot—to be the same comfort and support to you that you have been to me. May no evil (no real evil!) ever come nigh your dwelling, and when the temporary sorrows and anxieties—inseparable from even the happiest existence—come upon you, may God bless them to you and turn them into good.

That last day at Clandeboye was full of sweet and bitter thoughts to me. I walked round the lake, and took leave of all the old (and new) places! I sat upon a fallen tree at "the Mother's Seat," and looked long at the Tower,[36] the monument of your love. May all those objects be pleasant memories to you. I had a poignant thought of regret in thinking I should see them no more (at least with my earthly eyes), for I have occasional happy fancies of some sort of spiritual presence with those we love that may be permitted after death, and if so, how continually I shall be with my darling—alone—or in company—in your walks, or by your fireside;—the fervour of my love, my blessing—my whole soul—will surely encompass you!

---

[35] Note in Original Text: Harriot.

[36] Refers to Helen's Tower, a lookout tower built by Lord Dufferin and Clandeboye for his mother which featured a poem she had written for him. He also asked several contemporary poets to write poems about his mother and the tower—including Alfred, Lord Tennyson, Robert Browning, Thomas Carlyle, Rudyard Kipling, Sir Edwin Arnold, Richard Garnett, Wilfrid Scawen Blunt, and Lord Houghton--some of which were engraved in the tower with his mother's poem.

January 4th

What a freight that steamer held for me!—(you and Harriot and the three little ones). It was the first time I had been with you *all* under those circumstances, and my usual nervous anxieties beset me. I can't understand the frame of mind which prompts some people to say (speaking of some overwhelming catastrophe that should envelope themselves and friends) "at least we should all die together." To me it is an inexpressible comfort to think of you and yours continuing on this beautiful familiar earth when I shall have left it. It takes from death one of its great terrors—the sense of strangeness, the utter cutting off of all accustomed thoughts, hopes, fears. I keep up the sense of a posthumous share in this human life—(this first great, tangible *gift of God*, so fair in promise, so decorated with material and spiritual joys!)—when I project my thought into the coming years which I am not to see—when I look forward to your future earthly course, to my little Archie's youth and manhood, to my sweet Nelly's future grades and beauty and goodness! Why should so many religious writers seek to divide the two worlds by such an impassable barrier? Living or dying, are we not equally God's poor creatures, within reach of his love, within the compass of his mercy? Why are we "*to wean our thoughts from this Life*" on the approach of death, as if *Life* with all its small cares, and poor joys, and strong affections and tormenting fears, were not as much *His* good gift as Immortality itself? *Nothing*, while life and reason last, can wean my thoughts from you, my darling, my only child, my one consolation for many sorrows. No, nor from your human welfare during the days appointed to you on earth. I shall take with me to the brink of the grave the great love I bear you, and fervently hope not to be separated from it hereafter. It has been, *here*, almost a burden at times (so full of cares and fears), but there I trust nothing but Peace and Content unspeakable.

I enjoyed so much that soaky, splashy visit to Castle Kennedy with you both, my dear ones, though few people would have understood my pleasure in it. It was *taking a part* in your daily interests and pleasures which may not again be permitted to me. I mean that particular sort of interest and pleasure which we both derive from Beauty in Nature and in Art, and I enjoyed the journey, in spite of fatigue, and the come *Home* for ever, as I feel it is to be.

Hewett told me nothing new, nothing that I had not surmised before I saw him, but I will not deny that the *certainty* of the fatal nature of my malady, in its new form, was a slight shock during the first few minutes' but I am glad to think that you could have seen no trace of it when I went down to you in the garden. I told Hewett my reasons for wishing to withhold from you a knowledge which would have poisoned all the pleasant days we have spent together since we returned to England, which would have taken from you all the pleasure of the task you had set yourself in, "The letters on the state of Ireland," and perhaps diminished your powers of writing. One of the proofs of the instinct you unconsciously possess on the subject of my health was shown the other day in your saying to me when I was helping you to correct your M. S.—"this association with you in this little matter is such a pleasure to me—it will be a memory." I am always glad of these indices of the relaxing chain, (never to be broken) between us.

To be removed from you, for a time, is not "to part for ever," as it is so often called. I hope it is not presumptuous, but I feel so *certain* of a happier future existence than this—so safe in God's hands, whatever he may will it to be, that I cannot feel that dread of Death which so many better Christians than I are said to feel. I pray God that this dread may not come upon me later! I pray that pain may not be allowed to conquer me. I suffer a good deal, more than I let you see or know, and I am aware that this suffering must increase, and that death must be the cure, but, as yet, I am able to contemplate this certainty without the uneasiness of mind which I should think but natural in any other person. I can only attribute this to God's special and undeserved mercy towards me. I often think over the circumstances and arrangements that must follow my death, hoping that it may be in summer time—that my flight need not be in the winter—as I know my poor boy would forget all about cloaks and wraps at my funeral, and perhaps lay himself up with illness afterwards, but my dear little Harriot must promise to see to all that, and take care of him. One of my reasons for wishing to change my room is that you must have melancholy associations with this one, in which Archie was born, and which I trust will be your own. I mean to make this room as pleasant and gay-looking as I can.

My own darling, if it is convenient, and does not run counter to your views and feelings *in any degree*, I should wish to be buried in the little Church-yard at Friern Barnet, where the body of my poor Gifford rests. Had it been God's will to try me with the greatest of all human sorrows,—to see the order of nature reversed, and my only child taken from me in his prime, you know well that I should have asked not to be separated from you in Death, whom I have loved so infinitely beyond any other human being. (But He has been so merciful to me! I have you to comfort and support me through my last trial.) But *after* you, I have dearly loved my poor, affectionate, faithful Gifford, to whom I was the first object in life for many years. *For my sake*, I know you will not let his memory utterly perish. There are few who will care to keep it alive when I am gone. You will take care of his bust which I had made by Marochetti, and his books and casts and the seedling oak which he planted. If you approved, and if the thing could be done without inconvenience and without incurring any fooling expense, I should like a little project of mine carried out which I have often had in my thoughts;—that is, to have that beautiful monody written by Caroline on his death, placed on a tablet in the little Church at Friern Barnet.*[37] His poor name is "writ in water," for he never did anything in the world's eye, or was anything in its estimation, but this would at least preserve the memory of what he *might have been* under happier influences and circumstances. But, remember, my darling, that I leave all this entirely subject to your own views of what is right and convenient, and you are only to consider it in that light, and not as an express recommendation on my part.

I think I would wish the inscription on the stone over my grave to run something in this way, (always subject to your opinions and wishes):—"Helen Selina, widow of Price 4th Lord Dufferin and Clandeboye,—married secondly (13th October 1862) to George Earl of Gifford, and died—&c." (I wish I could have *mother* of Frederick Temple Lord D. & C., written above me, for *that* is my great "illustration," as the French call it, and the principal end and happiness of my earthly being. I purposely omit mention of my age in the inscription, as those who knew nothing of his sad story and long enduring affection would only see something to ridicule or criticize in the difference of years between Gifford and myself. None can enter into the sorrow of that time, but let it be buried with me. My life has not been a happy one, my darling; *you* have been the *one* joy belonging to it, but a joy that ought to outweigh *many* sorrows and privations, and a blessing far greater than I desired.

Thursday, January 24th

I feel so young in heart and spirit, in spite of this failing body, that I can hardly realize the fact that the end of earthly cares and pleasures is so near. I have exactly the same enjoyment in the things that best pleased me in youth— the aspect of nature, beautiful sights and sounds, books, pleasant conversations, my garden, and above and before all, your company, my own darling, which I have possessed for so large a portion of my life. As you often say in jest, "we have spent our youth together," and I cannot grow old while I see you by me looking young.

---

[37] Note in Original Text: The Rector of the Parish would not permit this to be done.

I walk about my dear garden and try to figure you all enjoying its pleasant terraces and flowers a year or two hence. I fear so much that *at first* you will not take much pleasure in it, connecting my remembrance too closely with everything you see, but that will not be the right way to view it. On the contrary, you must think how much enjoyment I have derived from it, how (even now, when I am aware that I shall hardly live long enough to see the fruits of our new alterations), my principal occupation and delight consists in decorating it, and preparing for the time you will live here *without me*. I can hardly prevent the words coming to my lips (when talking to you and Harriot about the arrangements of the new rooms, &c.), "Yes, but that will be one of your spare rooms next year." When you discuss the point of my comfort in going back to my old rooms again, I constantly catch myself beginning to give dear Lal instructions as to how she should best manage matters of this nature when there will no longer be a necessity for studying my convenience. I have been able to consult her tastes about the furniture, &c., which requires present decision, without any difficulty. I do hope I may live to see her through her confinement, and to give my blessing to another grandchild, but if that happiness is not allowed me, I bless her, and it most fervently, and pray God that the next little one may be as healthy and lovely and promising as the others, and that all your dear children may be the same blessing and comfort to you that you have ever been to me.

Thursday, January 31st

To-day I enjoyed so much going with you to Muswell Hill with H. and the little one, but I am angry with myself for a moment of weak emotion which I gave way to, and for which I could have beaten myself the next moment. I was merely expressing the pleasure I felt in being able still to take part in these every-day enjoyments, which seem such commonplace matters when one is strong and well, but which take on a character of rare festal delights when strength and health are gone, and then a mixed feeling of regret for lost occasions of the same simple pleasures and the thought that you would miss me sometimes in their recurrence hereafter, altogether overcame me, and I cried; but you will all that my foolish weakness passed off in a moment, and I shall take care to behave like a sensible old grannie in the future. Instead of regretting the past, I ought to be (and trust I am) thankful to God for giving me these present gleams of sunshine and renewed life.

Saturday, February 2nd

What a pleasure the children are! I cannot give an idea of the unutterable tenderness with which my heart swells while I watch their dear pretty looks and gestures—Archie above all. He seems to me two treasures in one lovely presence—he is in himself one of the most attractive children I ever saw, and he is the "eidolon" of your own dear childhood.

Monday, 4th

The honeysuckle is beginning to put out my feelers into the spring—actual leaves. I don't remember any spring in my existence when these first tender wakenings of glorious Nature did not send a thrill of intense happiness through my heart. The one pageant that never tires, the one pleasure that never falls upon us, is at hand. I thank God that I have never (at any moment of my life) been insensible to this great gift. I hope to be permitted to see the full glory of the summer this year.

Tuesday, 5th

Cossie Graham's presence is always a cheering, pleasant circumstance. I am in hopes that I succeed capitally in showing a brave front in this battle. I am resolved that pain shall not prevent my being gay and cheerful during our little evening meetings, and I flatter myself that I cheat at cards with as much depraved *aplomb* as if I were in full health and vigour, and exercise the usual spiteful supervision over Fred's frauds.

Wednesday, February 6th

To-day I had a crowd of visitors after my interview with Hewett—Bessie Wellington, Lady de Ros, Lady Sydney, and the Nugents—all so kind and sympathetic. But I sometimes feel so wear in spirit after discussions (kindly meant) about my health, in which I am bound to re-echo the hopeful expectations of amendment "when once the fine warm weather sets in." How I long to say, "Dear people! let me alone, let ill alone! What I have to do is die, and all the sunshine in the world won't defer that necessity, and all the kind wishes in the world won't make it less unpalatable or inevitable." Yet, why do I say *unpalatable*? Death in itself is not an evil; it is but the long looked for termination of a lease of certain faculties granted at God's will; why do we always meet it as if it were a cruel and unjustifiable "eviction?" There is no "Tenant-right" in this world's possessions, but we have" [sic] "Emigration," I trust, in view, and to a sweet and blessed country. My darling sees that here my thoughts take their colouring from certain "Letters in the *Times*," in which I take much pride!

Friday 8th

The good Duke and beloved little Duchess of Argyll came to luncheon yesterday. I spoke very openly to her about myself—always a relief with real friends. What a warm sympathetic heart she has; what good people they all are. I was so glad to hear of the improvement in her mother's health. Later, came the young Duchess of—, a splendid vision in blue velveteen. Poor dear little soul; how I wish her real happiness and peace amid all the unrealities of her pursuits—religion included.

Saturday 9th

I saw Hewett to-day, and told him that I saw plainly the rapid progress of my malady in spite of his efforts to check it, and he was honest, as he always is, and said nothing to remove the impression. Went afterwards to see my dear Lal's picture, which I like in its present state. Lizzie Ward, with gifts of violets and mandarin oranges, stood like Pomona on Swinton's threshold.

Sunday 10th

I wish I felt well enough to go to Church with my dear ones to-day. I hope that at least that much amendment may come with fine weather.

Monday, February 11th

My nights are very full of suffering. I get some quiet sleep towards morning, but I wake very little refreshed. It is a curious sensation, the watching (with full consciousness and power of appreciating every symptom of decay) the gradual approach of death. This great bugbear of mortal existence, *as yet*, has had no permission to daunt me. May my Gracious and Most Merciful Father still avert this *worst* of life's last trials.

Tuesday 12th

Ah! my poor boy! The time is approaching when I *must* tell you what will be such a heavy grief to your loving heart. To-day I put a very positive question to Mr. Hewett. I asked him if he thought I should live till summer. He answered with his usual kindly sincerity—"Yes, if no unforeseen contingency arises." I am glad of the chance this gives me of once more seeing the lovely summer time which has always been a joy to me, but this *approach* to *precision* as to the date of our parting brings a certain pang with it, though it has, in fact, thrown further off the term I myself had begun to think probable. I am so "torn with contending feelings" (as heroines of novels say of themselves) as to what is best and wisest to do about you. Surely it is but common humanity to spare you a painful knowledge as long as I can, and yet I dread so much that you should hereafter be vexed at this reticence on my part, and think you had a right to know the exact truth on a matter so near your heart! Oh, my darling, forgive me if I have erred about this. I would give one of the few months left me to spare you an hour's pain. Just as I was writing this sentence this morning, my darlings came to my bedside with a heap of merry Valentines, and I myself have been "fêted" by the gentle saint. It was a practical answer to my faithless doubt. Why should I deny myself or *you* any occasion of cheerful thought or innocent fun? As long as we can, let us be happy and merry together, as we have always been. We would not have had this pleasant Valentine's day together if I had blackened all your thoughts with my prospective sorrow.

Friday 15th

Lady Grey came to see me. I have always had a feeling of strong attraction towards her, but have seen less of her during our acquaintance than I always wished. Dear Janie Ellice was a mutual bond between us if circumstances had allowed more opportunities for cultivating a friendship which, I think, she was as much disposed to as I was. But early youth is the *sowing* season for friendship: in after life the ground gets hard and choked with cares and individual interests, the soft, receptive, germinating faculty ceases to act; we still plant, but with no genial spontaneity of love, and we are content with more meager harvests. I have been rich in friends, and still can count many very dear ones, but the most beloved are gone before me.

Saturday, February 16th

Went to town to-day, and shopped with Lal. Mrs. Hamilton came.

Sunday 17th

I was able to go with my darlings to church this morning. Georgey came. She means kindly, but it is not enlightened kindness to bring accounts of marvellous nostrums and wonderful Quack Doctors who profess to cure the incurable.

Monday 18th

Last night, when you bade me good night, my dearly beloved son, you said something very kind and soothing about my gaiety and cheerfulness during the evening (Johnnie,*[38] Gawen, Mrs. Hamilton). It pleased me the more because I had in reality been suffering much pain and discomfort, and I am always glad of these proofs of the power of my will over my human infirmities—always acknowledging with heart-felt thankfulness the help which I am *persuaded*, I am receiving from my gracious, merciful God.

Saturday 23rd

When we all set off to Muswell Hill, I left the dear things and went on to Friern Barnet. No one has been buried near my poor Gifford's grave (which fear has been haunting me lately), and I have Mrs. Blackbrow (the sexton's mother) a sovereign to take care of the stone and inscription, and promised another for every year that the place near it is kept unfilled. But *remember*, by [sic] beloved son, that the wish I have expressed to be buried there is to be *entirely subordinate* to your wishes and feelings. It signifies little where *the body* rests. Through Christ's mercy, I trust for my spirit's destination elsewhere.

---

[38] Note in Original Text: Lord John Hay.

Monday 25th

Mrs. Hamilton went away.

Tuesday 26th

* * * came to see me. Pour soul! she would fain show me affection and sympathy, but she hardly knows how. She did not even answer or notice in any way the only letter in which I (in a moment of impulsive confidence) opened my whole heart to her, and spoke of *my inmost feelings* about my situation. Oh, my darling, bring up the children not only *to love others, but to show their love by words and deeds and looks, and every evidence that can help to cheer and bind together the poor units of humanity.*

Wednesday, February 27th

Went to town to Hewett, and brought back dear Lizzie Ward. I feel worse than I have done yet, and was foolishly nervous in talking to you, my own darling about the arrangements for your study and the new rooms. I could not explain to you that all the while I was thinking of the fast approaching time when there would be only *too much* room in the house, in your dear eyes. God bless you, and your task to-night at the dinner for the children's hospital.

Thursday, February 28th

My last birth-day. All my darlings came to my bedside this morning with offerings of beautiful flowers, even the dear little Terence brought a bunch of primroses in his unconscious, fat little hands. It has been my *one superstition* through life that the year in which my birth-day passed without a gift of flowers of some sort (if only a daisy or a violet), the following year would be an unhappy one for me. I had never had so many as I go to-day, and I thankfully accept the omen. God grant me to meet death happily and peacefully, and that my beloved may not unchristianly lament me.

Friday, March 1st

Changes preparing in political affairs. Shall I live to see you in office again, my own darling? It would be a pleasure, but whether it be granted to me or not to live to see it, I *earnestly* hope that when the opportunity is offered to you, you will accept it. Work is good for you at all times (if managed prudently and with due regard to health), but you will especially need it now as an occupation for your thoughts.

Saturday 2nd

Great increase of suffering these two days. I think there must be some change preparing in my malady: it cannot be a good one. Sat a long time while outside to see the plants put in the lawn opposite the hall door. I rejoice in thinking how pretty and complete will be my darling's home here, and that I have contributed to render it so, which will, I know, be a pleasure for them to remember.

Monday 4th

Lizzie went away, to my regret. The Duchess of Cleveland sat a long while with me on the terrace, kind-hearted and cheery. Walden[39] and then Lord Gilford came. A suffering day.

Tuesday, March 5th

My beloved, my darling, some days my heart feels so dry and dead that even my love for you seems only a dumb pain added to my other pains, and I can only dwell on the sadness of our mutual position and speculate on the worst side of it, thinking how it will be with you when the time comes, and how I can possible mitigate or soften the blow to you, and recognize the futility of any effort of that sort, and groan over the hard necessity. But there came better and brighter moments, when I can trust all to my good and Gracious God, who will prepare and uphold you I do trust. But how gladly I would bear even an aggravation of my suffering, could I buy it with the *certainty* that you will accept this first great sorrow of your existence with entire resignation and composure. If I could but spare you the grief, death would be welcome to me.

---

[39] Note in Original Text: Lord Tweeddale's son.

Monday 11th

Cossie came. Ill, ill. Kept my bed.

Tuesday 12th

Got up to-day in order to receive Blanche Airlie and her father. Great discussion on the merits of Mrs. Craven's book. Le recit d'une soeur." [sic] I am charmed with it. It is sad and *fateful* as a Greek tragedy, but inspired by such a triumphant faith that it leaves, even on the coldest reader's mind, a sense of contagious holy joy and security. What good people they all were! How happy in their sorrows.

Wed. 13th

Amelia Blackwood and Lady Sydney came.

Thursday 14th

Great suffering every night now, and indeed never out of pain all day. This snow makes everything look so wintry and sad. I feel its depressing influences, and find it hard to keep up the cheerful manner I have hitherto succeeded in showing at our little dinner meetings. I pray that increasing weakness may not *dash* my courage and make me fretful and disagreeable to you all, my poor darlings!

Friday 15th

Last night I could hardly refrain from praying that this time of trial may not be greatly prolonged. But what am I that I presume to choose times and seasons for God's judgments or mercies. Only may I bear patiently what is appointed. Lizzie Ward comes back to-day. Her presence is a great comfort to me.

"The Useful Book. Compiled by Mrs. Warren" (1875)

Introduction

Mrs. Eliza Warren, editor of *The Ladies' Treasury*, presents to her middle-class readers an article on cancer that quotes heavily from *English Mechanic*. By reproducing the article with few editorial interruptions, Mrs. Warren demonstrates confidence that her women readers will find the information understandable and appropriate. The article contains two narratives of breast cancer, the first from a woman identified only by the initials J.E.P.S. and the second from a reader who signs his letter "Cotswold." In both cases, the women patients—J.E.P.S. and Cotswold's female relative—undergo nonsurgical treatments for breast cancer that include an asbestos and acid paste and poultice that eat through flesh and tumor to remove the cancer from the woman's body.

The Useful Book. Compiled by Mrs. Warren (*The Treasury of Literature and The Ladies Treasury*, 2 August 1875)

A Cure for Cancer.—A correspondence has been going on for some time in the *English Mechanic* relative to a cure for cancer, which it is there asserted can be cured without surgical operation. Cancer is such a deadly and much-dreaded disease that anyone knowing of a cure or not to keep it concealed. The following appeared in No. 533, June 11th, 1875:—*Cancer Cured without a Surgical Operation*—"Some time ago I inserted a query in this paper—*English Mechanic*—as to whether there was any cure for tumours but the knife, and was advised by 'M. A. B.' to apply to the Cancer Hospital at Brompton, 'where the disease, if it could by any means be arrested, would be done in the most merciful manner.' Having a repugnance to the knife I was induced to disregard this advice and place myself under a London surgeon, who made these cases his specialty, and treated them by other than the ordinary means. I do not give the name, that my motives in writing this letter may be open to no misconstruction; but for the benefit of others, I give a description of the means, adopted in my case, with the happiest results. The tumour from which I was suffering was in the breast, and of a considerable size. Having first carefully marked the size and shape on paper, and selected a glass mould of suitable form, the operator made a paste of asbestos and the strongest sulphuric acid, and filled the mould to the depth of about half-an-inch. This cake of substance being removed from the mould was placed upon the breast immediately over the tumour. It caused great pain for about ten minutes, after which time it became quite bearable, and it was not at any time severe enough to require the application of anæthetics. A colorless fluid oozed from beneath the paste and was sopped up continually with small balls of charpie, so as to prevent the action of the acid, extending the beyond the proper limits. In five or six hours the paste was removed and made up with fresh acid, and at night a few drops of acid were applied to the upper surface to restore its activity. This remained on the breast until the following morning, when all pain has ceased, and the paste was removed. Almost the worst part of the operation was the being obliged to lie in exactly the same position for so many hours. For five or six days, no further action took place, and I did not suffer even inconvenience from what had been done. At the end of that time suppuration set in, and was accelerated by poultices; day by day little pieces of the dead flesh were snipped off with a pair of scissors, till in about a week the whole tumour came away bodily, leaving, no trace of its presence remaining. The deep wound thus formed was kept open sometime by poultices, to insure every atom of the morbific growth being eliminated, and this done, it was slowly and carefully healed, the granulation of the new tissues, being regulated by the occasional application of a little caustic (giving me no pain), so as to form perfectly healthy flesh. In two months, the entire cure was complete, and I am now perfectly restored and in good health. My general health has never been impaired, and I have not been confined to bed, or even to the house, for more than the first two days. The shock to the system so severely felt after a surgical operation, (and particularly by females) is by this system entirely avoided, and the tumour having been so utterly burned out and destroyed, the chances against its return are enormously increased—indeed, rendered well-nigh impossible. All cases which can be cured by the knife will yield to this treatment, and many also in which the knife dare not be used. A lady of my acquaintance, who was affiliated with cancer, having consulted one of the most eminent London surgeons, was told of the operation was impossible and her case hopeless. As a last resort she placed herself under the treatment I have attempted to describe, and in two months she was perfectly cured. Of course the other surgeons oppose the system because it is an innovation, but its ultimate general adoption can only, I think, be a matter of time, for facts will speak for themselves. As far as I know, it is as yet practised by only one surgeon in this country; but this surely, for the credit of English surgery, will not long be the case. "J. E. P. S."

Whilst appreciating our correspondent's motive, we think this is an instance where the name of the surgeon might with propriety be given for the benefit of others. "J. E. P. S." will therefore, oblige us by sending the name, and leave it to our discretion to publish it or not.—Ed. *English Mechanic.*

We have looked unsuccessfully for a reply to the Editor's remarks, but in the number for July 2nd the following appeared:—"*Curing Cancer.*—It is not true as 'J. E. P. S.' (p. 353) supposes, that there is only one surgeon in England practising the method she describes. A relative of mine, a few months back, having cancer in the breast, placed herself under the care of a surgeon, and his mode of procedure was almost identical with that described by 'J. E. P. S.,' but occupying a longer time. She suffered but little constitutional disturbance during its progress, and her general health is now very good, she being able to attend to her ordinary household duties. The place it occupied is now covered with healthy skin, but there is considerable tenderness about the place, and great susceptibility to cold, but no other remaining signs of the presence of the disease. The same surgeon had treated other cases successfully, one person that had been cured having recommended the one I have referred to above. Thinking that if a possibility exists of curing so fearful a disease it ought to be extensively known is my sole motive in writing these few lines. The name of the surgeon is Dr. Turnbull, Regent Street, Cheltenham. "Cotswold."

Ladies' Guide in Health and Disease: Girlhood, Maidenhood, Wifehood, Motherhood by J. H. Kellogg (1883)

Introduction

In his preface, Dr. John Harvey Kellogg describes the need for this volume as "the very remarkable increase in the number and frequency of" diseases impacting women to the point that "a fashionable woman has her favorite gynecologist as well as her favorite milliner or dress-maker" (i). In the sections on common maladies facing women, he specifies that his work is not "a substitute for the physician, except so far as the physician fails to do his duty in instructing his patient in relation to the nature, causes, and rationale of cure of her maladies, information to which every intelligent woman is entitled" (iii). By explaining the subjects in "simple and untechnical" terms, Kellogg suggests women can manage ordinary ailments "in the absence of a competent physician" (iii) and can use the book in working with their own doctors to avoid "the reach of quackery" and "cooperate intelligently and efficiently in the effort to aid nature in effecting a cure" (iv). As is seen in Chap. 3, Kellogg suggested a direct connection between abortion and gynecological cancers.

Cancer of the Womb

The usual symptoms of this horrible and often incurable malady are as follows: Very profuse watery discharge, of a dirty, pale-green color, always offensive, usually putrescent; sudden, and, in the later stages, frequent attacks of hemorrhage; severe local pain at night at first, in later stages constant; disturbances of digestion, nausea and vomiting; irregular action of the bowels; great mental depression; rapidly increasing debility; sallow countenance; when examined, the womb is found to be enlarged, nodular, fixed by adhesions in the pelvis so as to be immovable.

Little is known of the cause of this disease. It has been observed, however, that a laceration of the neck of the womb is usually the starting-point of the malady. Death usually occurs within two years. …

Treatment: Almost every imaginable form of treatment has been adopted, but modern medical science is still completely baffled so far as a radical cure is concerned. The most that can be done is to palliate the patient's sufferings by such means as will relieve pain and check the hemorrhage. For this purpose the most efficient measures are those already recommended for use in fibroid tumors of the womb and hemorrhage.

The use of "clover tea," and "Chian turpentine,"—remedies which have become popular within the last few years, offer at least the advantage that they will do no harm if they do no good, which cannot be said of many other popular remedies. We usually allow patients to take "clover tea" freely, but cannot say that we ever saw a case in the least benefited by the remedy.

Something can be done by surgical operations to check the development of the disease, and occasional instances are met in which after thorough removal of the diseased tissue the malady does not reappear, hence a surgeon of experience and skill should be consulted in all cases of this sort. No reliance should be placed upon the pretentions of quacks or "cancer doctors." Their reputation is wholly gained by false pretences.

Tumors of the Breast

The female breast is subject to various morbid growths, such as fibrous and cystic tumors, fatty growths, and to simple overgrowth of the breast. The latter condition may be due to an overaccumulation of fat or to an actual overgrowth of the gland itself. The causes of fat accumulation are obesity and masturbation and other sexual excesses. Over-growth of the gland itself is due to the organ not diminishing in size after lactation. In the first variety of enlargement, the breast is large and soft. In the second, it contains nodular masses which are portions of the enlarged gland.

Fibrous and cystic growths begin as small nodules in the gland, which are easily movable, and do not become intimately connected with the gland or the skin covering it. These growths are not at all dangerous, never terminating fatally, although it is possible that their character may in time become changed; they are, however, usually the cause of much mental uneasiness on the part of the patient, who imagines that she has a cancer. It is sometimes not easy to distinguish a cystic or fibrous growth from a cancer, but usually there is a marked difference in the character of the pain, and the mode of growth. The former grows slowly, while the cancer grows rapidly, and usually occasions death within two or three years. The pain of a cystic tumor is of a neuralgic character if present, and is worse at the menstrual period. The pain of cancer is very severe, and of a sharp, lacerating character, shooting down the arm. When considerably developed, cancer shows its real character by the enlargement of the lymphatic glands of the neck and armpit of the affected side, and by retraction of the nipple, which does not occur in non-malignant tumors. Cancers seldom occur under thirty, while other tumors may appear at any age after puberty, and are most frequent under thirty and in single persons.

Treatment: For overgrowth of the gland, the causes should be removed and pressure applied to the breast by means of adhesive straps or a well placed bandage. Pressure is one of the best means of checking the growth of all forms of tumors of the breast, not excepting cancer. The best mode of applying pressure is by means of an air-bag held firmly in position by a bandage. Compressed sponge, that is, sponge dried under pressure, is also a useful means. In the absence of either, a simple pad of cotton or wool may be applied over the tumor. The application of ice-bags when there is much heat, is a commendable measure of treatment.

When the tumor becomes troublesome by reason of causing pain, or inconvenience on account of its size, it should be removed. This may often be done by a skillful surgeon in such a manner as to leave scarcely any trace of the operation.

Cancer of the Breast

This is one of the most frequent and most formidable of all the forms of cancer. The following are the leading symptoms: a sharp, throbbing, lacerating pain often shooting down the arm; a sense of weight in the breast; sometimes little or no pain; a hard swelling in the substance of the breast which is first moveable, afterward becoming fixed; nipple drawn in; tenderness to the touch; skin over tumor reddish, afterward becoming purple; in some cases the whole breast is moderately hard, there being no distinct tumor; after a time the glands of the neck and armpit become enlarged.

The leading points of difference between cancer and other morbid growths of the breast have been given in the description of "Tumors of the Breast." It is important to note these differences, as a failure to distinguish between a malignant and a non-malignant tumor of the breast has often been the cause of years of unhappiness, and has perhaps quite as often led patients to allow a disease possibly curable at an early stage to reach a degree of development at which all remedies are alike useless.

Treatment: The intractable nature of malignant disease in any part of the body, when well developed, makes it important that prompt measures should be taken upon the first discovery of any symptom affording ground for suspicion of cancer of the breast. The patient should not hesitate and temporize until the chances for a permanent cure are lost. The opinion of the best pathologists at the present day is that the disease is wholly a local affection in its early stages, so that if the diseased part is removed before other parts become infected, the patient has a chance to recover. There is only one method of treatment for use and recommendation in these cases, and that is, thorough removal of the diseased part as soon as suspicious symptoms occur. The earlier the removal can be effected, the better. Of the various methods which have been employed, the removal by the knife is in the majority of cases the best, as it is a thorough operation, and it can be made painless by means of anesthesia; it also possesses the advantages of giving the parts an opportunity for healing immediately, thus affording less opportunity for the disease to return. It has been clearly shown that the slow healing by granulation which follows the use of caustics favors the return of the disease. We have seen caustics employed in many cases, and in every instance in which the disease had shown distinct evidences of cancer, the malady returned in full vigor in a short time. No remedy is a positive cure, however, since the same depraved condition of the system which gave rise to the disease in the first place may cause a new outbreak, even though the first be entirely cured.

The public cannot be too frequently and earnestly warned against patronizing the numerous horde of cancer doctors who thrive upon the ignorance of the masses, lauding the virtues and advantages of so-called specifics which are warranted to cure every case. These wonderful (?) specifics, when of any value whatever, are standard remedies which are well known to the regular profession and have been for years. The apparent success which many of these quacks achieve is due to the fact that they do not hesitate to pronounce all forms of tumors to be cancers, notwithstanding the fact that the great majority of tumors are wholly benign.

A person finding a small, painful lump in the breast should consult a skillful surgeon at once, especially if there is any history of malignant disease in the family. In cases of cancer of the breast which are already very far advanced, ulceration having begun and infection of the system having taken place, as shown by the debilitated condition of the patient and enlargement of the glands under the arm, etc., removal of the breast may still be of advantage in prolonging the life of the patient, and adding to her comfort, although there may be no hope of effecting a cure.

The application of ice to the affected part in the form of iced compresses, or better, by means of rubber bags filled with iced water or small pieces of ice, is an excellent means for relieving the severe pain which characterizes the disease, and also for delaying its progress. Frequent freezing of the diseased parts by means of a mixture of salt and pounded ice, in proportion of one part of the former to two of the latter, applied by means of a muslin bag, has been very highly recommended for holding in check the progress of this terrible malady. These modes of applying cold are also useful in checking the hemorrhage which is often severe after the cancer becomes an open sore. Pressure made by means of air bags and a properly applied bandage, is useful as a means of retarding growth, but cannot be employed where there is much tenderness. When the breast is hot and swollen, support of the breast and the application of cold bags or compresses are indicated.

In the appendix will be found prescriptions for a number of useful applications for use in these cases to remove fetor and subdue pain. When the hemorrhage is not controlled by cold or pressure, soft sponges or absorbent cotton wrung out of hot water may be applied. In severe cases, a physician should be called.

"Willie" by Katharine Tynan (1898)

Introduction

Published in the 18 June 1898 issue of *The Speaker*, "Willie" tells the story of an impoverished mother with breast cancer as her local community faces an outbreak of diphtheria. The juxtaposition of the two illnesses makes the story unique, but each provides important connections. The diphtheria epidemics in London would be familiar to readers of *The Speaker* which published multiple essays on public health apparent in the year preceding Tynan's story.[40] In the decade before "Willie" was published, Tynan lost two friends and mentors, Christina Rossetti and Ellen O'Leary, to breast cancer and published memorial essays about each. The issue of diphtheria in children provides Tynan with an important basis (the affective appeal of a child) for talking about women undergoing medical examinations during which they disrobed and revealed that the symbols of maternal generosity and female beauty were also sites of disease and suffering.

"Willie" (*The Speaker,* 18 June 1898)

They are very poor in Oyster Creek, but poverty seems bearable there in the exquisite air and amid the beauty of sky and sea. All day the quiet thunder of the Atlantic rollers—for Oyster Creek is in the next parish to America—is booming in your ears. Green and purple and aquamarine sea, the fishing village basking in the sun between a couple of majestic headlands, a sky of magnificent clouds—that is Oyster Creek as I remember it. The men go out to sea in old leaky boats to catch the herring, and are poorly equipped in the race against the French and Cornish fishermen with their seaworthy boats and strong nets. The women stay at home, and are busy with a multitude of children, yet find a deal of time for gossiping with each other in the warm sun.

In the whole settlement of Oyster Creek there was only one child alone, and that was Judy Carroll's Willie, aged seven. You might distinguish him from the multitude of his fellows playing their interminable games on the shore by the fact that, at seven years of age, he was still in petticoats, which consorted oddly with his very masculine little personality. The fact was that Judy was the poorest of the poor. Her man had been drowned in a big storm the December following her marriage, and ever since she had had to provide for herself and the child, in spite of delicacy and an utter absence of equipment for the rough tasks that might come her way.

Still, Willie flourished, and was as merry as one of the little mountain lambs that frisked by their mothers up in the grey hills yonder. The pinch never actually reached him, though his mother might go to skin and bone. And like all the children in Oyster Creek, he was lovely, blue-eyed, golden-headed, with skin like the finest rose-leaf. That he was in petticoats hardly disturbed him, though he had the years for the trousers of manhood. He was so popular with

---

[40] For more on this story, its exploration of poverty and illness, and its relation to public health, see Patrick, "Breast Cancer in Short Fiction."

the other children—always the centre of their games, the ringleader in their adventures—that the most heedless respected his petticoats. Once only a jibe had been uttered, and then Willie had gone for his assailant, and having laid him in the sand had turned, quivering and flushed from his victory, and wiped away one or two bitter tears. If he had cried first perhaps the popular sympathies would not have gone with him so unanimously, but that he should first wipe out the insult, and then show the hurt to his tender little heart, ranged every budding man, ay and woman, in the place on his side. The offender against good manners and Willie was a marked infant till the time he had expiated his fault by repentance. Willie sobbed out the tears he had thrust back on his mother's breast.

"Never mind, my lamb," said Judy, sobbing with him. "Just wait till Miss Nora comes home, an' I'll ask her for a bit of the Colonel's homespun,[41] an' 'tis then you'll have the finest trousers in the place."

As she comforted him Judy felt once again the pain in her breast, sharper than an arrow. which had first stabbed her some weeks back. "Glory be to God!" she muttered, as she put down the child and wiped the perspiration from the face that had gone suddenly ashen. "I'll have to be droppin' in to Dr. Sharp when he comes to do the vaccination. I'll be no good at all if this goes on."

A week or two later the doctor came to Oyster Creek, and Judy was amongst the matrons, who came unwillingly, hugging their yet unhurt babies to their breasts.

"And what is the matter with you, Judy?" said the doctor, with a keen look at her, as he gave the last baby back to its wet-eyed mother. "That old neuralgia[42] again, eh?"

"Somethin' like it, doctor," said Judy humbly, following him into the inner room.

"Too much stewed tea and too little food, and rotting thatch and wet beds. That is why all you women suffer the same way," said the doctor.

But his face grew grave as Judy uncovered her breast. His young wife had died before the honeymoon was old, and he was compassionate to women. He looked at the white breast disfigured by an eruption.

"My poor Judy," he said. "You'll have to go to hospital. This thing has roots and will have to be taken away."

---

[41] A cotton fabric.
[42] Pain caused by damaged or irritated nerves

Judy trembled all over, and her eyes were like the eyes of a bird that has been shot. The terror of women had overtaken her, and she knew what it meant; for even in Oyster Creek women had died of cancer.

"But Willie, doctor," she said, helplessly sitting down in the chair he had placed for her. "What is to become of Willie?"

"He will be all right, the little rascal," said the doctor, turning his eyes from her. "He will be as happy as the day is long, and you'll be back to him in a few weeks' time. Be brave, Judy, my woman; we'll do our best for you."

"You'll cure me, doctor?"

"We'll do our best, Judy; be sure of that."

"I wouldn't mind," said Judy, wiping her cold face, "if only I'd last till Willie was man; I'd feel he was all right then for me to go from him."

"You'd never feel he was all right, Judy. It isn't the way with you women. However, we won't talk about that. We must get you into hospital as soon as possible, and make a cure of you."

He spoke with a confidence he was far from feeling. Judy went into hospital within the week and was operated on. The operation was satisfactory, and in a few weeks she was back again with Willie. She had obeyed the doctor humbly and implicitly, but in her own heart she had no great confidence. She had known other women to be cut for the cancer, and it had always come back.

"If it was the will of God," she said to herself, "to spare me a few years more to Willie, I'd go gladly. Sure it wouldn't be a strange country where Terence is, an' 'tisn't me 'ud be afraid of the road, But it is leavin' Willie troubles me. No matter how good they are to him, he won't have his own mother."

But for Willie, she would have hidden away her poor breast and let the cancer take its course. Like all her class, she had a deep horror of an operation, but since it promised at least a respite, she endured what they feel to be the degradation of being cut and maimed, for sake. But the operation seemed to have struck at the roots of life, for Judy was no more able for so much work as she had been accustomed to do. That was the year Mrs. Crosby died in Italy, and the family remained abroad. To go on "the relief"[43] was something Judy shrank from with terror. None of her family had ever eaten the poor bread, and though she would be dead and gone, the disgrace of it would stick to Willie. The neighbours, who knew now that Judy was a very sick woman, were good to her, and it was surprising how many sups of milk and trifles of

---

[43] Various acts and amendments to Britain's Poor Laws led to the creation of County and District Councils in the 1880s and 1890s to support the poor. While these changes made the support more humane, the stigma of accepting such support remained.

meal that this woman and that had no use for and would be obliged by Judy's accepting.

She got through the winter somehow, and spring smiled with its promise of better things. But Judy had hardly begun to take courage when what she had foreseen all along happened. The cancer started in the other breast.

But now Judy went no more to doctors. "It is the will of God," she said, "and I'll stay as I am till He calls me." And wrapping her little shawl across the breast that was eaten as by vultures, she set her eyes towards God and waited.

"'Tis myself," she said, "could bear it all easy, if it wasn't for l'avin' Willie; the cr'ature is lone in the world." And in those days she thought how she could have rejoiced now if he had died in his babyhood, and was waiting for her over yonder beyond the golden gleam of the setting sun with Terence.

"Leave him to God, child," said the priest, who knew all her trouble; and she strove hard to resign herself and trust the child with God, but her heart carried as fierce an ache as her breast in those days when every day brought her nearer the end of her pain.

Then one evening Willie came in and put his curly head in her lap. He had a headache, and his throat was sore, and his hands burned. Judy put him to bed, and gave him hot tea. It is the popular remedy for a cold in Oyster Creek. All night the child tossed and turned, and even her words had no power to soothe him. He was burning hot, and incessantly thirsty. In the morning, when the smoke of the first sticks began to rise from the hearthstones of Oyster Creek, Judy slipped out to the nearest neighbour's for drop of milk.

"Little Willie is that bad with a could," she said, "an' the druth" (*i.e.* drought) is on him, an' the red tay doesn't seem to do him any good. If you could spare a drop o' the goat's milk 'tis myself 'ud obliged, Mrs. Sweeney."

"To be sure, woman dear," said Mrs. Sweeney, who looked harassed. "But the childher here aren't rightly themselves at all. 'Tis the could runnin' through 'em, most likely, or they've been up to some tricks, the rascals, swimmin' in the Pooka's Hole, where it's could enough to perish the heart in you."

It was the same story everywhere. All the children were ill in Oyster Creek, where contagious illness had not been known within the memory man. It was not till the first child died, and that was Mrs. Murphy's Danny, that they thought sending a boy running for his life the eight miles to the town to fetch the doctor. Dr. Sharp came with all speed, and found Oyster Creek full of dead and dying children. It was diphtheria of a virulent type; and having sent for help, the doctor began round of the village, doing what he could to relieve the sick children. A few hours brought doctors and nurses, but before they came the village was full of the cries of bereaved mothers. Dr. Sharp was almost exhausted when he reached Judy's cabin, which a little outside the village. No smoke came from chimney, and the door stood partly open. The place had a deserted look.

Inside, Judy sat with Willie in her lap. She looked up as the doctor came in—"He's gone these two hours," she said tearfully. " I was by myself wid him all night, an' hard I prayed for God to take him. He suffered a dale for an innocent lamb like him. What is it has happened to us at all, doctor?"

"It's something you never heard of, my poor Judy," said the doctor, as he knelt to examine the child. "It's the diphtheria, though God knows how it ever got here, and not a drain within miles of you. Yes, he's gone, poor little man. Lay him down, Judy child, and let me look at yourself."

Judy laughed out, a strange sound in such a place. Then she suddenly flung the shawl from her breast.

"Look, doctor," she said, "'tis not long I'll be after him. 'Tis eating into my heart, it is now, and I won't have to leave Willie, after all. I've kept it to myself, afeard you'd want me to go to hospital again. I didn't want it to be cut. It's the breast Willie was fondest of when he was a baby."

The doctors and nurses came too late, and Oyster Creek was swept almost clear of children. When I have gone there since and have seen the quiet women, and the few children playing on the beach, I have always recalled Willie, a big boy in his petticoats, riotously leading his madcap little crowd.

Articles from *The People's Health Journal of Chicago* (1900–1901)

Introduction

The People's Health Journal of Chicago was a homeopathic monthly newspaper that appealed to a general audience. In the two pieces selected here, they consider the different treatment options for women's cancers. The first selection comes from their monthly advice section that invited readers to submit their "peculiar, obscure or troublesome complaint, or some question of great importance concerning health to be answered." The introduction repeated in each installment explains that they aim "to make it the best bureau of medical information in the world" by having the questions answered for free by the medical professionals employed by the paper. In this case, a woman inquires about a prolapsed uterus, which may also have a cancerous tumor. Though the paper focused on health and preventative medicine, the doctors here recommended a surgical treatment. In the second selection, Dr. John Ellis Gilman reports on new applications of recently discovered x-ray technology as a treatment for cancer, citing two cases of reported cures.

Free Consultations: Case 60 (*The People's Health Journal of Chicago*, 15 January 1900)

I am a farmer's wife, age 62. have eight children. I have prolapsus of the womb so bad it comes out almost all, it looks purple and red and has a small lump in the end. When I am doing my work on my feet it seems like it pulls my bladder down. I am troubled with my bowels, nothing passes without physic. I have to press it back to let the urine pass. At night after I lay for some time it all goes back and then I can pass the urine all right. I was examined by our family physician a few days ago, he thought it was a small tumor or it might be cancer. It has a little dripping of a glue nature when I am on my feet and it bleeds a little. The doctor said, if I would make up my mind to let him cut a piece of it off he would have it analyzed and see what it is. This trouble started twelve years ago and I have always been on my feet and worked hard. Can anything be done to relieve me, and if so, what would it be.

We would advise the complete removal of the uterus. Her age makes it a useless organ. Its dislocation makes it very inconvenient. It is doubtful if any supporter can be adjusted so as to give satisfaction. The possibility of cancer developing is considerable, if it has not already started. Its prompt removal is safe and wise, and it would be a justifiable operation. The danger to life from the operation would not be very great. If she did well she need not be confined to bed more than two weeks. She, of course, should go into a hospital and have an experienced surgeon perform the operation.

Cancer and X-Ray by J. E. Gilman (*The People's Health Journal of Chicago*, 15 November 1901)

CARCINOMA CURED.—Four years ago a nodule appeared in the left breast of Mrs. O. W. Potter[44] of Chicago. It increased in size steadily and with considerable pain. A year ago the nodule began to break down and showed all the characteristics of an encephaloid cancer.

On July 24th, 1900, its size was 7½ by 5½ inches. The tumor itself was bloodred; the nodular margin was blue, hard, and distended, extending under

---

[44] Note in Original Text: Mrs. O. W. Potter, who is well known in this city, consents to the publication of her name as a further guarantee of the genuineness of the cure.

the arm. The axillary lymph nodes were enlarged. In the center of the tumor was an open crater, 2 inches in diameter and 1½ inches deep, whose margin recurved outward like a mushroom. From this there had been three hemorrhages one of which was so severe as to endanger the patient's life. The pain was very severe; sharp, lancinating and burning; making her days and nights a torture. There was considerable discharge having a very foul odor, necessitating a redressing every two hours. The patient was anemic. A blood test was made by Dr. W. H. Wilson from which he diagnosed carcinoma. No microscopic examination of the cancerous tissue was made.

The patient was told by her attendant physician that her case was absolutely hopeless, and that she probably could not live more than three or four months.[45]

The treatment was exposure to the X-ray for ten minutes every other day, with an intensity just short of burning (X-ray dermatitis). This was done at the Illinois X-ray and Therapeutical laboratory, with a low vacuum tube excited by a coil, The medicinal treatment consisted in the administration of tissue remedies to induce marked glandular activity and active excretion. Under the combined treatment the foul odor of the cancer rapidly disappeared; the discharge took on the character of ordinary pus; some of the nodules melted away, while the worst ones discharged pus and healed by granulation; the pain gradually diminished; and in three months from the beginning of the treatment every trace of the cancer was gone and the breast was healed.

It is, of course, too early to say that there will be no return. But a return has now no terrors for the patient.

SCIRRHOUS CANCER CURED.—Mrs. M. of Kenwood, age 73, was referred to me by Dr. Charles W. Crary[46] for treatment. Her right breast was a shapeless mass of hard nodules. The axillary nodes were as large as hen's eggs. The induration extended from the border of the clavicle to the lower margin of the ribs. Dr. A. H. Ferguson, Surgeon of the Chicago Hospital,[47] pronounced cancer and advised its removal.

Treatment was begun April 13th, 1901. It consisted of tissue remedies aimed at cell nutrition and increased assimilation; and exposure for 10 or 12 minutes every second day to the X-rays from a low vacuum tube at the Illinois

---

[45] Ellen Owen Potter died from cancer four years later on 19 June 1904.

[46] Dr. Charles Wesley Crary served as a surgeon in the union army during the Civil War and later established his practice in Chicago where he was a member of the Board of Examining Surgeons.

[47] Dr. Alexander Hugh Ferguson was professor and was a professor and chair of surgery at multiple medical schools in Chicago. He developed multiple surgical instruments and an operation for the cure of hernia, which is still known by his name.

laboratory. The pain, which was considerable, gradually diminished. The induration softened and decreased in size for three weeks, then discharged pus freely, and rapidly healed. On July 15th the only remaining evidence of the cancer was two small nodules in the breast. August 14th the cure was absolute complete.

I think that in the X-ray we have an absolute panacea for cancer. A patient undergoing this treatment may die, then or later, from anemia or other results of the cancer. But if he has strength to overcome these other conditions that exist when the X-ray treatment is begun, he has every prospect of being completely cured.

Manual of Health for Women: Plain Advice in Sickness and Health by Peter J. Latz (1906)

Introduction

In the Preface to the volume, Dr. Peter J. Latz explains his belief that women should understand the diseases common among them enough to live a healthy life and to consult their doctors when they need treatment. His larger purpose is on the ability of women to procreate, as "a sickly mother cannot give birth to healthy, vigorous children" (7). For many of the conditions included, Latz concludes the section with advice on whether a patient should consider marriage. Chapter XXVII focuses entirely on marriage and includes the following a full-page that reinforces the message from the Preface: "no one should enter the married state who is not in perfect good health and who can not reasonably hope to have healthy children" (175). The sections below include gynecological cancers but the volume makes no mention of cancer or tumors in the breast.

Cancer of the Womb (Carcinoma uteri)

Cancerous tumors form a sharp contrast to those just described. While the myoma seldom endangers life, cancer is generally fatal. This dreaded malady has been studied closely by physicians at all times and is defined in our days as a proliferation of the epithelial cells of the womb, leading to ulcerous degeneration, decay, and serious general disease.

Every woman who, after the cessation of her monthly flow at the change of life suffers from irregular hemorrhages, should at once consult a physician, because under such conditions there is always danger of cancer.

Causes: Little is known of the real cause of cancer. Heredity, syphilis, gonorrhoea, mental depressions, etc., have been assigned as causes; but physicians as a rule unite in believing that the true nature of the disease is yet to be discovered.

It is a fact that cases of cancer of the womb have increased of late in a frightful manner, and perhaps not without reason; the increased consumption of meat is blamed for this.

Cancer is most often observed between the ages of 35 to 55; seldom in younger persons.

Symptoms: The symptoms of cancer of the womb are so uncertain in the beginning that ordinarily when its existence is discovered it is too late to offer any hope of a cure. Yet in some cases, there is a characteristic early discharge from the vagina, a discharge that is bloody and sanious, rather than purulent. When the cancerous tumor once is formed, discharges and hemorrhages are abundant, often being caused by the slightest irritation, such as produced by intercourse, or straining at stool.

Frequently a brine-like liquid is discharged with the blood from the vagina. This is likely to be the case when the growth has the shape of a cauliflower. As the disease progresses all vaginal discharges have a disagreeable, putrid odor. The acridity of the discharge causes inflammation of the vagina, of the outer genital parts and of the groins, especially in patients who neglect to observe strict cleanliness.

Sometimes the cancerous tumor presses on the rectum and causes difficult evacuation; at other times it may cause inflammation of the mucous membrane of the rectum, followed by bloody, purulent diarrhoea.

Where cancer has attached the bladder there is frequent desire to urinate and the passage of the urine, which at times is bloody and purulent, is extremely painful.

Patients complain but little in the beginning; as a rule the pains begin when the tumor enlarges and the womb presses upon surrounding organs, or when the inflammation extends to the peritoneum. These pains may become excessive and are described as piercing, like labor pains or those of colic. They may radiate towards the back, the external genital parts, and the groins. By pressure on the large blood vessels, dropsical swellings may appear in the lower limbs, the external genitals, and the lower abdomen.

The general condition of the patient is at first little disturbed; she lacks appetite, however, looks sickly, and grows thin. As a rule there is no fever. The duration of the disease varies greatly, generally it lasts two years, but cases of four and five years standing have also been observed. Death comes in various ways. Hemorrhage, peritonitis, general debility, toxic absorption, any of these clinical conditions may bring on the end.

Hygienic Measures: When cancer of the womb has been discovered, a surgical operation should follow as soon as possible, providing of course an operation can be performed. It is of prime importance that the operation be performed early, as this offers the best hope for life. The delay, while one remedy after another is tried, only raises false hopes in the mind of the patient and her friends, and lessens the chances of a cure by operation.

Whether favorable results may be obtained by the natural curative method, has not as yet been demonstrated.

Where a complete extirpation of the cancer cannot be accomplished the patient is to be treated according to symptoms present. For the pains wet warm bandages over the abdomen, to be renewed every two or three hours are advisable. If they do not give relief, lukewarm sitz baths, lasting from a quarter to half an hour may be tried. Should they also fail, steaming poultices over the abdomen and small of the back, of ten minutes duration, repeated four to six times, may help. A wet towel may be placed over the abdomen, and over it a hot water bag, to prevent loss of heat, and over all a woolen blanket.

Sometimes, especially where the cancer is situated in the vagina and neck of the womb, repeated injections of hot water, 110° F., will relieve the pain.

If all these measures are unavailing, the physician will necessarily apply anodyne remedies.

For hemorrhages and offensive discharges, when no pains are felt, cold compresses over the abdomen, to be renewed every three to five minutes, and repeated cold sitz baths, lasting from one half to one minute, may be used.

Vaginal injections at 77° F. of a decoction of oak bark are especially beneficial. Of greatest service, however, is a systematic tamponing of the vagina with absorbent cotton previously dipped into boiled water, after it has cooled off. It may be necessary to change these tampons twice or three times a day.

In more serious cases of hemorrhage, and foul smelling discharges where the odor of the secretions remains offensive, these tampons may be dipped into a strong decoction of oak bark or in diluted lemon juice.

The bowels should move more freely, because constipation increases pains in the womb. Stewed prunes, or apples, raw fruit, graham breast with fruit or honey, buttermilk, clabber, etc., will be of service. On account of the odor the sick room should be large and frequently aired.

It is hardly worth mentioning that a person suffering from cancer of the womb must not marry under any circumstance.

Sarcoma of the Womb (Sarcoma uteri)

Sarcoma is a malignant tumor of the connective tissue, which is of rare occurrence, and in the beginning shows much similarity to benign growths. A thorough diagnosis is possible only be the aid of a microscopical examination. A rapid growth of the womb in young people is suspicious.

Causes: The cause of sarcoma is not known.

Symptoms: They are similar to those of cancer, with this difference, that pain is frequently absent, and general debility and sanious discharges set in later than in cancer.

Hygienic Measures: The only treatment is a surgical operation as soon as possible. It may at least prolong the life of the patient for a few years.

As to hygienic measures for particular symptoms, they are the same as given for cancer of the womb.

Sarcoma belongs, as has been mentioned above, to the class of malignant tumors, and in such cases marriage is to be absolutely interdicted.

Ovarian Tumors

Tumors of the ovaries are of frequent occurrence, as no organ of the female body is so inclined to new growths of all kinds as the ovaries. They occur most frequently between the ages of thirty and forty, but younger women may likewise be subject to them.

According to their origin, we distinguish three kinds of ovarian tumors: (1) cysts, consisting of a vesicle or sac filled with a thin liquid, forming round tumors, and arising from glandular elements; (2) dermoid tumors, such as are formed from growth of included epithelium. On the inside of such tumors are found sweat and sebaceous glands, long hair, and often also bones and cartilage and teeth. (3) Solid neoplasms as fibroma, sarcoma and carcinoma.

Causes: The origin of ovarian tumors is unknown.

Symptoms: The symptoms are very variable. There may be no indication whatever of the malady, or the symptoms may be very obscure. Small tumors ordinarily cause trouble only when they are of inflammatory character. Again there may be severe manifestations from the beginning, such as intense radiating pains, urinary troubles, constipation, enlargement of the abdomen, etc.

In some cases menstruation is interrupted or irregular. In its further development the tumor may increase enormously in size, and so cause serious symptoms. By pressing the diaphragm upwards and compressing the lungs, breathing may become difficult. Pressure of the tumor on the veins of the kidney may cause congestion of this organ, or albuminuria.

Add to this stomach troubles, such as nausea, which interfere seriously with the general nutrition. Usually the patient is sterile although conception is possible if only one ovary is affected.

A timely operation is almost invariably followed by complete recovery. If neglected a twisting of the pevicle maybe followed by fatal peritonitis, there may be chills, emaciation, and often dropsy. Simple or dermoid cysts offer the best chance of recovery.

Hygienic Measures: Where an ovarian tumor has been diagnosed the patient must avoid everything that is likely to bring about a congestion in the pelvic organs, for instance, immoderate intercourse, and hard work during the monthly flow. The patient should have regular daily evacuations of the bowels and bladder.

In every case of ovarian tumors their surgical removal is to be recommended; especially in medium sized, very movable tumors, because in such cases there is danger of twisting of the pedicle, followed by peritonitis, i. e., inflammation of the covering of the bowels. In this case the advocate of the natural method of healing must advise a timely surgical operation, unless he desires to assume a gross responsibility.

Whether a person with an ovarian tumor ought to marry depends upon the character of the growth. Marriage is absolutely proscribed when the tumor is malignant. Even with benign growths of the ovary, marriage may not be advisable, since these tumors not infrequently become malignant. It goes without saying that a person afflicted with an ovarian tumor should, when contemplating marriage, consult a conscientious gynecologist. In doubtful cases marriage ought not to be thought of.

"A Protest Against the Surgical Invasion of Cancers and Tumors" (1917)

Introduction

This essay from *Current Opinion* presents for a more general audience a debate about surgical treatments for cancer based on a note from Dr. Haven G. Emerson (New York City's health commissioner and public-health physician) in the 27 January 1917 issue of *The Medical Record* and the response from Dr. Thomas L. Stedman (medical doctor and editor of *The Medical*

Record) in the 17 February 1917 issue. The article sides with Stedman and considers risks of a two-part procedure that would first remove a portion of a tumor for biopsy and diagnosis and in a second operation remove the cancer and in order as treatment. Though the essay is unsigned and "the health commissioner of the greatest city in the land" and "the editor of *The Medical Record*" are not named, the article cites by name Dr. Joseph C. Bloodgood, surgeon at Johns Hopkins Hospital where he worked with Dr. William S. Halsted, who pioneered the radical mastectomy. *Current Opinion* was a popular American illustrated monthly news magazine.

A Protest Against the Surgical Invasion of Cancers and Tumors (*Current Opinion*, November 1917)

Emphatic as have been the warnings of eminent surgeons in the recent past against the practice of operating upon cancers and tumors on general principles, the tendency has not, according to The Medical Record (New York), been adequately checked. An instance we are told, is afforded by "a most ill-advised suggestion" of the health commissioner of the greatest city in the land regarding the excision of suspected cancerous tissue for diagnostic purposes. When the danger inherent in this advice was pointed out to him, he replied that the editor of *The Medical Record* is apparently unaware of the report of a committee for the control of cancer on the very question raised by the controversy. The commissioner says:

> The scheme lends itself particularly to the early diagnosis of superficial and other accessible cancers—the lips, tongue, cervix, breast, etc., but is no less applicable to the investigation and diagnosis of all suspicious lesions from which it is possible to remove small particles of tissue for microscopic examination. In these the operation is free from danger…and the result of microscopic investigation is practically always such as to determine the diagnosis with scientific exactitude….It is hoped that the plan will commend itself most strongly in connection: with the diagnosis of malignant growths….Specimens in which an immediate diagnosis is imperative should be sent directly to the Research Laboratories,…and a report based upon examination of frozen sections will be sent by letter or telephone within 24 or 36 hours. Otherwise specimens may be left at the nearest collecting stations, and will be reported upon within two or three days, or sooner, if practicable.

The commissioner's recommendation is, as a matter of fact, condemned by the very report to which he appeals, says the medical organ. The advantage in the way of diagnosis sometimes gained by microscopical examination of a piece of suspected tissue is counterbalanced by the danger of aggravating the disease through the resultant wound. That is what the committee for the control of cancer reported. To cut through the skin into a malignant tumor of the breast, the committee said, and to remove a piece for examination is generally discountenanced. Not a few errors in diagnosis result from the excision of inflamed tissue on the edge of a tumor, the malignant area being missed. In general, it may be said, according to the committee, that incisions into actively growing, deep-seated malignant tumors should, if possible, be avoided. The result might be to disseminate tumor cells through the vessels or to permit unnecessary extension to the skin or surrounding tissues, or to accelerate growth by relief of a capsular tension.

No surgeon, according to the well-known authority, Dr. J. C. Bloodgood, should remove a lump in the breast for microscopic study, delay a few days or weeks and then perform the complete operation for cancer if the tissues studied microscopically should prove malignant, because the patient whose chances to be cured were at least eighty per cent., will by such a procedure be almost doomed to death. In the very early stages of cancer the surgeon often employs a method for diagnosis—excision of a piece—which is dangerous before undertaking an operation. It would be of advantage to the patient, according to another high authority quoted, if each questionable tumor of the breast, for example, could be regarded as a high explosive, the least manipulation of which should be absolutely avoided both prior to and during the operation. The organ of the New York medical profession concludes:

> In case of doubt, and after all other means of diagnosis have been exhausted, it may be permissible or even advisable to remove scrapings from ulcerated mucous or cutaneous surfaces and examine them under the microscope. Such an examination will usually, but not always, establish the diagnosis. But it should be realized that one who harpoons or excises a piece of tissue from a tumor with unbroken cutaneous or mucous surface, especially an encapsulated tumor, and then waits a day or two while the specimen is being examined, will almost inevitably destroy the patient's chance of recovery by operation. The health commissioner's unqualified recommendation to physicians, who are responsible for the lives of their patients, to resort to indiscriminate digging into all tumors on the chance of thereby reaching a diagnosis, which can usually be made by safer measures and which moreover is not always absolutely necessary, is positively wicked, and a physician acting on this advice would have no defense whatever if the heirs of his patient should bring a malpractice suit.

The House on the Bogs by Katharine Tynan (1922)

Introduction

In this 1922 novel, Katharine Tynan draws her portrayal of breast cancer heavily on Maria Edgeworth's *Belinda*, again illustrating the ways that fear of breast cancer could make women susceptible to be tricked and made ill by unqualified or dishonest caregivers. In the excerpts presented here, the protagonist Doreen O'Kelly finds her friend and benefactor Peggy Hamilton sick with breast cancer and being treated by her servant Margot. Like Lady Delacour in *Belinda*, Peggy Hamilton is afraid to seek treatment with a licensed or professional doctor both because she fears a mastectomy and because she worries about mental illness. Doreen's training in nursing connects her to the established medical field and allows her to see the realities of Peggy's condition and begin treating her.

Excerpts from Chapter X: The Lit House

"Eat something now. I shall not eat more than half of this omelette."

"Oh, I couldn't," Miss Hamilton said, with a greedy look at the omelette. "Such food would be poison to me. I never eat meat of any kind, nor eggs. My diet is kept very low. I must not see such food or I could not resist eating it."[48]

"Why, I believe you are starved," said Doreen, indignantly. "It was time I came. That is why you are so thin."

"Ah, no," said Miss Hamilton, and laid a hand on her breast. "There is something here—a growth of some kind. I have had the gnawing pain for many months now. Margot is certain it is a growth."

"Have you seen a doctor?"

"No; I am afraid of doctors. The last one I saw told Margot that I ought to be in an asylum. I couldn't bear that. I would rather be dead a thousand times."

"I don't believe any doctor would say such a thing," said Doreen. "Come! You are starved. Eat some of the omelette."

...

"Margot said that heating foods were bad. They simply feed the thing that is eating me up. It is true that I feel no worse for the omelette and the wine, but better, much better. I may be worse later. We shall see."

---

[48] Starvation diets were commonly advised throughout the nineteenth and early twentieth centuries as part of treatment for cancer.

"If you are not worse you will consent to take more food?"

"If I am not worse. Why, I long for food. I am sick for it. I have told Margot so. She says it is the growth that is hungry. I have enough to live on in the biscuits, the thin gruel for breakfast, the baked apples."

"I don't believe you have a growth at all," said Doreen, greatly daring. In her own mind she believed she was right. Miss Hamilton looked rather a starved woman than a sick woman. The skin had not changed colour although it was dry and parched-looking. She remembered an old nun at the Abbey who had a growth—the heavy yellow darkness of her skin and complexion.

"Margot looks as though she had a growth," she said.

"She is not healthy," Miss Hamilton agreed. "I do not like her about me, but I cannot do without her. After all, they have saved me from the mad-house."

Her eyes dilated. A wild fear came into her expression.

Excerpts from Chapter XII: The Poison of Jealousy

With such alternations of courage and weakness in Miss Hamilton Doreen had to contend, while the autumn went on and the leaves fell and the bogs and a distant line of hills hitherto hidden, came into view.

She had discovered what lay at the root of Miss Hamilton's subjection to her hideous nurse. The poor thing believed herself doomed to a death from cancer. The trouble had begun with acute pain in the breast. For this Margot had treated her mistress with stupes, poultices and blisters of one kind or another, which had but added to the suffering, for apparently sores and terrible eruptions had broken out following this treatment.

"I ought to have sent you away at first, Doreen," she said one day, weeping, "before you had become so necessary and dear to me. It is selfish of me to let you stay now, but, when things get worse, you must go. Do you remember when you came first and I thought of going back into the world for your sake? I wish it had been possible. But this pain tells me I am a dying woman. A little more and you must leave me to die alone."

"I wish you would see a doctor," pleaded Doreen, for the hundredth time. "I cannot believe there is anything malignant. You have put on flesh wonderfully since I came and insisted on your being fed—for which Margot hates me. You are not the same woman. You have pain in your face, but otherwise it is healthy. It is not like a woman of your strength of mind to allow yourself to be treated by an ignorant old quack like this Frenchwoman."

…

"Ah, she would not like to hear that said of her. Not that she often leaves her kitchen. If there was anyone there, it must have been Pierre. You are sure the door is closed? You were talking about a doctor, Doreen, but I am weary of telling you I will not have a doctor. I won't be cut to pieces. Moreover, a doctor might certify me insane."

…

She was oppressed by the futility of her efforts to induce Miss Hamilton to see a doctor. She had been hoping that with returning health and strength, for both had come under her regime, Miss Hamilton would come to her senses and free herself from the domination of Margot. But so far there had been no such result. Doreen had her moments of despair, in which she felt that Miss Hamilton's belief in her own imminent death must have a fatal effect.

Miss Hamilton's face was turned on her, with a strange light upon it.

"I ought to tell you that at a certain stage of my illness you must go," she said, "but it means so much to me that you are willing to stay; it means the whole world of difference. I should like to tell you that when I am gone, everything will be yours—with adequate provision for the servants, and a few bequests to charity. I have no relatives to grudge it to you…"

…

Miss Hamilton, after a little protest, drank the wine.

"Margot would say I was poisoning myself," she said, putting down the glass. "Meat and wine, she always said, are poison for me, food for the trouble here," she laid her hand on her breast. "I am beginning to believe Margot is wrong. I am better than when you came and took me off the starvation diet. Margot has always over-eaten. She had no pity for me."

The colour came back to her cheeks. She certainly looked as though the tears, or the confession she had made, had relieved her.

Excerpts from Chapter XVIII: Fear

If a cold chill came to the high heart, remembering that Peggy Hamilton believed herself to have a mortal disease, she quickly recovered. She would not believe that there was not happiness yet left for the woman whose life had been poisoned at its prime. She was determined to take the sick woman to a Dublin specialist away from the irresponsible servant who had doubtless been using quack medicines, so aggravating the trouble, whatever it might be. Once out of Moat they were not going to return till the whole place had been purged and cleansed from the malign influences about it.

…

A whisper came from the great four-poster bed, in the darkness.

"Is it you, Doreen? I have been calling you, and calling you, and you did not come."

"Yes, it is I," said Doreen. "I came as soon as I could. Why, what has happened to you? I have not been a week away?"

"Bolt—the—door," said Miss Hamilton, lifting her head from the pillows and staring with dilated eyes towards the door.

Doreen obeyed and came back.

"Open a window!"

She let up the blind with a jerk and opened the window up and down as far as it would go. The fresh cold air came pouring in, the afternoon light showing the neglected room. The fire in the grate was grey ash and the turf ash, fine and powdery was over everything. On the table by the bed were various cups and glasses, all unwashed, with one or two medicine bottles. The dreariness of a neglected sick-room, in addition to the disorder which follows human occupation and needs incessant putting in order, was over everything.

Excerpts from Chapter XX: Child's Play

Very gently Doreen uncovered the place Peggy Hamilton had indicated as the seat of a mortal disease. There was bandage after bandage, which she handled deftly. Why on earth were there all these bandages? There was no sign of a suppurating sore that she could perceive; but, after the sixth or seventh bandage had been taken off, there was a dark stain on the linen and a smell she thought she recognised. Madame Thekla had dangled it as a bait before Doreen, that if she stayed on at Klosterberg she should nurse the dear sick.[49] It was a nursing talent, a *nerveille*[50] which Doreen possessed. A thousand pities it should be lost or be only for the few.

Miss Hamilton was lying back, very pale and with closed eyes, while Doreen removed the bandages. "It is horrible, Doreen," she murmured. "You should not have to attend to such a thing, child. It is not fit for you. I should not permit it."

---

[49] Doreen's studies in Germany, funded by Peggy, included some nursing.
[50] This literally translates as "to the nerves," but suggests that Doreen has strong nerves in dealing with illness.

"Ah, bella-donna!"[51] said Doreen, having got off the last bandage. She had located the smell—beneath the last bandage lay a bella-donna plaster of considerable thickness.

"This has got to come off," she said gently. "I shall hurt you as little as possible. I hope it will come quite easily."

The kettle was boiling on the fire. She poured water into a basin and began stuping the plaster, lifting it by infinitesimal bits as she proceeded. At last the plaster was off, with very little suffering to the patient, but, as it was lifted, Miss Hamilton groaned with a spiritual pain.

"Ts it horrible, Doreen?" she asked, and, glancing at her face, Doreen saw that a sweat had come out upon it. The place indeed looked horrible enough, but she had no disgust. It was one of the inestimable qualifications for nursing, Madame Thekla had said, that Doreen had no disgust where the sick were concerned; or disgust was lost in compassion.

She laid a fold of clean linen gently over the place, while she fetched clean water and a boracic wash. When she had cleaned the sore place, her eyes were very angry and her mouth stern.

"Why did you let that ignorant woman treat you, Peg?" she asked hotly. "It is as I anticipated. For one with your colour bella-donna is poisonous. It has been eating through your skin. It says a deal for your power of resistance, that the place is not much worse."

Miss Hamilton's eyes opened wide. The colour flooded her face.

"It is not cancer———?" she said, with a cry.

"Cancer; no! The irritation once removed, it will heal. It is external. I believe the pain you suffered from was merely intercostal neuralgia. That wretched woman! She deserves to suffer!"

Deliberately she spoke with that air of confidence. The intercostal neuralgia had been an after-thought. A nun at the Abbey had suffered agonies of pain from what a Vienna specialist had diagnosed as intercostal neuralgia, not cancer, as the poor nun had feared.

"You blessed child!" Peggy Hamilton broke into sobbing. "Are you sure, Doreen? It would be terrible to be relieved from that agony only to take it on again."

"I am sure about the bella-donna."

She remembered the Herr Doktor standing up by the nun's bed and saying: "Not bella-donna with her complexion. It would eat the skin into holes."

---

[51] Belladonna is a plant used as part of homeopathic and alternative medical treatments. It has also been used as a poison.

"As soon as I can move you out of this, you will see a doctor. By that time this place will be healed."

"Oh Doreen, you don't know what you have done for me," Peggy Hamilton said, her face bright, despite the tears. "You have opened new life to me. When I am able we shall go away from this place. We shall travel. I am not an old woman. There should be some happiness in life left for me yet, for us, Doreen."

"The Prevention of Cancer" by James Ewing (1927)

Introduction

In this essay from *The Forum*, Dr. James Ewing explains current medical understandings of cancer for a general audience, describing differences in the various parts of the body. In the section on breast and uterine cancer, he describes the connections between reproductive behaviors and the incidence of cancer. Ewing was one of the foremost cancer doctors of the early twentieth century and helped to found the American Society for Control of Cancer (now the American Cancer Society) and Memorial Hospital (now Memorial Sloan Kettering Cancer Center). *The Forum* was a widely read monthly American journal, which included fiction and poetry as well as essays on contemporary social and political issues (sometimes by American presidents).

The Prevention of Cancer (*The Forum*, March 1927)

How shall we protect ourselves against cancer, the greatest of all the natural hazards in the adventure of living? For cancer is generally like old age, the result of the wear and tear of the tissues, due to the natural stresses of living. Unlike senility, cancer attacks the young much more frequently than is commonly realized and it plays the greater havoc the younger the subject. If an ounce of prevention is generally worth a pound of cure, who may measure the value of cancer prevention? Yet prevention does not form a prominent chapter in the literature of cancer. It has not been dignified, like cancer therapy, by decades of acrimonious debate in medical societies. Nevertheless there is a great deal to be done for the prevention of cancer, and most of it must be done by the person himself.

There are two main reasons for this neglect of the prophylaxis of cancer. In order to prevent a disease one must know its causes, and every one has been told again and again that the ultimate cause of cancer is unknown. There is a very venerable and widespread belief, in and out of the medical profession, that cancer is caused by some mysterious microscopic parasite. Every month or so, one reads of the discovery of this parasite, and often of cancer cures based upon the new discovery. If cancer really is caused by an unknown parasite, then prevention is not to be considered; and we are not much better off than the ancient Egyptians, since we may at any time be stung to death by this hobgoblin parasite in its own mysterious way. The distressing difference in favor of the Egyptians is that they were beautifully embalmed like Tut-ankh-Amen, and we are not.

To-day, however, the scientific evidence is against the parasitic theory of cancer. It is a fortunate fact that most cancers are caused by various forms of chronic irritation, many of which we can detect and eliminate and thus prevent cancer. What the scientists mean by the cause of cancer is the ultimate cause of cell growth, and this we shall probably never know. What people want to know are the effective, exciting factors in cancer, and of these we have much useful knowledge.

…

Cancer of the breast is one of the most urgent problems in the entire file of malignant tumors. Until recently there has been very little to say about its prevention. The interest of the medical profession has been directed toward its earlier recognition and treatment. It has long been known that breast cancer is much more frequent in women who have not nursed children than in others, and since it occurs mainly after forty years of age it has been vaguely attributed to abnormal processes connected with the natural atrophy of the breast and the loss of its functions. Yet the disease frequently occurs in young women, from twenty to thirty years of age. Recently new light seems to have been thrown on the causation of breast cancer by the discovery that in mice breast cancer can readily be produced by withdrawing the young at birth and allowing the breast to become swollen with retained and decomposing milk. Ligating the ducts on one side of the mouse has led to cancer in four of the six breasts on the ligated side, while no cancers developed on the nursed side. That stagnation of milk and other secretions occurs in striking degree in many cases of human breast cancer has long been known, so that the recent experimental observations are supported by much former knowledge of the disease. Such experimental results require repetition and verification before they can be assumed to apply to the human subject; but if they do prove to be applicable, as seems extremely probable, then we have a basis for the prevention of cancer of the breast.

Contrary to previous notions, it thus appears that the breast will not always take care of itself, but must be watched and cared for intelligently by women themselves, directed by sound medical advice. Secretions accumulate in the ducts of the breast during monthly periods of congestion, as the result of miscarriages and abortions, and especially when the normal periods of nursing are reduced or eliminated. Massage and the regular use of the breast pump are available to correct these conditions, but our present knowledge does not warrant a definite statement of the best methods of establishing a normal hygiene of the breast. This is the task of the well-informed family physician. It is notably safe to assert that the habit of early and abrupt weaning of infants conduces to cancer of the breast. Comparatively few women who develop breast cancer give a history of normal lactation.

The domestic cow is milked every morning and every evening, and the last vestiges of milk are "stripped". No one hears of breast cancer in this animal. After all, we humans are not so far removed from our lower animal friends that we may not learn something from their experiences.

It must not be assumed that stagnation is the only factor concerned in the causation of mammary cancer or that the hygiene of the breast ends with attention to this matter. Diseases of the skin of the breast, infections of the nipple, abcesses of the breast, congenital and probably inherited anomalies in the structure of the organ, and some benign tumors, all occasionally lead to cancer, and should, as far as possible, be guarded against.

Cancer of the breast is sometimes preceded by the appearance of a lump in the breast or by bleeding from the nipple. Both of these conditions call for immediate examination by a physician.

Cancer of the uterus (womb) is by far the most frequent form of the disease in women, and is responsible for about thirty to thirty-five per cent of the deaths from cancer in the female. It is one of the forms of cancer which is probably increasing in frequency. It is much more frequent in women who have borne children than in those who have not; and there is general agreement among physicians that the uterine lacerations occurring in childbirth are a very important factor in its causation. It is especially when the lacerations, often slight, are not properly repaired and fully healed that cancer is prone to develop. About these neglected, unhealed wounds, inflammation and infection become established, abnormal discharges appear, and in the course of time, sometimes relatively short, cancer develops and generally makes rapid headway. The remedy is rather simple and easily applied, but only periodical examinations by a competent physician can determine when and how to apply the remedy. There seems to be no other means of preventing uterine cancer than recognizing it early, for if the patient waits until the bleeding occurs, it is often too late. There is a most pernicious belief among women that the change of life is accompanied by bleeding. Abnormal discharge, or any bleeding in a woman after forty years of age, calls for immediate examination by a competent physician. Very early cancer of the uterus frequently gives no detectable symptoms and can be recognized only through a physical examination by a physician. To further this end, clinics for free examination of women for breast and uterine cancer, and for the conditions that lead to them, have been established in a few cities. It is obviously the duty of women of intelligence to consult their private physicians on this important matter.

In another considerable group of cases, cancer affects the body of the uterus, and here the causes are more numerous and less clear. The whole matter of the prevention of uterine cancer reduces itself to periodical examinations by a competent physician at least once a year, and the maintenance of a proper hygiene of this organ.

It thus appears that the major forms of cancer which cause most of the deaths are due to controllable factors, generally some form of chronic irritation. There is a sound basis for the effort to prevent cancer by such public propaganda as is conducted by the American Society for the Control of Cancer and by increased medical efficiency. This belief is strongly supported by the fact that cancer does not as a rule develop suddenly in previously normal tissues, but nearly always slowly in tissues that have been altered by inflammation and disease. The changes that precede cancer are called "precancerous", and it is an important fact that they require time to become cancer. During this time both patient and physician usually have definite and ample warning of approaching danger. Absence of pain is probably the chief reason why the danger signs are not more generally heeded. The fact that they are not generally heeded is one of the great anomalies of modern life.

...

Finally, the analytical reader will probably notice that most of the factors tending to produce cancer belong among the personal habits of the individual, which are more or less necessitated by the stress of modern civilized life. The most effective plan of avoiding cancer is to practise moderation in all things, to live as simple a life as possible, to attend to any minor persistent disturbances in the functions of one's organs, and to consult a physician at least once a year, with specific reference to the hazards of cancer.

References

American Cancer Society. Breast Cancer Facts & Figures 2022–2024. Atlanta: American Cancer Society, Inc. 2022. https://www.cancer.org/content/dam/cancer-org/research/cancer-facts-and-statistics/breast-cancer-facts-and-figures/2022-2024-breast-cancer-fact-figures-acs.pdf

Aronowitz, Robert A. 2007. *Unnatural History: Breast Cancer and American Society.* Cambridge: Cambridge University Press.

"Breast Cancer Statistics and Resources." Breast Cancer Research Foundation. https://www.bcrf.org/breast-cancer-statistics-and-resources/ Accessed 26 Jan 2023.

Couser, G. Thomas. 1997. *Recovering Bodies: Illness, Disability, and Life Writing.* Madison: University of Wisconsin Press.

DeShazer, Mary K. 2013. *Mammographies: The Cultural Discourses of Breast Cancer Narratives.* Ann Arbor: University of Michigan Press.

Ferlay, Jacques, et al. 2020. Global Cancer Observatory: Cancer Today. International Agency for Research on Cancer. https://gco.iarc.fr/today

Gardner, Kirsten E. 2006. *Early Detection: Women, Cancer, and Awareness Campaigns in the Twentieth-Century United States.* Chapel Hill: University of North Carolina Press.

Kaartinen, Marjo. 2016. *Breast Cancer in the Eighteenth Century.* London: Routledge.

Knopf-Newman, Marcy Jane. 2004. *Beyond Slash, Burn, and Poison: Transforming Breast Cancer Stories into Action.* New Brunswick: Rutgers University Press.

Leopold, Ellen. 1999. *A Darker Ribbon: Breast Cancer, Women, and their Doctors in the Twentieth Century.* Boston: Beacon Press.

Lerner, Barron H. 2001. *The Breast Cancer Wars: Hope, Fear, and the Pursuit of a Cure in Twentieth-Century America.* Oxford: Oxford University Press.

Löwy, Ilana. 2011. *A Woman's Disease: The History of Cervical Cancer.* Oxford: Oxford University Press.

Montini, Theresa, and Sheryl Ruzek. 1989. Overturning Orthodoxy: The Emergence of Breast Cancer Treatment Policy. *Research in the Sociology of Health Care* 8: 3–32.

Morantz-Sanchez, Regina. 2000. *Sympathy and Science: Women Physicians in American Medicine.* Chapel Hill: University of North Carolina Press.

Moscucci, Ornella. 2016. *Gender and cancer in England, 1860–1948.* London: Palgrave Macmillan.

Nielsen, Emilia. 2019. *Disrupting Breast Cancer Narratives: Stories of Rage and Repair.* Toronto: University of Toronto Press.

Olson, James S. 2002. *Bathsheba's Breast: Women, Cancer, and History.* Baltimore: Johns Hopkins University Press.

Index[1]

A

Abortifacient, 11, 196, 202, 204, 280, 284
Abortion Act of 1967, 1, 202
Abortionist, 204, 214, 224, 231, 240, 241, 246, 302, 374, 376
Abstinence, 195, 196, 203, 251
Accoucheurs, 17, 21, 56, 59, 63, 65, 69, 71, 76, 91–96, 161, 220, 363, 376
Adams, John, 356, 358–361
Advertisements, 212, 219, 231, 234, 235, 237, 238, 240, 294, 296, 322
Advice books and articles, 348
Allbutt, Henry Arthur, 24, 115–121, 247
Alternative medicine, 350
American Cancer Society (American Society for the Control of Cancer), 341n1, 445, 448
Anesthesia, 4, 5, 16, 19–22, 24, 82–88, 169, 170, 172, 342, 344, 347, 348, 350, 395n29, 424
Antiseptic, 4, 22, 152, 204, 342, 345, 350, 388
Autobiography, 8, 97, 259, 264

B

Bakewell, Robert Hall, 24, 88–97
Bell, Pearl Doles, 284–287
Birth control, 5, 196–199, 203, 204, 212, 258, 287, 289–297, 310, 312
Blackwell, Elizabeth, 374–376
Blackwood, Helen, Lady Dufferin and Claneboye, Countess of Gifford, 406–418
Blatch, Harriot Stanton, 251–258
Breastfeeding, 197
Brown, John, 351, 397–405

---

[1] Note: Page numbers followed by 'n' refer to notes.

© The Author(s), under exclusive license to Springer Nature Switzerland AG 2023
A. Patrick, *Women's Health in Britain and America*, Humanities and Healthcare: Practical and Pedagogical Guides, https://doi.org/10.1007/978-3-031-41257-8

C

Caesarean section, 21, 22
Cancer
　breast, 6, 9, 12, 341–345, 341n1, 342n2, 344n3, 347n4, 348, 349, 351, 354, 356–361, 382–397, 406, 419, 425, 426, 440, 445–448
　cervical, 6, 12, 341, 342, 344, 345
　ovarian, 6, 12, 341, 345
　uterine, 12, 341, 344, 345, 374, 445, 448
　vaginal, 341
Charlotte, Princess, 56–64
Chloroform, 20, 21, 24, 80, 82–88, 95, 147, 155, 169, 284, 344, 395, 395n29, 400
Chopin, Kate, 24, 136–141, 153–155
Coitus interruptus, 195–197
Comstock, Anthony, 202, 204, 214, 215, 218–220, 287, 292–298, 312
Comstock Laws, 6, 218
Costello, Madame, 221, 223, 224, 231, 238
Criminal charges, 201–202, 216–219, 231–232, 238–247, 267–268, 293–294
Croft, Sir Richard, 56, 57, 59, 61–63, 104

D

D'Arblay, Frances Burney, 361–373
Dilation and curettage (D&C), 199, 328
Dobbs *vs.* Jackson Women's Health Organization, 6
Doyle, Arthur Conan, 11, 142
DuBois, W. E. B., 310–311

E

Ether, 21, 24, 78–80, 82–86, 144, 169, 172, 329, 334, 344, 395n29
Ewing, James, 445–448

F

Fallen women, 336
Family planning and limitation, 196, 199–200, 225–229, 287–292, 298–299, 334–338
Fitzgerald, F. Scott, 312–313
Forceps, 4, 16, 21, 22, 65, 168

G

Gilman, Charlotte Perkins, 121–136
Godwin, William, 36–43
Gosse, Edmund, 383–396, 387n25, 392n27
Gosse, Emily, 383–396
Gosse, Philip Henry, 383–396
Granville-Barker, Harvey, 271–280
Gynecology, 11, 19, 151, 153

H

Halsted, William Stewart, 345, 347, 438
Hardy, Thomas, 107–115, 280–284
Harper, Ida Husted, 156–158
Hemingway, Ernest, 323–327
Hendrick, Burton J., 166–174
Herbs and herbal treatments, 195
Homeopathy, 430
Hopkins, Mary Alden, 287–301
Humours or humoral theory, 29, 342, 342n2, 343, 352
Hunt, Leigh, 68–69
Hunter, William, 16
Hysterectomy (radical hysterectomy), 12, 345, 346

I

Infant Life (Preservation) Act (1929), 201
Infant mortality, 16, 174, 175, 180, 182, 184, 287, 289, 291, 310, 311

Infertility, 19–20, 208
Informed consent, 348

J

Jacobs, Harriett, 97–102
Jewett, Charles, 151–153
Johnson, Georgia Douglas, 310, 311

K

Kellogg, John Harvey, 238–247, 350, 421–425
Kittoe, W. Hamilton, 69–78, 220–221, 376–381
Knowlton, Charles, 208–211

L

Latz, Peter J., 268–270, 433–437
Laws and legal restrictions, 212, 220
Letters or epistolary correspondence, 8, 34, 46, 60–62, 85, 108, 117, 157, 165–167, 189, 201, 218, 222, 226–230, 233, 238, 250n6, 255, 276, 289, 290, 294, 295, 303, 304, 306, 310, 315, 316, 335, 348, 354–362, 361n8, 368, 374–376, 404, 409, 413, 416, 419, 438
Leupp, Constance, 166–174
Life writing, 4, 8–11
Locock, Charles, 20, 83n23, 86, 87
Lord Ellenborough Act (1803), 201
Lord Lansdowne Act (1828), 201
Lying-in hospitals, 18, 22, 95, 103, 172, 179

M

Marriage and marital relations, 55, 56, 85, 106, 122, 140, 143, 156, 179, 201, 204, 208, 226, 228–230, 257, 258, 270, 292, 299, 302, 307, 310–312, 355, 426, 433, 436, 437
Martin, Anne, 180–190
Mastectomy (radical mastectomy), 12, 342–349, 438
Maternal mortality, viii, 1, 5, 12, 15, 22–25, 65, 102, 184, 185, 190, 191, 200
Medical education, 233, 234, 238
Medical students, 18, 102–106, 161, 163, 179, 397
Mental health (postpartum depression), 7
Mesmerism, 382–383
Midwifery and midwives, 4, 11, 16–18, 21, 24, 38, 65–68, 75, 80, 81, 88, 90–92, 92n25, 96, 102–106, 115, 163, 173, 177, 178, 232, 235, 268
Mifepristone/RU-486, 6, 198, 199, 199n3
Miscarriage, 1, 7, 12, 15, 19–20, 22, 71–75, 89, 90, 115–117, 197, 199, 200, 220, 223–230, 245, 447
Misoprostol, 6
Mitchell, Silas Weir, 121, 126
Morton, William, 20

N

Narrative medicine, 8
Novels, 10–11, 31, 32, 40, 107, 153, 154, 192, 205, 207, 284, 302, 312, 354, 414, 440

O

Obstetrics, 16, 17, 20, 21, 65, 83–86, 102, 151–153, 163, 173, 174, 176–179, 313
Our Bodies, Ourselves, 1, 10, 346

P

Pain, 10, 15, 19–21, 24, 28, 29, 31, 35, 37, 43, 44, 51n16, 54, 62, 68, 69, 72, 74, 76, 77, 79–86, 89, 90, 92, 94–97, 99, 116–119, 123, 142, 149, 153, 155, 157, 164, 166, 168–173, 192, 265, 266, 311, 313, 331, 333, 337, 347, 353, 355–358, 362–364, 367, 370, 371, 377, 379–383, 385–394, 399, 400, 403, 409, 412, 414, 415, 417, 418, 420, 422–425, 427, 427n42, 429, 431–436, 440, 441, 444, 448
Parker, Dorothy, 314–323
Periodicals, magazines, newspapers, 8, 9, 11, 20, 21, 24, 48, 49, 56–64, 70, 82–88, 102, 151, 156, 161, 168, 180, 185, 196, 203, 212–221, 231, 238, 240, 258, 266, 287, 290, 291, 310, 328, 346, 347n4, 348, 349, 351, 364, 382, 383, 405, 430, 438, 447, 448
Pessary, 197, 250
Pharmaceutical, 196–199
Plan B, 198
Poetry, 10–11, 192, 260, 445
Politics, viii, 255
Poverty, 5, 33, 252, 269, 281, 287, 289, 351, 426, 426n40
Puerperal fever, 16, 22, 23, 30–31, 47, 49n14, 90, 95, 96, 102, 104, 105, 165, 175, 266

Q

Quickening, 20, 70, 71, 159–160, 200–202, 221

R

Race, 84, 85, 139, 152, 181, 199, 202, 240, 243, 252, 253, 255–259, 262, 301, 426

Religion, 28, 41, 85, 86, 217, 272, 298, 355, 413
Rest cure, 121, 135
Restell, Madame (Ann Trow Lohman), 212–220, 231, 234, 238, 312, 374, 376
Rhythm method, 196, 197
Richardson, Anna Steese, 174–180
Roe vs. Wade, 1, 6, 202
Rowson, Susanna, 31–36
Rush, Benjamin, 356–361, 361n8

S

Sanger, Margaret, 198, 201, 203
Seduction, 32, 207, 293
Short fiction, 10–11
Simpson, James, 20, 79, 81, 82, 84–86, 395, 395n29
Sims, J. Marion, 19
Slesinger, Tess, 327–339
Smellie, William, 16
Smith, Abigail Adams, 147, 356–361, 361n8
Smyth, Maria, 354–356
Snow, John, 20, 87
Social class, 350
Solis-Cohen, Myer, 159–166
Somerset, Lady Henry, 258–266
Sponge, 73, 121, 164, 197, 209, 249, 251, 369, 387, 423, 425
Surgery and surgical treatment, 4, 20, 21, 67, 76, 85, 106, 151, 153, 169, 174, 195, 284, 342–350, 420, 430, 437

T

Tumor, 159, 342–344, 346, 347, 357, 358, 419, 422–425, 430–434, 436–439, 446, 447
Twilight sleep, 21, 24, 166–174, 176, 177, 192
Tynan, Katharine, 425–430, 440–445

U

Unmarried mothers, 158
Unplanned pregnancy, 284

V

Victoria, Queen, 20, 24, 82–88, 106, 384n22
Voluntary motherhood, 201, 203, 251, 253
Voluntary sterility, 269–270

W

Wharton, Edith, 192–193, 302–310
Wollstonecraft, Mary, 36, 42, 43, 205–208
Wray, George, 36, 42–68
Wright, Henry Clarke, 225–230

Y

Yuzpe, Albert, 198

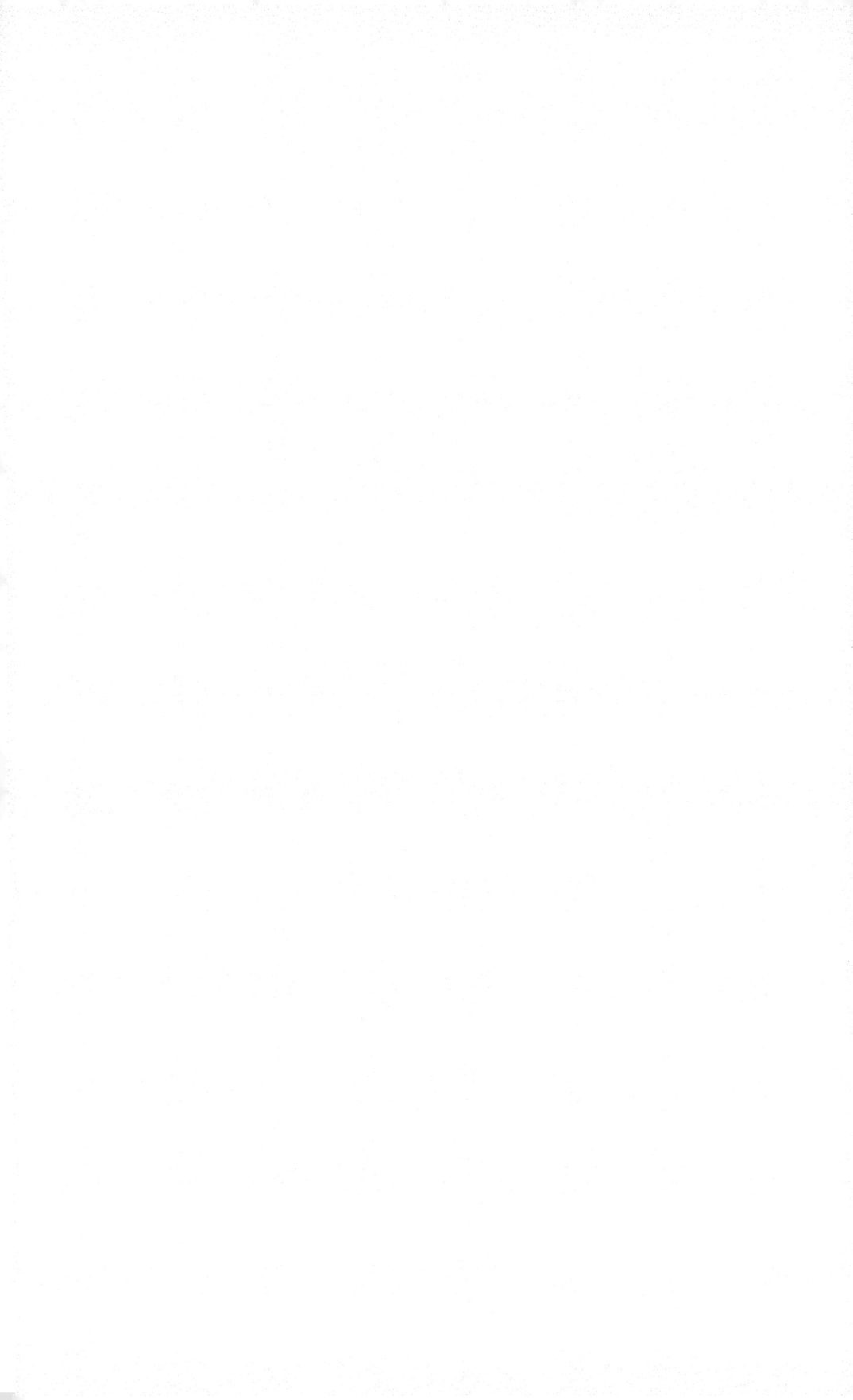

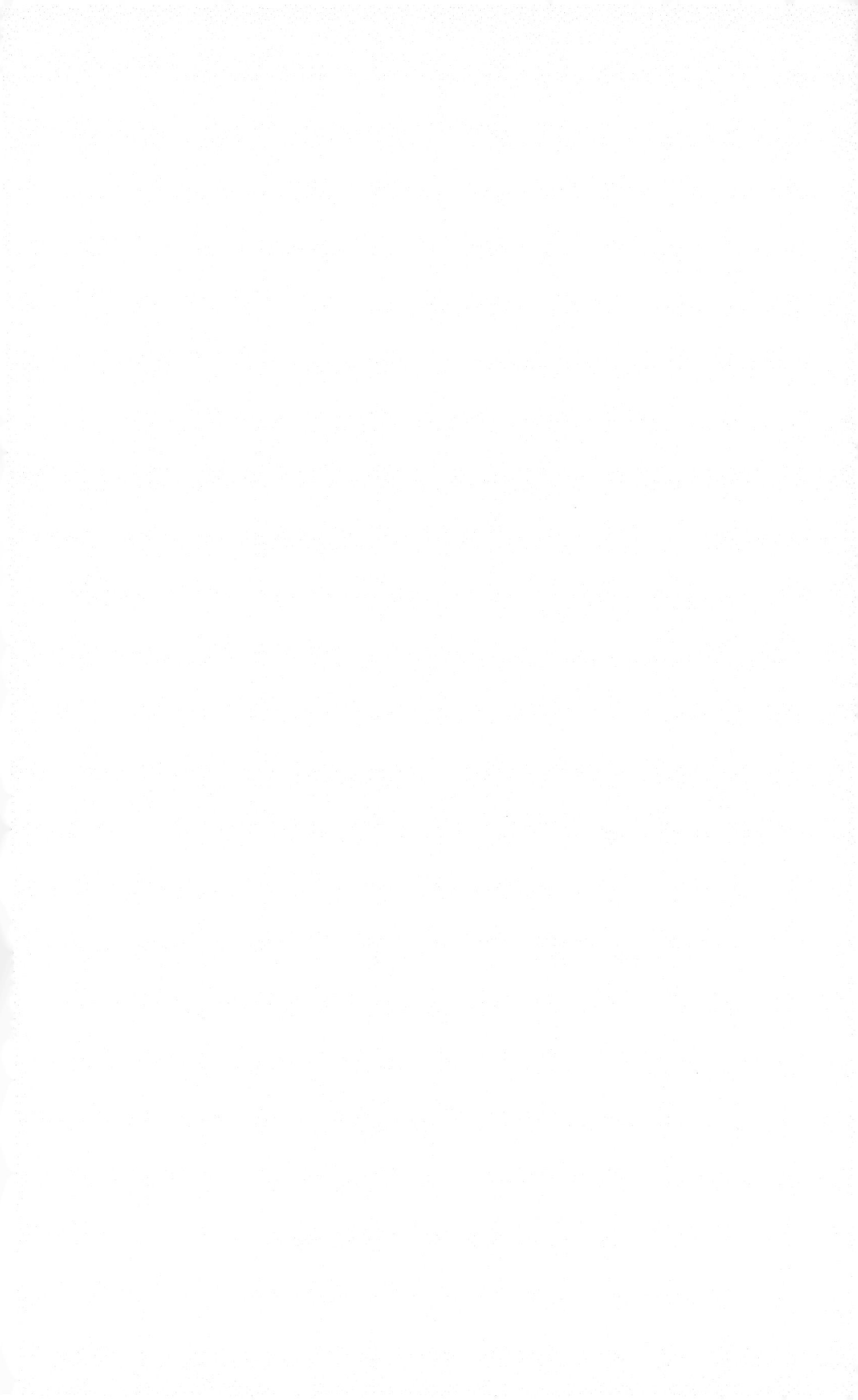

Printed by Printforce, United Kingdom